USMLE Step Mock Exam 2

2nd edition

Adam Brochert, MD

Staff Radiologist
Eisenhower Medical Center
Rancho Mirage, CA

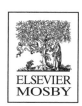

ELSEVIER
MOSBY

HANLEY & BELFUS, INC.
An Imprint of Elsevier

The Curtis Center
Independence Square West
Philadelphia, Pennsylvania 19106

Note to the reader: Although the information in this book has been carefully reviewed for correctness of dosage and indications, neither the author nor the publisher can accept any legal responsibility for any errors or omissions that may be made. Neither the publisher nor the editor makes any warranty, expressed or implied, with respect to the material contained herein. Before prescribing any drug, the reader must review the manufacturer's current product information (package inserts) for accepted indications, absolute dosage recommendations, and other information pertinent to the safe and effective use of the product described. This is especially important when drugs are given in combination or as an adjunct to other forms of therapy.

Library of Congress Control Number: 2004103676

ISBN-13: 978-1-56053-610-9

ISBN-10: 1-56053-610-1

USMLE STEP 2 MOCK EXAM

Permissions may be sought directly from Elsevier's Health Sciences Rights
Department in Philadelphia, PA, USA: phone: (+1) 215 239 3804, fax: (+1) 215 239 3805,
e-mail: healthpermissions@elsevier.com. You may also complete your request on-line
via the Elsevier homepage (http://www.elsevier.com), by selecting 'Customer Support'
and then 'Obtaining Permissions'.

Printed in the United States of America

Last digit is the print number: 9   8   7   6   5   4   3

TABLE OF CONTENTS

INTRODUCTION

Mock Boards is intended to give you a realistic idea of the types of questions you can expect to see on the USMLE Step 2 boards examination. Some of these concepts are recycled every year because certain core concepts must be learned by those hoping to practice medicine. Almost all of the concepts contained within have appeared on recent boards. Although the format of the boards is constantly changing (remember taking exams with a pencil and paper?), the patients still have the same problems and diseases.

I will not tell you how to take the examination because most of you reading this have already passed Step 1 or, for IMGs, another comparable examination. I want to pass on a few tips, however:

- Many of the questions and passages are quite long. Sometimes you will read a passage that is a half-page long, and the question has little to do with the passage you just read (strange, but true) or can be answered without reading the whole passage. If you see a long passage, try reading the question first, then going back and reading the rest of the passage if you need to. Doing this also helps you focus on the relevant aspects of the passage.

- It is just as important to know when something is normal or needs only observation as it is to know when to intervene. Do not order an MRI of the brain in a 1-year-old who cannot say "mama" yet (without more information to support its use), and do not get more history if a person has stopped breathing (establish an airway).

- Knowing the approximate reference ranges of common laboratory values (complete blood count and basic chemistry [chem 7] profile) saves a lot of time. Being able to plow through a list of normal laboratory values quickly without having to check the normal range makes you a faster passage reader. Time is precious for many during the exam.

I wish all of you the best on the examination and in your future endeavors.

REFERENCE RANGES FOR LABORATORY VALUES (IN ADULT SERUM)
(to be used on all portions of the examination)

Albumin	3.5–5.0 g/dL
Amylase	53–123 U/L
Arterial blood gases	
pH	7.38–7.42
PaO_2	80–100 mmHg
$PaCO_2$	38–42 mmHg
HCO_3	24–28 mEq/L
Bilirubin, direct	0–0.4 mg/dL
Bilirubin, total	0.1–1.0 mg/dL
Calcium	8.5–10.5 mg/dL
Carbon dioxide content (CO_2)	24–30 mEq/L
Cholesterol	120–220 mg/dL
Chloride	100–108 mmol/L
Creatinine	0.6–1.5 mg/dL
Glucose	70–110 mg/dL (fasting)
Hematocrit	
Females	37–48%
Males	45–52%
Hemoglobin	
Females	12–16 g/dL
Males	14–18 g/dL
Leukocyte count	4500–11,000/μL
Lipase	4–24 U/dL
Magnesium	1.5–2.0 mEq/L
Mean corpuscular volume	80–100 μm/cell
Phosphorus	3.0–4.5 mg/dL
Platelet count	150,000–400,000/μL
Potassium	3.5–5.0 mEq/L
Protein, total	6.0–8.4 g/dL
Red blood cell count	4.2–5.9 million/μL
Sodium	135–145 mEq/L
Transaminases	
Aspartate aminotransferase (AST, SGOT)	7–27 U/L
Alanine aminotransferase (ALT, SGPT)	1–21 U/L
Triglycerides	40–150 mg/dL
Blood urea nitrogen (BUN)	8–25 mg/dL
Uric acid	3.0–7.0 mg/dL

EXAM
QUESTIONS

BLOCK 1

50 QUESTIONS

TIME ALLOWED: 60 MINUTES

Question 1

A 22-year-old thin man comes into the office complaining of almost constant daytime sleepiness. He claims to sleep well, averaging about 8 hours of sleep per night, although he has a fairly common sensation of "being frozen" when he wakes up. He also mentions "involuntary naps," which consist of sleep that comes on suddenly and without warning, often in the middle of some type of activity, such as walking. The sudden naps happen once every day or two. The patient almost always falls asleep when the attacks come on, only to be woken by a friend or coworker. The patient works as an office manager and relates no chemical exposure. Which treatment is most likely to help this patient?

(A) Nortriptyline
(B) Fluoxetine
(C) Diazepam
(D) Modafinil
(E) Continuous positive airway pressure breathing device

Question 2

A 21-year-old woman comes to the office complaining of sore throat, rash, and fatigue. The sore throat and fatigue began roughly 8 days ago, accompanied by a subjective fever (temperature not recorded). Three days before this visit, the patient visited an urgent care center and was given amoxicillin for her symptoms. A "rash" subsequently developed. The patient denies any drug allergies and remembers taking penicillin several years ago without having a problem. Her sore throat and fatigue did not improve with the amoxicillin. Vital signs are as follows:

Temperature	99.6°F
Blood pressure	126/82 mmHg
Pulse rate	88 beats/min
Respirations	14/min

On examination, the patient has a maculopapular rash on her trunk and marked pharyngeal erythema. What is the most likely cause of the patient's symptoms?

(A) *Streptococcus agalactiae*
(B) Epstein-Barr virus
(C) *Streptococcus pyogenes*
(D) *Staphylococcus aureus*
(E) Allergic reaction to amoxicillin

Question 3

A mother brings in her 10-year-old son because she is concerned about repetitive grunting noises that the child makes. On further questioning of the mother, you learn that the child began having unusually frequent eye blinking on a daily basis a few years earlier. The child is described as fairly hyperactive and unable to control his impulses. Which of the following might you expect the child to develop?

(A) Intermittent bursts of swearing
(B) Fire setting and cruelty to animals
(C) Bed-wetting
(D) Unwillingness to go to school because of fears of abandonment
(E) Paralysis

Question 4

A 29-year-old woman comes into the office at the request of her boss. She works as a secretary and claims her boss has noticed a recent change in her, although she thinks that "he is just jealous of my new plans." On further questioning, the woman tells you of her plan to open a new internet magazine, with herself as the president, editor, and lead writer. She has recently purchased $25,000 worth of office equipment and business learning tapes on several credit cards because she has no experience in business or writing. She speaks quickly and with few pauses, not waiting for replies. After a few minutes, she begins to smile seductively and mentions that she finds you quite attractive, inviting you to an all-expense-paid trip to the Bahamas. The woman has not slept in several days because "there is too much to do." Which of the following statements is true about this woman's most likely condition?

(A) She is unlikely to become depressed in the future.
(B) The most effective treatment would be an anxiolytic, such as buspirone.
(C) This personality disorder often responds to treatment with lithium.
(D) Relatives are unlikely to have any psychiatric conditions.
(E) An antipsychotic may be required in the treatment of this condition.

Question 5

A patient comes into the emergency department after an automobile accident in which he was unrestrained. He says his chest hurts, but he does not remember the accident. He is breathing rapid, shallow breaths because of pain and shortness of breath. His vital signs are as follows:

Temperature	98.9°F
Blood pressure	110/60 mmHg
Pulse rate	108 beats/min
Respirations	24/min

On examination, the neck veins are not distended; the anterior chest wall has a bruise in the right midclavicular area, and the underlying 4th, 5th, and 6th ribs are markedly tender to palpation. On auscultation of the chest, there is fairly poor air movement because the patient refuses to take a deep breath, with absent breath sounds on the right. The left side is clear to auscultation. On the right side of the chest, there is marked hyperresonance with percussion compared with the left. During the examination, the patient begins to get restless, his breathing becomes more labored, and his neck veins start to become distended. What is the appropriate intervention at this time?

(A) CT scan of the chest with contrast enhancement
(B) Pericardiocentesis
(C) Lateral and posteroanterior chest films done in the radiology department to ensure adequate film quality
(D) Intubation with positive-pressure ventilation
(E) Needle thoracentesis

Question 6

A 45-year-old man is brought to the emergency department after being stabbed during a bar fight. He is delirious and cannot answer questions. The emergency medical technician that brought him in says he was talking coherently when picked up but became incoherent during the ride to the hospital. The patient was given 2 L of normal saline en route. Vital signs from the scene and currently are listed as follows:

	At the scene	Currently
Temperature	98.6°F	97.9°F
Blood pressure	120/80 mmHg	94/60 mmHg
Pulse rate	110 beats/min	140 beats/min
Respirations	20/min	32/min

The technician estimates the patient has lost only about 500 mL of blood. On examination, the neck veins are distended, breath sounds are clear to auscultation, and chest percussion notes are normal bilaterally. There is a stab wound just to the left of the sternum at the fourth intercostal space with little bleeding. The heart sounds are distant, and the pulse is faint. The patient is somnolent and making little sense. What is the appropriate intervention at this time?

(A) Pericardiocentesis
(B) Portable chest radiograph
(C) Electrocardiogram
(D) CT scan of the chest
(E) Needle thoracentesis

Question 7

A woman brings in her 6-year-old daughter for a painful arm after the child fell out of her chair. The child has a recent linear bruise across the left forearm that is tender to palpation. When you ask the child how she fell out of the chair, the child looks at her mother, and the mother explains how the child was reaching for the salt shaker and fell off her chair. You ask the child to remove her shirt and notice an old, fairly large bruise in the small of her back. The child has poor eye contact and tends to stare at her feet. You suspect the patient may have been abused. Which of the following is true about child abuse?

(A) Children commonly get bruised in these areas during falls, and care should be taken not to suspect child abuse too readily in a case like this.
(B) The interaction between mother and child as well as the interaction between the child and you does not support a suspicion of child abuse.
(C) A history of premature delivery or low birth weight in abused children is common.
(D) Women are rarely the culprits in child abuse cases.
(E) Proof is required before reporting the mother for suspected abuse.

Question 8

An 18-year-old healthy male athlete comes to the office with his mother after passing out while playing basketball. The mother's husband (the boy's father) died suddenly at age 26 while jogging. The patient says the spell was "no big deal" and admits to a few previous episodes during basketball games that resolved without incident. The peripheral pulse is brisk and the chest is clear to auscultation.

On cardiac examination, the apical impulse has a markedly sustained thrust and is located in the mid-clavicular line in the fifth intercostal space. A grade 3/6, nonradiating, systolic ejection murmur is heard best at the left sternal border in the fourth intercostal space. The murmur increases with the Valsalva maneuver. A loud S4 can be appreciated. Which of the following should be **avoided** in the workup and treatment of the most likely diagnosis?

(A) Echocardiography
(B) Antibiotic prophylaxis before dental procedures
(C) Propranolol
(D) Verapamil
(E) Digoxin

Question 9

What is the most likely location of an intracerebral bleed resulting from hypertension?

(A) Parietal lobe
(B) Basal ganglia
(C) Occipital lobe
(D) Frontal lobe
(E) Medulla

Question 10

A 27-year-old man presents with an acutely painful, swollen, erythematous left knee in the absence of any trauma or previous arthritis history. In the patient's social history, he admits to occasional "binge" drinking and has multiple sexual partners. He has never used IV drugs. If culture of the joint fluid from the affected knee is performed, which organism is likely to grow?

(A) *Salmonella*
(B) *Staphylococcus*
(C) *Neisseria*
(D) *Treponema*
(E) *Streptococcus*

Question 11

Which of the following is **least** likely to be seen with osteoarthritis?

(A) Bone spurs on radiograph
(B) Heberden's nodes
(C) Worsening of symptoms after use
(D) Swollen, erythematous joints
(E) Bouchard's nodes

Question 12

Which of the following should generally be **avoided** during an acute attack of gout?

(A) Indomethacin
(B) Injection of corticosteroids into the affected joint
(C) Allopurinol
(D) High levels of fluid intake
(E) Colchicine

Question 13

A 31-year-old woman develops a fever of 101.8°F on postpartum day 1. She has mild uterine tenderness to palpation, and the decision is made to start broad-spectrum antibiotics. After 6 days of therapy with piperacillin and gentamicin, the fever persists and peaks at around 102.4°F. A CT scan of the pelvis is negative for abscess. The patient complains of abdominal fullness and vague pain but is no longer tender to palpation on abdominal or pelvic examination. There has been no vaginal discharge or bleeding in the last 2 days. What is the next step in the treatment of this patient?

(A) Add fluconazole to the other antibiotics to cover fungi.
(B) Continue with another week of broad-spectrum antibiotics at an increased dose.
(C) Do a uterine dilation and curettage with aerobic and anaerobic cultures.
(D) Administer heparin.
(E) Do a transvaginal hysterectomy, leaving the ovaries in place.

Question 14

What condition should you suspect if a patient has an anaphylactic reaction to immunoglobulin therapy?

(A) Emphysema
(B) Leukemia
(C) IgA deficiency
(D) Severe combined immunodeficiency
(E) DiGeorge's syndrome

Question 15

An obese 32-year-old woman brings her 1-month-old child in for a routine checkup after requiring a cesarean section for dystocia. She received no prenatal care. Her infant boy weighed 4700 gm (10 lb, 6 oz) at birth after a 37-week pregnancy and appears healthy at this time. Which of the following is true?

(A) Regular prenatal care most likely would have resulted in an infant of lower birth weight.
(B) The woman likely had preeclampsia during her pregnancy.
(C) The woman probably has a small, male-shaped pelvis.
(D) The infant likely has Down syndrome.
(E) The infant should be put on a strict, low-fat diet so that he does not become obese as an adult.

Question 16

You are called to see a newborn reported to be in distress. On arrival to the neonatal care area, the nurse reports the infants's vital signs as follows:

Temperature	96.7°F
Blood pressure	70/30 mmHg
Pulse rate	196 beats/min
Respirations	42/min

Laboratory tests reveal the following:

Hemoglobin	20 gm/dL (normal: 17–22)
White blood cell count	6000/mL (normal: 2000–7400)
Sodium	128 mEq/L (normal: 133–146)
Potassium	6.5 mEq/L (normal: 3.2–5.5)
Chloride	90 mEq/L (normal: 96–111)
Glucose	40 mg/dL (normal: 55–115)

On physical examination, the infant is lethargic, tachycardic, and tachypneic, with good bilateral breath sounds, no evidence of consolidation in the lungs, and a tachycardic, regular rhythm of the heart. You notice that the genitalia are ambiguous, with what appears to be a large, hypertrophied clitoris. What should your next step be?

(A) Administer corticosteroids.
(B) Acquire buccal smear for Barr body analysis.
(C) Give hypertonic saline.
(D) Call the infant's mother to ask about family history of ambiguous genitalia.
(E) Measure a 24-hour urine for 17-ketosteroids.

Question 17

A mother brings in her 11-year-old son because of frustration with his behavior. Apparently the child was caught torturing the family dog, the latest in a series of destructive behaviors. According to the mother, the child lies repeatedly, steals money from her purse, and has been caught drinking beer, which the mother suspects he stole from a neighbor's garage. He has no friends because he tends to manipulate and abuse other children. The mother is a single parent; the child's father, an alcoholic, left before the child was born. The child denies any problem and smiles as he responds to the allegations, "I'm a pretty good kid if you ask me." Assuming the mother is telling the truth, which of the following is **false**?

(A) Little in the way of treatment has been found to be effective.
(B) Antipsychotics are not indicated.
(C) The child most likely has oppositional defiant disorder.
(D) The child has an increased risk of becoming an alcoholic as an adult.
(E) The child has an increased risk of developing somatization disorder as an adult.

Question 18

A 58-year-old man comes to the emergency department because of pain in the lower left abdomen and nausea. The patient has not been to a physician in more than 10 years and reports no medical problems or current medications. The patient says that these symptoms happened once before in the past and resolved on their own, but this time his wife demanded that he seek help. He admits to some loose stools and mild chills over the past 2 days. His vital signs are as follows:

Temperature	99.9°F
Blood pressure	164/96 mmHg
Pulse rate	84 beats/min
Respirations	14/min

Physical examination is normal except for the presence of left lower quadrant tenderness on palpation. Stool testing reveals no evidence of gross or occult blood, and no masses are appreciated on rectal examination. There is no guarding or rebound tenderness. Which of the following is true regarding the most likely diagnosis?

(A) Colectomy is the treatment of choice in this patient.
(B) Intravenous fluid containing 5% dextrose and water should be administered.
(C) Colonoscopy should be performed as soon as possible to confirm the diagnosis and allow prompt intervention.
(D) A barium enema done 2 weeks after symptoms resolve is usually adequate to confirm the diagnosis.
(E) Empirical antibiotics are likely to make this condition worse.

Question 19

A woman brings in her 3-month-old infant with a complaint of poor feeding and weakness in the infant that began yesterday afternoon and is getting worse. Before yesterday, the infant was healthy and active, as he has been on previous visits. The infant's diet consists of breast milk and occasional formula feedings and spoonfuls of honey "to keep my little sweetie sweet." On examination, the infant has markedly decreased muscle tone in all four extremities, hyporeflexia in all four extremities, lethargy, and apathy. Which of the following is the most likely cause of these symptoms?

(A) Degeneration of anterior horn cells in the spinal cord
(B) Neglect
(C) Infection with a toxin-producing species of *Streptococcus*
(D) Decreased levels of thyroid hormone
(E) Gut colonization with *Clostridium botulinum*

Question 20

A 45-year-old woman comes to the office complaining of fatigue and weakness. Medical history includes hypertension, diabetes, obesity, and severe asthma. Her daily medications include enalapril, metformin, glipizide, prednisone, a salmeterol inhaler, and an albuterol inhaler used when needed. Vital signs are as follows:

Temperature	99.2°F
Blood pressure	162/92 mmHg
Pulse rate	80 beats/min
Respirations	16/min

On examination, there is some mild wasting in the extremities, truncal obesity, pigmented lines radiating out from the navel on the skin of the abdomen, mild pedal edema bilaterally, and several small bruises on both shins. A finger-stick reveals a glucose level of 268. Which of the following is **false** regarding the patient's use of prednisone?

(A) Prednisone can cause wasting in the extremities.

(B) Prednisone can worsen the patient's diabetes.

(C) Prednisone may be the cause of the patient's fatigue and weakness symptoms.

(D) Prednisone may be the cause of the changes on the skin of the abdominal wall.

(E) Prednisone tends to protect against the development of osteoporosis.

Question 21

A 38-year-old man comes to the emergency department with his girlfriend complaining of a severe, constant headache that started 4 hours ago. The girlfriend states that the patient was walking up a flight of stairs when he suddenly collapsed and became unresponsive for roughly 2 minutes. He then woke up confused and has had the headache since, with two episodes of vomiting. The patient does not get headaches normally. Past medical and social history are unremarkable. Family history is significant for a mother and 36-year-old brother with early adult onset of kidney failure requiring dialysis.

Vital signs are within normal limits. Neurologic examination is within normal limits other than mild confusion and an unwillingness of the patient to move the neck because of pain, which also is a new symptom according to the girlfriend. Which of the following is most likely to be true?

(A) Lumbar puncture would reveal numerous neutrophils and a high bacterial count.

(B) The carotid arteries contain critical stenoses bilaterally.

(C) The patient's kidneys contain multiple large cysts.

(D) Echocardiography would clinch the diagnosis.

(E) Anticoagulation with heparin would improve symptoms.

Question 22

A woman brings in her 3-month-old daughter because she noticed the child does not seem to be gaining much weight. The woman also notices a salty taste when she kisses her infant and read in a magazine that this could mean the infant has cystic fibrosis. She vehemently denies any family history of cystic fibrosis in her or her husband's family. She wants to know whether or not the infant has cystic fibrosis and the likelihood she has "defective DNA," because this is her first child. Which of the following is true regarding cystic fibrosis?

(A) It is an autosomal dominant disease; either the woman's or her husband's DNA could be "at fault."

(B) It is an X-linked recessive disease; the woman and her husband must have genetic mutations for the child to get the disease.

(C) If the child has cystic fibrosis, there is a 50% chance that the next child the woman has will develop cystic fibrosis.

(D) The diagnosis can be made presumptively if the potassium concentration in sweat is elevated markedly.

(E) If the child has cystic fibrosis, she still may be able to give her mother normal, healthy grandchildren if she survives to adulthood.

Question 23

Which of the following is **false** concerning cystic fibrosis?

(A) Life expectancy is reduced.
(B) Affected infants are at an increased risk for rectal prolapse and meconium ileus.
(C) Frequent respiratory infections most commonly are due to *Klebsiella*.
(D) Pancreatic insufficiency is common in cystic fibrosis.
(E) Inheritance is autosomal recessive.

Question 24

A 34-year-old married woman comes to the office complaining of a vaginal discharge. Her medical history includes diet-controlled diabetes. She says the discharge started 1 week ago, shortly after her husband returned from a trip to the Caribbean. On speculum examination, you note a malodorous, thin, frothy, grayish discharge with no erythema or irritation present. A potassium hydroxide preparation of a discharge specimen is negative, although you notice a fishlike odor when the potassium hydroxide is applied. A saline preparation of the discharge reveals multiple epithelial cells with a granular appearance. Which of the following is true regarding this patient's condition?

(A) The patient's diabetes most likely has been poorly controlled.
(B) The discharge is likely due to bacterial overgrowth, not an infection.
(C) The patient and her husband need to be treated with antibiotics.
(D) Without treatment, this infection frequently leads to pelvic inflammatory disease.
(E) The treatment of choice is tetracycline.

Question 25

A 34-year-old woman complains of gradually worsening weakness and fatigue over the past 2 months. She notes that she especially has trouble getting out of a chair. When asked about depression, the patient shrugs her shoulders and says she's tired more than anything else. Past medical history is insignificant. Vital signs are within normal limits. Physical examination reveals marked symmetric weakness of the shoulder muscles and hip flexors. These muscles are also tender to palpation. There is mild periorbital edema with a slight purple color in the upper eyelids. Laboratory tests reveal the following:

Hemoglobin	10 gm/dL
Mean corpuscular volume	86 μm/cell
Platelets	450,000/μL
Creatine kinase	1500 U/L (normal = 10–80)

Which of the following is true regarding the most likely cause of the woman's symptoms?

(A) The cause is most likely a subclinical depression.
(B) An electrocardiogram should be done immediately to rule out a silent myocardial infarction.
(C) Muscle biopsy most likely would be normal.
(D) Electromyography would be expected to show spontaneous fibrillations and irritability.
(E) The woman has about a 95% chance of developing a malignancy during her lifetime.

Question 26

A 28-year-old woman comes to the office because of pains in her knees, fatigue, and skin problems. She has a rash over both cheeks in a butterfly pattern that has been present for 3 days. The rash came about suddenly after the woman was at the beach for several hours and got a mild sunburn. Her knee joints have been sore for about 3 weeks now but recently got worse, and the pain is no longer controlled by ibuprofen. Both knee joints are slightly swollen, with some erythema and pain on passive range of motion. You suspect systemic lupus erythematosus. Which of the following points would **not** increase your suspicion of the diagnosis?

(A) The patient has been taking procainamide for an atrial arrhythmia.
(B) The patient has been on tuberculosis prophylaxis.
(C) The patient had a positive blood test for gonorrhea.
(D) The patient was losing some of her hair.
(E) The patient had noticed some weight loss.

Question 27

A 54-year-old man comes to see you because of abdominal "heaviness." Medical history is significant for impotence for the past 5 years and arthritis of the knees and hands, for which he has never seen a doctor. The patient takes no medications and has never used alcohol or other drugs. On examination, the skin on the face and neck has a grayish hue to it. Abdominal examination reveals firm, smooth hepatomegaly without discrete mass. Laboratory tests reveal the following:

Hemoglobin	17 gm/dL
Ferritin	4000 ng/mL
	(normal = 10–200)
Transferrin saturation	95% (normal = 20–40%)
AST	40 U/L (normal = 7–27)
ALT	60 U/L (normal = 1–21)

Which of the following is true of the most likely underlying condition?

(A) This patient has a markedly increased risk of dying from cirrhosis or hepatocellular carcinoma.

(B) Bone marrow transplant is curative.

(C) Women usually are affected at a younger age by this condition.

(D) Ocular involvement is a prominent feature of this condition.

(E) The pattern of liver enzyme abnormality indicates that the patient most likely has been drinking alcohol.

Question 28

A 72-year-old woman complains of loss of vision in the right eye that happened suddenly this morning while the woman was eating breakfast. The woman relates a history of pain and stiffness in the shoulders as well as jaw muscle pain and fatigue after chewing for the past 2 weeks. Vital signs are remarkable only for a temperature of 100.9° F. There are no skin rashes. The right pupil does not respond well to light, although there is an intact consensual response in the right pupil. Funduscopic examination reveals a pale fundus and optic disk on the right with a small red spot in the area of the fovea. The patient has scalp tenderness to palpation, more on the right than the left side. Musculoskeletal examination shows intact strength but some tenderness in the shoulder muscles with movement against resistance. Laboratory tests reveal the following:

White blood cell count	4500/μL
Sedimentation rate	100 mm/h (normal = 1–20)
AST	15 U/L
Creatinine	0.8 mg/dL
Potassium	4.2 mEq/L

What is the best thing to do next?

(A) Administer corticosteroids.
(B) Check an antinuclear antibody (ANA) titer.
(C) Refer the patient for a temporal artery biopsy.
(D) Refer the patient for a muscle biopsy.
(E) Order blood and urine cultures.

Question 29

A 66-year-old man presents to the emergency department with a chief complaint of transient blindness in the right eye that lasted 2 minutes and subsequently resolved before he reached the emergency department. He describes the vision loss as "someone pulling a shade down in front of my eye." Medical history is significant for long-standing hypertension, diabetes, a myocardial infarction 6 months ago, and tobacco abuse. His medications include amlodipine, glipizide, and pioglitazone. Vital signs and physical examination are within normal limits other than obesity. Laboratory tests reveal the following:

Hemoglobin	16 gm/dL
Mean corpuscular volume	90 µm/cell
Creatinine	1.3 mg/dL
BUN	15 mg/dL
Sodium	140 mEq/L
Potassium	4.1 mEq/L
Chloride	106 mEq/L
CO_2	27 mEq/L

Which of the following is **false**?

(A) A carotid duplex scan (ultrasound) should be ordered.
(B) The patient should have a fasting lipid profile analysis done.
(C) The patient should be put on an angiotensin-converting enzyme inhibitor, such as captopril.
(D) The patient should undergo urgent carotid endarterectomy for the best long-term prognosis.
(E) The patient likely would benefit from being put on a beta blocker, such as metoprolol.

Question 30

A 34-year-old woman comes to the office complaining of pain and blurry vision in the right eye. She says it feels as though she has something in her eye. Visual acuity is 20/20 in the left eye and 20/100 in the right eye. The patient has never had vision problems before and does not wear glasses. The patient pain and discomfort in the right eye when you shine a light into her pupils. The right eye shows marked conjunctival hyperemia and excessive lacrimation. When fluorescein dye is applied to the cornea, you note a branching lesion on the cornea with knoblike terminations. What should you do next?

(A) Prescribe erythromycin eye drops and see the patient back in 3 days to reassess the eye.
(B) Prescribe corticosteroid drops and see the patient back in 1 week to reassess the eye.
(C) Refer the patient to an optometrist for glasses.
(D) Cover the eye with a patch and see the patient again in 48 hours to reassess the eye.
(E) Refer the patient to an ophthalmologist promptly for further treatment.

Question 31

A 25-year-old woman with cystic fibrosis comes to the office complaining of worsening night vision and dry eyes. On examination, the patient is quite thin and has scattered crackles on lung auscultation. The skin is dry and flaky, and the eyes appear dry. Chest radiograph reveals diffuse osteopenia and bilateral scarring of the lungs with no acute abnormalities. The patient was hospitalized 2 months ago for a respiratory infection, which was treated successfully with 3 weeks of broad-spectrum antibiotics. She has a history of noncompliance. Which of the following is true?

(A) The patient's current complaints likely are due to malabsorption.
(B) The patient needs a second course of antibiotics.
(C) The patient most likely has developed psoriasis.
(D) The patient would be treated best with daily iron therapy.
(E) The patient is likely to be in an acutely hypercoagulable state.

Question 32

A 32-year-old woman is brought to see you by her husband for bizarre behavior. The woman has been accusing neighbors of stealing water from her garden hose and using the water to grow plants with the ability to take over the world. The woman has a resting tremor, which has been present for the last 4 years. She has not seen a physician since childhood. On examination, the woman is uncooperative, paranoid, and refuses to answer questions. You notice a coarse resting tremor of the upper extremities and note the woman's clumsiness when she undoes the buttons of her jacket. She has marked ataxia on testing. The liver is enlarged and nodular with a firm liver edge. Laboratory tests reveal the following:

Ceruloplasmin	Undetectable (normal = 23–43 mg/dL)
AST	60 U/L (normal = 7–27)
ALT	84 U/L (normal = 1–21)
Hepatitis B surface antigen	Negative
Hepatitis B surface antibody	Positive

Which of the following is true regarding diagnosis and treatment of the most likely disorder?

(A) Progression of cirrhosis can be slowed by antiviral treatment.
(B) Iron supplements commonly are used to slow progression of the disorder.
(C) An abnormal serum copper level is the gold standard test to confirm the diagnosis.
(D) Penicillamine often is the treatment of choice.
(E) The patient could not have received the hepatitis B vaccine.

Question 33

A 17-year-old male presents with a facial port wine stain.

Which of the following conditions is most closely associated with this finding?

(A) Sturge-Weber syndrome
(B) Cystic fibrosis
(C) Congenital rubella syndrome
(D) Neurofibromatosis
(E) Tuberous sclerosis

Question 34

Which of the following factors is **least** likely to cause deep venous thrombosis?

(A) Immobility
(B) Heart failure with an ejection fraction of 15%
(C) Trauma
(D) Malignancy
(E) Hypertension

Question 35

A 35-year-old woman comes to the office complaining of numbness and tingling in the fingers of both of her hands and around her mouth. When the nurse takes her blood pressure, the patient's hand closes involuntarily and starts to have painful spasms. The nurse removes the blood pressure cuff and attempts to take the blood pressure from the other arm, and the same thing happens. Which of the following is correct concerning this woman's condition?

(A) Electrocardiogram probably will show QT interval shortening.
(B) You should ask about a recent history of thyroid surgery.
(C) She most likely has Graves' disease.
(D) Voluntary hyperventilation may improve symptoms.
(E) The patient requires high-dose corticosteroids.

Question 36

A 59-year-old male housepainter comes to the office complaining of numbness and weakness in his dominant right hand. He says he started to get numbness and tingling in the right hand 3 months ago, "like the pins and needles when your foot falls asleep," and occasionally wakes up in the middle of the night with pain and tingling. The patient rarely gets weakness ("like a clumsiness") in the right hand and has dropped his paintbrush a few times at work because of this. Tapping on the volar (palm side) surface of the wrist in the midline causes a reproduction of the tingling sensation, which is in a median nerve distribution. The patient has not been to see a doctor in 20 years. Which of the following is the best answer given the clinical scenario?

(A) Schedule the patient for a routine barium enema.
(B) Refer the patient for bilateral wrist surgery.
(C) Measure a vasoactive intestinal peptide level.
(D) Get an MRI of the brain.
(E) Prescribe allopurinol.

Question 37

A 16-year-old boy presents to the emergency department with abdominal pain. A crampy pain started in the periumbilical area yesterday afternoon after 8 hours of nausea with one episode of vomiting. The pain subsequently migrated into the lower right portion of the abdomen and became more intense and sharp. The patient has no appetite, is nauseous, and has vomited twice since being in the emergency department. He is lying still in the bed because he says it hurts to move. His vital signs are as follows:

Temperature	101.6° F
Blood pressure	110/70 mmHg
Pulse rate	106 beats/min
Respirations	16/min

Laboratory tests reveal the following:

Hemoglobin	15 gm/dL
White blood cell count	16,000/μL
Creatinine	1.0 mg/dL

Which of the following do you expect to be present on physical examination?

(A) Rovsing's sign
(B) Trousseau's sign
(C) Kernig's sign
(D) Murphy's sign
(E) Grey Turner's sign

Question 38

An 18-year-old man presents to the office with a chief complaint of severe testicular pain that started suddenly 2 hours ago after lifting weights. He says the pain is a 10 out of 10 and is constant; he also reports nausea. The patient has no significant medical history and is on no medications. He reports no recent urinary symptoms or illnesses and is not sexually active. On examination, the patient has some scrotal wall edema and erythema as well as marked testicular tenderness to palpation. The testicular pain is not decreased by manual testicular elevation. There is no evidence of direct or indirect hernia. Which of the following is true?

(A) The patient requires immediate referral to a urologist.
(B) The patient requires antibiotics to cover possible chlamydial infection and follow-up in 2 weeks.
(C) The patient requires an exploratory laparotomy.
(D) The patient should use scrotal ice packs and nonsteroidal anti-inflammatory drugs and follow-up in 48 hours.
(E) The patient probably has mumps.

Question 39

Which of the following laboratory or physiologic values **decreases** in the second trimester of a normal pregnancy?

(A) Heart rate
(B) Minute ventilation
(C) BUN
(D) Erythrocyte sedimentation rate
(E) Sodium
(F) Hematocrit
(G) Both C and D
(H) Both D and F
(I) Both C and F
(J) Choices A, B and D

Question 40

Which of the following laboratory or physiologic values **increases** in the second trimester of a normal pregnancy?

(A) Heart rate
(B) Minute ventilation
(C) BUN
(D) Erythrocyte sedimentation rate
(E) Sodium
(F) Hematocrit
(G) Both C and D
(H) Both D and F
(I) Both C and F
(J) Choices A, B and D

Question 41

Which of the following laboratory or physiologic values remains unchanged in the second trimester of a normal pregnancy?

(A) Heart rate
(B) Minute ventilation
(C) BUN
(D) Erythrocyte sedimentation rate
(E) Sodium
(F) Hematocrit
(G) Both C and D
(H) Both D and F
(I) Both C and F
(J) Choices A, B and D

Question 42

Which of the following factors in a patient with schizophrenia implies an **improved** prognosis?

(A) Married
(B) Late age at onset
(C) No precipitating factors
(D) Family history of schizophrenia
(E) Predominance of positive symptoms, such as hallucinations, delusions, and bizarre behavior
(F) Predominance of negative symptoms, such as flattened affect, loss of motivation, and anhedonia
(G) Choices A, B and E
(H) Choices A, B, C, and E
(I) Choices C, D, and F
(J) Choices D and F

Question 43

Which of the following factors in a patient with schizophrenia implies a **poorer** prognosis?

(A) Married
(B) Late age at onset
(C) No precipitating factors
(D) Family history of schizophrenia
(E) Predominance of positive symptoms, such as hallucinations, delusions, and bizarre behavior
(F) Predominance of negative symptoms, such as flattened affect, loss of motivation, and anhedonia
(G) Choices A, B and E
(H) Choices A, B, C, and E
(I) Choices C, D, and F
(J) Choices D and F

Question 44

A 36-year-old African American woman presents with a chief complaint of heavy periods. Past medical history is unremarkable. On exam, the uterus is significantly enlarged. Ultrasound reveals numerous scattered uterine masses. A hysterectomy is performed. The uterus contains multiple smooth masses. A sample histologic section of the uterus is shown, which reveals an additional tumor (labeled "T" in the figure) not appreciated grossly. The tumor was noted to be surrounded by normal myometrium (labeled "M" in the figure).

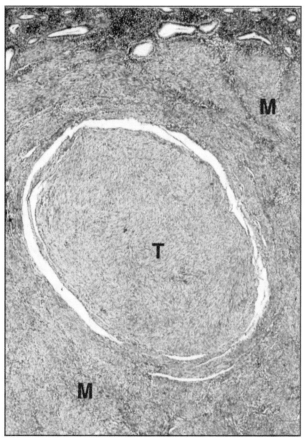

Which of the following is **false** regarding the underlying neoplastic disorder?

(A) Hysterectomy is a required part of treatment for these tumors to exclude extrauterine extension.
(B) The risk of malignant transformation is less than 1%.
(C) It is the most common gynecologic neoplasm.
(D) These neoplasms are often hormonally responsive.
(E) The subserosal subtype is unlikely to cause menstrual disturbances.

Question 45

A 59-year-old man with a history of hypertension presents to the emergency room with severe, ripping chest pain that radiates through to his back. A chest x-ray is performed and reveals a widened mediastinum. The patient dies suddenly. An autopsy is performed and a section of the patient's thoracic aorta is shown.

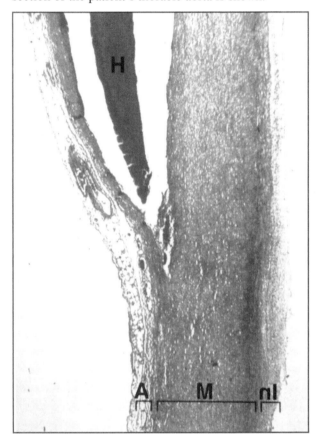

Which of the following is true regarding the condition shown in the figure?

(A) The patient most likely had Marfan syndrome.
(B) This disorder is more common in women.
(C) It is unlikely to be related to the patient's death.
(D) In almost all cases involving the thoracic aorta, immediate surgical management is required.
(E) Hypertension is strongly associated with this condition.

Question 46

Which of the following infectious agents is most highly associated with nasopharyngeal carcinoma?

(A) Adenovirus
(B) Epstein-Barr virus
(C) Hepatitis C virus
(D) Herpes simplex virus
(E) Human herpesvirus 8
(F) Human papillomavirus
(G) Mumps virus
(H) None of the above

Question 47

Which of the following infectious agents is most highly associated with anal carcinoma?

(A) Adenovirus
(B) Epstein-Barr virus
(C) Hepatitis C virus
(D) Herpes simplex virus
(E) Human herpesvirus 8
(F) Human papillomavirus
(G) Mumps virus
(H) None of the above

Question 48

Which of the following infectious agents is most highly associated with Kaposi's sarcoma?

(A) Adenovirus
(B) Epstein-Barr virus
(C) Hepatitis C virus
(D) Herpes simplex virus
(E) Human herpesvirus 8
(F) Human papillomavirus
(G) Mumps virus
(H) None of the above

Question 49

Which of the following infectious agents is most highly associated with African Burkitt lymphoma?

(A) Adenovirus
(B) Epstein-Barr virus
(C) Hepatitis C virus
(D) Herpes simplex virus
(E) Human herpesvirus 8
(F) Human papillomavirus
(G) Mumps virus
(H) None of the above

Question 50

Which of the following infectious agents is most highly associated with hepaocellular carcinoma?

(A) Adenovirus
(B) Epstein-Barr virus
(C) Hepatitis C virus
(D) Herpes simplex virus
(E) Human herpesvirus 8
(F) Human papillomavirus
(G) Mumps virus
(H) None of the above

BLOCK 1 ANSWER KEY

1. D	11. D	21. C	31. A	41. E
2. B	12. C	22. E	32. D	42. G
3. A	13. D	23. C	33. A	43. I
4. E	14. C	24. B	34. E	44. A
5. E	15. A	25. D	35. B	45. E
6. A	16. A	26. C	36. A	46. B
7. C	17. C	27. A	37. A	47. F
8. E	18. D	28. A	38. A	48. E
9. B	19. E	29. D	39. I	49. B
10. C	20. E	30. E	40. J	50. C

Refer to Answers and Explanations Section for Block 1

Pages 197–205

Figure credits

Question 44: Stevens A, et al: Female reproductive system. In Stevens A, et al (eds): Wheater's Basic Histopathology, 4th ed. New York, Churchill Livingstone, 2002, pp 198–215.

Question 45: Stevens A, et al: Cardiovascular system. In Stevens A, et al: Wheater's Basic Histopathology, 4th ed New York, Churchill Livingstone, 2002, pp 110–121.

BLOCK 2

50 QUESTIONS

TIME ALLOWED:
60 MINUTES

Question 51

A 65-year-old man complains of impotence for the last 6 months. He has difficulty achieving an erection when highly aroused and is unable to maintain the erection when he rarely achieves one. On questioning, the patient reports a lack of morning erections and an inability to achieve erection with masturbation. The patient is a long-time smoker, but the social and psychiatric history are otherwise unremarkable. Examination reveals moderate to severe atrophy of the buttock muscles. The patient tells you he frequently feels pain in his buttocks after walking for more than 2 or 3 minutes at a time. On extremity examination, the pedal and popliteal pulses are not palpable, and the skin covering the shins is cool, shiny, and hairless. What is the most likely cause of the patent's impotence?

(A) Aortoiliac occlusive disease
(B) Psychological anxiety
(C) Alcoholism
(D) Heart failure
(E) Depression

Question 52

A 9-year-old girl is brought to the emergency department after being in a high-speed automobile accident and suffering blunt abdominal trauma. She is crying quietly and complaining of abdominal pain and pain in the left shoulder. She received 1.5 L of normal saline on the way to the hospital. Vital signs are as follows:

Temperature	98.0°F
Blood pressure	60/40 mmHg
Pulse rate	148 beats/min
Respirations	26/min

The girl appears pale and now is complaining of dizziness. Two large-bore intravenous catheters are in place with lactated Ringer's solution being infused. Her skin is cool and pale. Her peripheral pulses are weak and becoming faster. Her abdomen is tender to palpation mostly in the left upper quadrant. The left shoulder is not tender to palpation and has a full range of passive motion without pain. Laboratory samples have been drawn (complete blood count and chemistry profiles) and are pending. The girl begins to get drowsy and starts to talk to her mother, who is not in the room. What is the next best course of action?

(A) Begin packed red blood cell transfusion with type O positive blood.
(B) Take the patient to the operating room for an emergency exploratory laparotomy.
(C) Start emergency cardiopulmonary resuscitation (CPR).
(D) Check the results of the complete blood count to see if a transfusion is required.
(E) Perform a mini-mental status examination.

Question 53

A 36-year-old woman complains of right leg pain. She has just returned from Tokyo, an 18-hour flight, and says the pain started as she was walking out of the airport. Medical history is significant for peptic ulcer disease and heavy smoking (2 packs per day). Medications include ranitidine, birth control pills, and multivitamins. She denies trauma to the leg, chest pain, or ever experiencing anything similar before. The patient's right thigh and calf are slightly edematous and erythematous when compared with the left side. Pedal pulses are intact bilaterally and symmetric. On dorsiflexion of the ankle with the knee straight, the patient has no increase in calf pain. Laboratory tests reveal the following:

Hemoglobin	15 gm/dL
Mean corpuscular volume	90 mm/cell
White blood cell count	6000/μL
Sodium	140 mEq/L
Potassium	4.2 mEq/L
Chloride	106 mEq/L
CO_2	25 mEq/L
BUN	10 mg/dL
Creatinine	1.0 mg/dL
Prothrombin time	10 sec (normal = 8–12)
Partial thromboplastin time	30 sec (normal = 25–38)
International normalized ratio (INR)	0.8
AST	10 U/L (normal = 7–27)

Which of the following is appropriate or true related to the most likely condition affecting this patient?

(A) Limited venography of the right calf veins should be ordered.

(B) The patient will likely need to stop taking birth control pills.

(C) The patient's smoking was unrelated to the development of this condition.

(D) The patient has cellulitis and should receive an antibiotic to cover *Streptococcus* and *Staphylococcus* species.

(E) Deep venous thrombosis is unlikely because of a negative Homan's sign.

Question 54

A 42-year-old man is brought to the emergency department after sustaining a closed head injury and being knocked unconscious. He is intubated when you see him in the emergency department. A CT scan of the head is performed and is negative for intracranial bleed or fracture. A few hours later, the patient wakes up and extubates himself. His oxygen saturation remains stable after extubation, his disorientation clears, and the patient claims to be fine other than "one heckuva headache." A few hours later, the nurse calls you because the patient has developed high blood pressure. When you go to see the patient, you look over the vital signs from admission and compare them with the current values:

	Initial	*Current*
Temperature	98.6°F	99.1°F
Blood pressure	124/80 mmHg	198/118 mmHg
Pulse rate	110 beats/min	50 beats/min
Respirations	16/min	6/min

The patient's respirations are irregular, with rapid respirations interspersed with random cessation of respirations for several seconds, then at other times, slow respirations. The patient is disoriented. What is the most likely underlying pathophysiologic abnormality?

(A) Infection

(B) Hypoxia

(C) Increased intracranial pressure

(D) Acute cocaine withdrawal with delirium

(E) Intensive care unit–induced delirium

Question 55

A 58-year-old man has been feeling "down" and has lost his appetite over the last 3 months. He estimates a 30 lb. weight loss in the last 2 to 3 months without trying. He has no urinary or bowel habit changes, but mentions dark-colored urine. Six months ago, the patient felt perfectly healthy. He has smoked 2 packs of cigarettes a day for the last 30. Medical history is significant for gout and diet-controlled diabetes.

On examination, the patient has mild scleral icterus and is cachectic appearing. No lymphadenopathy or jugular venous distention is appreciated. On abdominal examination, a soft round mass consistent with a distended gallbladder is appreciated under the right rib cage, distinct from the barely palpable liver edge. The spleen is not palpable. Laboratory tests reveal the following:

Hemoglobin	12 gm/dL
Mean corpuscular volume	86 μm/cell
White blood cell count	7500/μL
AST	30 U/L (normal = 7–27)
ALT	36 U/L (normal = 1–21)
Alkaline phosphatase	900 U/L (normal = 13–39)
Total bilirubin	5.0 mg/dL (normal = 0.1–1)
Direct bilirubin	4.0 mg/dL (normal = 0–0.4)
5′-Nucleotidase	750 U/L (normal = 1–11)

A chest radiograph is within normal limits. What is the most likely cause of the patient's symptoms?

(A) Occult lung cancer with metastases
(B) Pancreatic cancer
(C) Primary bone malignancy
(D) Hemochromatosis with cirrhosis
(E) Primary sclerosing cholangitis

Question 56

A 46-year-old woman comes to the emergency department with abdominal pain, fever and chills. The pain started 48 hours ago as a dull, crampy pain and has gotten progressively worse, with the development of fever and shaking chills 8 hours ago. The patient also complains of nausea. She has had minor bouts of the crampy pain before that went away on their own within an hour. Medical history is significant for hypertension, obesity, and sleep apnea. Vital signs are as follows:

Temperature	103.2°F
Blood pressure	98/64 mmHg
Pulse rate	114 beats/min
Respirations	22/min

On examination, the patient has mild scleral icterus, and her skin is warm, flushed, and moist. Chest and cardiac examinations are notable only for tachypnea and tachycardia. On abdominal examination, the patient has marked tenderness to palpation in the right upper quadrant. The rest of the examination is unremarkable. Laboratory tests reveal the following:

Hemoglobin	16 gm/dL
Mean corpuscular volume	88 μm/cell
White blood cell count	26,000/mL
AST	30 U/L (normal = 7–27)
ALT	20 U/L (normal = 1–21)
Alkaline phosphatase	380 U/L (normal = 13–39)
Total bilirubin	3.0 mg/dL (normal = 0.1–1)
Direct bilirubin	2.0 mg/dL (normal = 0–0.4)

Abdominal ultrasound reveals a significantly dilated common bile duct and gallstones within the gallbladder. What is the best thing to do at this point?

(A) Begin intravenous fluids and broad-spectrum antibiotics.
(B) Order a CT scan of the abdomen with contrast enhancement.
(C) Proceed to the operating room for emergent exploratory laparotomy.
(D) Administer bile acids, such as ursodeoxycholic acid, to dissolve the gallstones.
(E) Repeat the complete blood count to follow the white blood cell count.

Question 57

You are called to do a routine well-baby examination in the nursery on a female newborn who was born to a 46-year-old woman without delivery complications. On examination, the infant is placid and has microcephaly. The infant's eyes are slanted, the bridge of her nose is flattened, and she has moderate muscular hypotonicity. Both palms have a single palmar crease. When looking at the eyes more closely, you notice whitish spots around the periphery of the iris that resemble grains of salt. Which of the following is most likely to be true?

(A) The infant has a markedly increased risk of leukemia.
(B) The infant probably will die of renal disease.
(C) The infant will have a normal to above-average IQ.
(D) The infant's karyotype is 45 XO.
(E) The infant is likely to have ambiguous genitalia.

Question 58

A mother brings in her 14-year-old son after she noticed his appearance at the beach. She asks her son to show you and proceeds to leave the room. The boy, clearly embarrassed, takes off his shirt to reveal moderate asymmetric gynecomastia. He has no medical history and is on no medications. Review of systems is negative. On examination, the breast tissue is mildly tender to palpation bilaterally without masses, discharge, or overlying skin changes. The boy is at Tanner stage 3 in terms of development. The mother knocks, then comes back in the room and asks what the treatment options are. What should you tell her?

(A) The boy may have breast cancer and needs further workup.
(B) The boy may have a pituitary tumor and needs further workup.
(C) The boy may have a testicular tumor and needs further workup.
(D) The boy is going through normal development.
(E) The boy should have breast reduction surgery to obtain a good cosmetic result.

Question 59

What is the best preventive measure in regard to decubitus ulcers in paralyzed or debilitated patients?

(A) Prophylactic antibiotics
(B) Frequent turning
(C) Artificial skin applied to pressure points
(D) Daily multivitamins
(E) Hyperalimentation to ensure adequate nutritional status

Question 60

A 16-month-old male infant is brought in by his grandmother for a checkup. When asked about the child's mother and father, the woman rolls her eyes and says, "Next topic, please. I guess I'm his mother." The infant is unable to say any words and does not respond well to your voice. You notice that the infant has mild microcephaly, small eyes with short palpebral fissures, thin lips, and a wide and flattened philtrum. On cardiac examination, you hear a harsh 3/6 systolic murmur to the left of the sternum. The grandmother tells you that the infant has a "hole in his heart" that was diagnosed at birth. Which of the following is likely to be true regarding this infant?

(A) His karyotype involves trisomy 13.
(B) His biologic mother drank moderate to heavy amounts of alcohol during the pregnancy.
(C) He is likely to catch up with his peers in terms of cognitive development around the age of 6.
(D) His karyotype involves trisomy 18.
(E) He is likely to have Barr bodies on a buccal smear.

Question 61

Which of the following is thought to be the most common cause of pelvic inflammatory disease?
(A) *Chlamydia trachomatis*
(B) *Neisseria gonorrhoeae*
(C) Herpes simplex virus
(D) *Treponema pallidum*
(E) Human papillomavirus
(F) *Trichomonas vaginalis*

Question 62

Which of the following is a leading cause of blindness in developing countries?
(A) *Chlamydia trachomatis*
(B) *Neisseria gonnorrhoeae*
(C) Herpes simplex virus
(D) *Treponema pallidum*
(E) Human papillomavirus
(F) *Trichomonas vaginalis*

Question 63

Which of the following is most likely to cause neonatal conjunctivitis 5 to 14 days after birth?
(A) *Chlamydia trachomatis*
(B) *Neisseria gonorrhoeae*
(C) Herpes simplex virus
(D) *Treponema pallidum*
(E) Human papillomavirus
(F) *Trichomonas vaginalis*

Question 64

Which of the following causes condyloma lata?
(A) *Chlamydia trachomatis*
(B) *Neisseria gonnorhoeae*
(C) Herpes simplex virus
(D) *Treponema pallidum*
(E) Human papillomavirus
(F) *Trichomonas vaginalis*

Question 65

Which of the following causes lymphogranuloma venereum?
(A) *Chlamydia trachomatis*
(B) *Neisseria gonorrhoeae*
(C) Herpes simplex virus
(D) *Treponema pallidum*
(E) Human papillomavirus
(F) *Trichomonas vaginalis*

Question 66

Which of the following should be treated with metronidazole?
(A) *Chlamydia trachomatis*
(B) *Neisseria gonorrhoeae*
(C) Herpes simplex virus
(D) *Treponema pallidum*
(E) Human papillomavirus
(F) *Trichomonas vaginalis*

Question 67

A woman brings in a 6-month-old African American female infant for fever and swollen hands. The woman is a neighbor who is babysitting the infant for the mother, who is out of town and currently unreachable. The woman noticed the infant was irritable and crying excessively this morning and felt warm. Subsequently the infant's hands swelled up and seemed tender to the touch. The woman does not think the infant has any medical problems, and the infant does not take any medications. The woman remembers that there is a family history of anemia. Vital signs are as follows:

Temperature	100.2°F
Blood pressure	90/60 mmHg
Pulse rate	130 beats/min
Respirations	20/min

On examination, the infant is slightly small for her age. Both hands and feet are symmetrically swollen, warm, and markedly tender to the touch. The sclera and mucous membranes are pale. No other abnormalities are detected. Which of the following is most likely to be correct?

(A) The infant is a victim of abuse.
(B) Broad-spectrum antibiotics would improve this condition.
(C) The infant should be treated with acetaminophen and sent home.
(D) The cause of this condition is a virus.
(E) The infant has abnormal hemoglobin.

Question 68

Which of the following is **not** one of the four hallmark signs of a basilar skull fracture?

(A) Periorbital ecchymosis
(B) Scalp ecchymosis
(C) Postauricular ecchymosis
(D) Hemotympanum
(E) Cerebrospinal fluid rhinorrhea

Question 69

A 67-year-old woman comes to the office complaining of pain and stiffness in both hands for the last 3 years, which tends to be worse at the end of the day or after gardening. The patient has peptic ulcer disease, which was complicated by a "bleeding ulcer" that required multiple transfusions. The patient now avoids aspirin and takes only acetaminophen and lansoprazole. She claims the acetaminophen is no longer controlling her pain.

On examination, you note that several fingers on both hands have hard, painless nodules on the dorsolateral aspects of the distal interphalangeal joints. The joints are not warm or erythematous. The rest of the physical examination and review of systems is negative. Which of the following is true regarding the patient's arthritis?

(A) Antinuclear antibody and/or rheumatoid factor titers are likely to be positive.

(B) The patient should be put on a trial of indomethacin.

(C) Aspiration of the distal interphalangeal digit of the right third finger should be performed.

(D) The patient is likely to be HLA-B27 positive.

(E) The patient would be a good candidate for a trial of celecoxib or rofecoxib.

Question 70

A 29-year-old woman comes to the office complaining of pain in her joints. She says the pain started roughly 2 months ago in both her hands and is worse in the morning or after inactivity, with accompanying stiffness. She decided to consult you when both her wrists and ankles also started to hurt 2 weeks previously and her energy level continued to decline, with marked fatigue by the end of the day. The woman has been a competitive soccer player for the last 15 years and now cannot play because of her fatigue and ankle pain. She is sexually active only with her partner of 10 years. On examination, the metacarpophalangeal and multiple proximal interphalangeal joints are warm, swollen, and edematous bilaterally. Both ankle joints are slightly warm and swollen, but not erythematous. Each of these affected joints is tender to palpation, and pain occurs with active range of motion of the affected joints. Analysis of the synovial fluid from arthrocentesis of the left metacarpophalangeal joint reveals the following:

White blood cells	32,000/µL
Neutrophils	50%
Crystal examination	Negative for crystals
Gram stain	Negative for organisms
Bacterial culture	Pending

Which of the following is the best choice regarding the most likely cause of this woman's arthritis?

(A) She is unlikely to have a positive rheumatoid factor.

(B) Broad-spectrum antibiotics should be given until the culture comes back negative.

(C) Culture for *Mycobacterium tuberculosis* is an important part of the work up.

(D) She may develop inflammation of serosal linings outside of her joints.

(E) Meals rich in protein or excessive alcohol consumption commonly precipitate arthritis attacks in this condition.

Question 71

Which of the following is true regarding plain abdominal radiographs?

(A) Nephrolithiasis is more likely to be detected than cholelithiasis.

(B) Free air under the diaphragm usually means a pneumothorax is present.

(C) The psoas shadow on the right often becomes more pronounced with appendicitis.

(D) Early colon cancer usually is seen as a hazy mass on abdominal radiographs.

(E) Multiple air-fluid levels in a markedly dilated small bowel usually mean the patient has infectious diarrhea.

Question 72

A 54-year-old alcoholic homeless man comes to the emergency department complaining of low back pain for the last 15 years and requests narcotics to relieve the pain. He is unaware of his medical history and smells of alcohol. On examination, the patient is unkempt and has tenderness to palpation in the right upper quadrant with an enlarged liver. Chest, cardiac, back, and neurologic examinations are within normal limits. Laboratory tests reveal the following:

Hemoglobin	11 gm/dL
Mean corpuscular volume	112 µm/cell
Sodium	140 mEq/L
Potassium	4.0 mEq/L
Chloride	108 mEq/dL
CO_2	27 mEq/L
BUN	6 mg/dL
Creatinine	1.0 mg/dL
AST	58 U/L (normal = 7–27)
ALT	20 U/L (normal = 1–21)
Total bilirubin	1.2 mg/dL (normal = 0.1–1)
Albumin	3.2 mg/dL (normal = 3.5–5.0)

Which of the following is true regarding this patient?

(A) The pattern of liver function tests indicates probable viral hepatitis.

(B) Folate deficiency is likely to be the cause of the anemia.

(C) Vitamin B_{12} deficiency is likely to be the cause of the anemia.

(D) He should receive narcotics for back pain.

(E) His back pain most likely is due to metastatic cancer.

Question 73

A 27-year-old woman comes to the office complaining of weakness and fatigue for the past month. She has no significant medical history. On examination, the sclera are pale. The chest, cardiac, abdominal, pelvic, and neurologic examinations are all within normal limits, as is a review of systems. A rectal examination reveals stool that is negative for occult blood. Laboratory tests reveal the following:

Hemoglobin	10 gm/dL
Mean corpuscular volume	76 mm/cell
Reticulocyte count	1%
Peripheral smear	Red blood cells are hypochromic
Haptoglobin	300 mg/dL (normal = 40–336)
Ferritin	10 ng/dL (normal = 15–350)
Iron:	12 µg/L (normal = 50–150)
Iron binding capacity	520 µg/L (normal = 250–410)
Lactate dehydrogenase	58 U/L (normal = 45–90)

What is the most likely cause of this patient's anemia?

(A) Menstrual blood loss

(B) Chronic inflammation

(C) Thalassemia

(D) Intravascular hemolysis

(E) Extravascular hemolysis

Question 74

A 68-year-old male patient you have been caring for has been diagnosed with terminal pancreatic cancer. After a discussion between the two of you about his condition, the patient decided to draft a living will. The will states that he is not to be intubated or given CPR under any circumstances. Three weeks later, the patient's wife, who is upset, calls you to the emergency department. When you arrive in the emergency department, the patient has extremely labored respirations, tachycardia, and delirium. The emergency department physician refused to perform aggressive intervention because of the diagnosis and living will. The wife demands that you save the patient's life, including putting him on a respirator. She does not care about the living will. She threatens to sue if prompt intervention is not performed. What should you do?

(A) Intubate the patient temporarily until you can contact an attorney.
(B) Tell the woman her behavior is inappropriate and leave the emergency department.
(C) Tell the woman you understand why she is upset but refuse to intubate the patient.
(D) Respect the wife's wishes and intubate the patient. Later, schedule elective extubation after the wife has come to accept the patient's terminal condition.
(E) Schedule an emergency family meeting and have them vote on the issue.

Question 75

A 55-year-old woman is scheduled to undergo a cholecystectomy for symptomatic gallstones, and you are asked to provide preoperative clearance. The patient has no significant medical history, and a routine physical examination done 1 year ago was within normal limits. Family history is significant for a father who died of lung cancer. The patient is currently on no medications. A review of systems and physical examination are within normal limits other than mild obesity. Routine laboratory tests reveal the following:

Hemoglobin	14 gm/dL
Mean corpuscular volume	88 μm/cell
Sodium	140 mEq/L
Potassium	7.9 mEq/L
Chloride	105 mEq/L
CO_2	26 mEq/L
BUN	8 mg/dL
Creatinine	0.9 mg/dL
Total bilirubin	0.5 mg/dL (normal = 0.1–1)
Indirect bilirubin	0.4 mg/dL (normal = 0.1–0.8)

Electrocardiogram and chest radiograph are within normal limits. Which of the following is true regarding the patient's potassium level?

(A) It likely is due to intrinsic renal disease.
(B) It likely is due to a problem within the adrenal glands.
(C) You should call the laboratory and ask about hemolysis of the specimen.
(D) It most likely represents early multiple myeloma.
(E) Urgent treatment is needed.

Question 76

Which of the following is the most common cause of new-onset sensorineural hearing loss in adults?

(A) Presbyacusis
(B) Viral infection
(C) Otosclerosis
(D) Meningitis
(E) Aminoglycosides

Question 77

A 42-year-old man comes to the emergency department complaining of severe abdominal pain. The pain started this morning, is constant, is located in the epigastric area, and radiates to the back. The patient also vomited a small amount of material that looked like "coffee grounds" according to him. The patient has a medical history significant for peptic ulcer disease and alcoholism. He thinks he may have high blood pressure as well. Vital signs reveal tachycardia with a rate of 112 beats/min and temperature of 99.6°F, with a normal blood pressure and respiratory rate. On examination, the patient is slightly tremulous. Abdominal examination reveals extreme tenderness to palpation in the epigastrium with some rebound tenderness and decreased bowel sounds. No masses are palpable, and the liver is mildly enlarged. Abdominal radiograph reveals a small amount of free air under the right diaphragm. Laboratory tests reveal the following:

Hemoglobin	12 gm/dL
Mean corpuscular volume	98 µm/cell
White blood cell count	10,000/mL
Amylase	160 U/L (normal = 53–123)
AST	32 U/L (normal = 7–27)
ALT	16 U/L (normal = 1–21)
Total bilirubin	1.0 mg/dL(normal = 0.1–1.0)
Sodium	136 mEq/L
Potassium	4.2 mEq/L
Chloride	104 mEq/L
CO_2	25 mEq/L
BUN	8 mg/dL
Creatinine	1.0 mg/dL

What is the most likely cause of the patient's symptoms?

(A) Pancreatitis
(B) Pancreatic abscess
(C) Hepatic abscess
(D) Viral hepatitis
(E) Perforated peptic ulcer

Question 78

A 27-year-old asymptomatic woman is referred to you for abnormal findings on routine laboratory examination. Medical history is significant for irregular periods over the past 2 years. Review of systems is negative. The laboratory data, done at another clinic, are as follows:

Alkaline phosphatase	235 U/L (normal = 13–39)
5′-Nucleotidase	5 U/L (normal = 1–11)
AST	12 U/L (normal = 7–27)
ALT	10 U/L (normal = 1–21)
Total bilirubin	0.5 mg/dL (normal = 0.1–1.0)
Direct bilirubin	0.1 mg/dL (normal = 0–0.4)

Of the following choices, which is the most likely cause of this patient's laboratory abnormality?

(A) Chronic viral hepatitis
(B) Bile duct obstruction
(C) Pancreatic cancer
(D) Bone disease
(E) Cholecystitis

Question 79

A 42 year-old woman with a medical history significant only for alcoholism presents to the office complaining of weakness for the last 2 weeks. She admits to still drinking heavily and declines treatment for her alcohol abuse at this time. Physical examination and vital signs are within normal limits. Laboratory tests reveal the following:

Sodium	140 mEq/L
Potassium	3.0 mEq/L
Chloride	104 mEq/L
CO_2	25 mEq/L
BUN	9 mg/dL
Creatinine	1.0 mg/dL

You give the patient some intravenous potassium as well as some oral potassium supplements and schedule a follow-up visit in 1 week. If, in 1 week, the laboratory values are exactly the same, which of the following should you do first for workup of the patient's hypokalemia?

(A) Check a magnesium level.
(B) Obtain an abdominal CT scan with contrast enhancement.
(C) Do a captopril stimulation test to check for renal artery stenosis.
(D) Administer high-dose potassium supplements and see the patient 1 week later.
(E) Administer corticosteroids.

Question 80

A 42-year-old obese woman presents with shortness of breath. She noticed that she has been unable to catch her breath for the last 2 hours. Although her medical history is significant for asthma, the patient claims this is not her asthma, as she has used her albuterol inhaler multiple times since this morning without relief. Vital signs are as follows:

Temperature	99.2°F
Blood pressure	90/58 mmHg
Pulse rate	102 beats/min
Respirations	26/min

On examination, the patient has moderate tachypnea and appears somewhat anxious. Lungs are clear to auscultation with good air movement, and the cardiac examination is normal other than mild tachycardia. On extremity examination, the right calf is slightly swollen and mildly tender to palpation. Neurologic examination is within normal limits. Chest radiograph, electrolytes and renal function tests are within normal limits. Arterial blood gas measurements done on room air are as follows:

pH	7.47 (normal = 7.35–7.45)
PaO_2	65 mmHg (normal = 80–100)
$PaCO_2$	30 mmHg (normal = 35–45)
HCO_3	25 mEq/L (normal = 22–28)
Hemoglobin	15 g/dL

What should you order next for workup of the patient's dyspnea?

(A) High resolution non-contrast CT scan of the chest
(B) Expiratory chest radiograph
(C) Thoracotomy with embolectomy
(D) Ventilation-perfusion nuclear lung scan
(E) Pulmonary function testing

Question 81

An 18-year-old man comes to the office for a routine health examination. He has no current complaints. Medical history is significant only for asthma and an appendectomy. Medications include an albuterol inhaler and zafirlukast. Physical examination reveals nasal polyps, lungs that are clear to auscultation, a surgical scar in the right lower quadrant of the abdomen, and a scar on the left shin, which the patient attributes to old trauma. The rest of the examination is within normal limits. The patient does not drink alcohol or smoke, although he has tried both as well as trying marijuana "once or twice." His affect and mood are within normal limits. Which of the following is true concerning this patient?

(A) He most likely has antisocial personality disorder.
(B) He should avoid aspirin.
(C) He has a substance abuse disorder.
(D) He needs to stop taking zafirlukast.
(E) The most common cause of death in his age group is suicide.

Question 82

A woman brings in her 3-year-old daughter for severe nausea and vomiting. The child had a "cold" that started about 1 week ago with low-grade fever, sore throat, runny nose, and malaise. The mother had been giving the child aspirin for the fever and aches over the last 4 days with some relief. The mother says the child developed severe nausea and vomiting this morning and seems to be acting "out of sorts."

On examination, the child appears dehydrated and retches several times during the examination. Vital signs are within normal limits except for a slight tachycardia and slightly low blood pressure. She is lethargic and confused, not responding to your questions or attempts at interaction. Meningeal signs are absent. Lumbar puncture is performed and is within normal limits except for a decreased glucose level of 35 mg/dL. Laboratory tests reveal the following:

Hemoglobin	16 gm/dL
AST	503 U/L (normal = 7–27)
ALT	599 U/L (normal = 1–21)
Glucose	50 mg/dL (normal = 70–110)
Ammonia	82 mmol/L (normal = 12–55)

What is the most likely underlying cause of the child's condition?

(A) Reye's syndrome
(B) Hypoglycemia
(C) Subacute meningitis
(D) Brain tumor
(E) Meningococcemia

Question 83

In which of the following effects is there a difference between aspirin and acetaminophen?

(A) Antipyretic effects
(B) Vomiting with overdose
(C) Analgesic effects
(D) Antiplatelet effects
(E) Useful in osteoarthritis

Question 84

A 29-year-old woman comes to you concerned about the risks versus the benefits of oral contraceptive pills for birth control. Which of the following is true regarding oral contraceptive pills?

(A) They usually worsen dysmenorrhea.
(B) They commonly cause weight loss.
(C) They reduce the incidence of ovarian cancer.
(D) They reduce the incidence of hypertension.
(E) They are often given to women with active liver disease because they tend to lessen liver inflammation.

Question 85

A G1P1, 29-year-old woman comes to the office for her annual Pap smear. She has no significant medical history. Her only medications are oral contraceptive pills, started 6 months ago (after delivery of her daughter), and multivitamins. She has no complaints. Vital signs are as follows:

Temperature	98.7°F
Blood pressure	158/92 mmHg
Pulse rate	72 beats/min
Respirations	14/min

The patient has never had high blood pressure before. Repeat blood pressure 5 minutes later on the other arm is unchanged. Physical examination is within normal limits, and a Pap smear is performed. Which of the following is true?

(A) The patient should be asked to reduce salt intake and begin an exercise regimen.
(B) The patient should be put on hydralazine.
(C) The patient should stop taking birth control pills and have her blood pressure remeasured in a month.
(D) The patient should be scheduled for a repeat blood pressure check in 1 month, and if she is still hypertensive, medication should be started.
(E) The patient should be allowed 6 months of lifestyle changes, and if her blood pressure is still elevated, medication should be started.

Question 86

Which of the following medications is most likely to cause a clinically significant induction of liver enzymes, potentially resulting in increased metabolism of other drugs?

(A) Cimetidine
(B) Penicillin
(C) Phenobarbital
(D) Lansoprazole
(E) Fluoxetine

Question 87

You follow a difficult 42-year-old male patient for arthritis of both knees, confirmed by radiographs showing severe degenerative changes, secondary to old sports injuries. He requires frequent follow-up visits and often calls you in the middle of the night because of pain. He is in your office today for routine follow-up after you decided to try an experiment. You gave him a bottle full of sugar pills and told him they were a powerful new antiarthritis medication because you suspect a strong psychological component to the pain. The patient reports that the sugar pills have worked well, and he asks for a refill. Which of the following is true?

(A) You should give the patient more sugar pills but not tell him what they are.
(B) The pain is psychological.
(C) The patient responded to placebo.
(D) The patient is most likely malingering.
(E) You should give the patient more sugar pills but tell him that the pills are made simply of sugar.

Question 88

A 35-year-old man is dropped off in front of the emergency department unconscious, and no history is obtainable. Vital signs are as follows:

Temperature	98.2°F
Blood pressure	110/80 mmHg
Pulse rate	90 beats/min
Respirations	10/min

The pupils are small but reactive to light bilaterally, and the patient does not respond to painful stimuli. Which of the following is **not** an appropriate initial intervention?

(A) Administration of naloxone
(B) Administration of oxygen
(C) Administration of glucose
(D) Intravenous access using a large-bore catheter
(E) Administration of sodium bicarbonate

Question 89

A 34-year-old woman complains of fatigue and abdominal pain. She says the fatigue started roughly 3 weeks ago and has been getting progressively worse. The abdominal pain started this morning. It is intermittent, sharp yet crampy, located on the right side of her abdomen with some radiation down into the groin area, and associated with nausea when the pain becomes severe. The patient has never experienced pain like this in the past. She has no significant medical history and takes no medications. Vital signs are within normal limits. Physical examination reveals a tender right flank but is otherwise unremarkable. Laboratory tests reveal the following:

Sodium	140 mEq/L
Potassium	4.3 mEq/L
Chloride	102 mEq/L
CO_2	27 mEq/L
BUN	10 mg/dL
Creatinine	1.0 mg/dL
Albumin	4.2 g/dL (normal = 3.5–5)
Calcium	12.7 mg/dL (normal = 8.5–10.5)

An abdominal radiograph is pending. Initial patient management should include which of the following?

(A) Furosemide
(B) Hydrochlorothiazide
(C) Intravenous normal saline
(D) Fluid restriction
(E) Pamidronate

Question 90

An HIV positive 40-year-old homosexual man with AIDS presents for follow-up and a second opinion regarding a rash on his torso that began 7 months ago. The man was told that the rash was inflammatory and has been treated with a number of drugs, including penicillin, antifungals, and topical and oral steroids over the past 6 months with no improvement. Additionally, new lesions have appeared. The man has been losing some weight and is frustrated at the lack of improvement in the lesions. The appearance of these nonpruritic, nontender lesions is shown below. The man is not acutely ill appearing and has no other complaints.

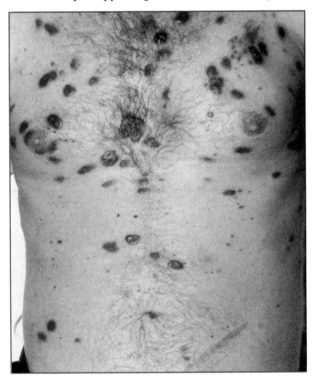

Which of the following is true regarding this AIDS-related condition?

(A) It is associated with human herpesvirus-8 infection
(B) It is related to reactivation of the same virus that causes chickenpox
(C) The lesions typically regress spontaneously
(D) Biopsy would likely reveal caseous necrosis
(E) It represents a disseminated form of human papillomavirus infection

Question 91

A 27-year-old woman presents complaining of a rash on both her elbows for the last month. The lesions are well-demarcated, raised and erythematous, with a silvery scale. The lesions do not itch. A slide from a biopsy of one of the lesions is shown below.

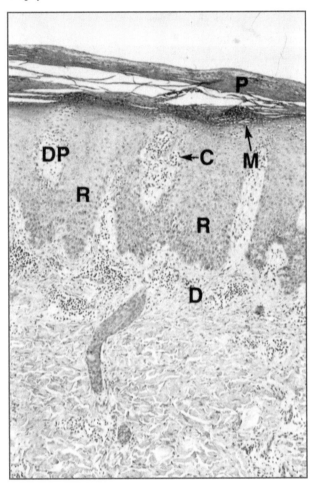

Which of the following is true regarding the most likely condition?

(A) Excisional biopsy is the treatment of choice.
(B) A course of oral fluconazole would cause complete regression of the lesions but would take several weeks of therapy.
(C) The patient is at a high risk for visceral malignancy.
(D) A family history of similar lesions is fairly common.
(E) In most cases, the lesions have a "Christmas tree" appearance on the back.

Question 92

What is the most common malignancy in people younger than 20?

(A) Brain tumors
(B) Leukemia
(C) Kidney tumors
(D) Peripheral nerve tumors
(E) Ocular tumors

Question 93

Deficiency of which of the following vitamins can cause petechial bleeding?

(A) Vitamin B_1 (thiamine)
(B) Vitamin B_{12} (cobalamin)
(C) Folate
(D) Vitamin C
(E) Vitamin K

Question 94

Which of the following substances is **not** generally associated with thrombocytopenia?

(A) Alcohol
(B) Aspirin
(C) Sulfonamides
(D) Heparin
(E) Quinidine

Question 95

Which of the following associations between a medication or disease and its effect on clotting function tests is correct?

(A) Enoxaparin—prolongs partial thromboplastin time
(B) Warfarin—prolongs prothrombin time and bleeding time
(C) Aspirin—prolongs prothrombin time
(D) von Willebrand's disease—prolongs bleeding time and slightly prolongs partial thromboplastin time
(E) Hemophilia—primarily prolongs prothrombin time

Question 96

A 42-year-old woman comes to the emergency department with confusion. She also has a nosebleed in the absence of trauma according to her husband. She has no recent sick contacts, is on no medications, and has no medical history. Her temperature is 102° F. Examination reveals no specific deficits other than confusion and mild disorientation. CT scan of the head and chest radiograph are negative. Laboratory tests include the following:

Hemoglobin	10 gm/dL
Mean corpuscular volume	94 µm/cell
White blood cell count	8000/µL
Platelet count	33,000/µL
Peripheral smear	4+ schistocytes, 3+ helmet cells, 2+ polychromasia
Reticulocyte count	7% (normal = 0.5–2.5)
Lactate dehydrogenase	812 U/L (normal = 45–90)
Prothrombin time	Normal
Partial thromboplastin time	Normal
ALT	18 U/L (normal = 1–21)
Creatinine	1.2 mg/dL
Urinalysis	Within normal limits
Blood culture	Pending, but Gram stain is negative

Which of the following is likely to improve the outcome in this patient?

(A) Bone marrow biopsy
(B) Empirical intravenous acyclovir
(C) Platelet transfusion
(D) Packed red blood cell transfusion
(E) Plasmapheresis

Question 97

A 24-year-old man presents with a chief complaint of chest pain. He states that this retrosternal, sharp pain began last night, is fairly constant, and is aggravated by lying down or coughing and relieved by sitting up. The patient had "a cold" roughly 1 week ago with runny nose, sore throat, and dry cough. He has no significant medical history but notes that his father had a heart attack at the age of 62 and his grandmother died of a heart attack around age 70. He is not currently taking any medications and has never used drugs or alcohol. Vital signs are as follows:

Temperature	99.8°F
Blood pressure	128/86 mmHg
Pulse rate	90 beats/min
Respirations	18/min

The patient is athletic appearing and in no apparent distress. He has mild pharyngeal erythema without exudate, no lymphadenopathy, and no jugular venous distention. His lungs sound clear to auscultation, although the patient is unable to inspire deeply secondary to pain. On cardiac examination, the rate and rhythm are regular, but you hear a scratchy, scraping noise throughout most of the cardiac cycle in the left parasternal area. Which of the following is true?

(A) The patient needs a cardiac stress test given his strong family history.
(B) Nonsteroidal anti-inflammatory drugs such as indomethacin are the treatment of choice.
(C) The most likely cause of this patient's symptoms is a streptococcal infection.
(D) The patient most likely had a previously damaged heart valve.
(E) You would expect Q waves in the precordial leads on an electrocardiogram.

Question 98

Which of the following is an advantage of chorionic villus sampling over amniocentesis for detection of fetal abnormalities?

(A) Can be performed earlier in the pregnancy
(B) Can detect neural tube defects with greater accuracy
(C) Lower miscarriage rate
(D) Abortion usually performed at the same time as the test
(E) None of the above

Question 99

Which of the following is a cause for a high maternal serum alpha fetoprotein level performed at 17 weeks' gestation?

(A) Trisomy 18
(B) Down syndrome
(C) Intrauterine growth retardation
(D) Anencephaly
(E) Inaccurate dates with an actual gestation of only 14 weeks

Question 100

A 4-year-old child presents with scalp itching, and you note the presence of lice on several hair shafts. Which of the following is true regarding treatment?

(A) Lindane is preferred over permethrin because of potential neurotoxicity with permethrin.
(B) This disorder is quite rare in children with good hygiene.
(C) Decontamination of bed sheets and clothing is required.
(D) You should report the parents for probable child abuse.
(E) Lice are a common cause of failure to thrive and short stature.

BLOCK 2 ANSWER KEY

51. A	61. A	71. A	81. B	91. D
52. B	62. A	72. B	82. A	92. B
53. B	63. A	73. A	83. D	93. D
54. C	64. D	74. C	84. C	94. B
55. B	65. A	75. C	85. C	95. D
56. A	66. F	76. A	86. C	96. E
57. A	67. E	77. E	87. C	97. B
58. D	68. B	78. D	88. E	98. A
59. B	69. E	79. A	89. C	99. D
60. B	70. D	80. D	90. A	100. C

Refer to Answers and Explanations Section for Block 2

Pages 207–215

Figure credits

Question 90: Hoffbrand AV, Pettit JE: Benign disorders of leukocytes. In Hoffbrand AV, Pettit JE Color Atlas of Clinical Hematology, 3rd ed. St. Louis, Mosby, 2000, pp 117–138.

Question 91: Stevens A, et al: Skin. In Stevens A, et al (eds): Wheater's Basic Histopathology, 4th ed. New York, Churchill Livingstone, 2000, pp. 242–257.

50 QUESTIONS

**TIME ALLOWED:
60 MINUTES**

Question 101

A 76-year-old woman is admitted to the hospital for weight loss and back pain. She is found to have metastatic breast cancer. The family is waiting outside the room when you are on your way to inform the woman of the diagnosis. The family asks you not to tell the patient. "It would devastate her," the patient's daughter tells you. You tell the family that you feel it is your obligation to inform the patient of the diagnosis, and they get upset because they "know the patient much better" than you do and know what is best for her. What should you do?

(A) Respect the family's wishes.
(B) Tell the patient the diagnosis anyway.
(C) Ask the family what their concerns are about revealing the diagnosis.
(D) Have each of the family members vote on whether or not they want the patient informed of her diagnosis.
(E) Call the hospital attorney to discuss the matter.

Question 102

Which of the following agents has **not** been associated with autoimmune phenomenon as a potential side effect?

(A) Isoniazid
(B) Procainamide
(C) Omeprazole
(D) Methyldopa
(E) Hydralazine

Question 103

Which of the following is true concerning Apgar scores in the newborn?

(A) When done at 1 minute after birth, it is the first assessment of how well the newborn is doing.
(B) It is a general measure of well-being based on five different categories.
(C) The maximum score is 5, with a minimum score of 1.
(D) Categories include respirations, heart rate, grasp reflex, muscle tone, and reflex irritability.
(E) Newborns with low Apgar scores are more likely to be healthy at 1 year than newborns with high Apgar scores.

Question 104

Minutes after a spontaneous vaginal vertex delivery of a male infant at 40 weeks' gestation, you are called to evaluate the newborn for swelling of the scalp. On examination, the child is alert and responsive. There is edema of the scalp with mild ecchymosis extending across the midline and overlying part of both parietal bones and the occipital area. The rest of your examination is within normal limits. What is the next best step in the workup?

(A) Ultrasound of the cranium
(B) Skull radiograph
(C) Aspiration of the subcutaneous space
(D) CT scan of the head
(E) None of the above

Question 105

A 17-year-old woman complains of gradual onset of blurry vision. She says that she is unable to see the chalkboard at school unless she sits in the front row of the classroom. She has no significant medical history, does not see a physician regularly, and is on no medications. She smokes 10 to 15 cigarettes a day and has been sexually active with multiple partners over the past 2-3 years. On examination, the pupils are equally round and reactive to light and accommodation. Funduscopic examination is within normal limits, and the disk margins are sharp. There are no apparent visual field deficits. On visual acuity testing, near vision is within normal limits, but distance vision is 20/50 in the right eye and 20/40 in the left eye. The rest of the physical examination is within normal limits. What should you do next?

(A) Make urgent referral to an ophthalmologist to prevent blindness.
(B) Start corticosteroid eye drops and place a patch over the left eye, instructing the patient to return in 24 hours for follow-up.
(C) Perform a Pap smear.
(D) Give the patient standard reading glasses.
(E) Check rheumatoid factor and antinuclear antibody titers.

Question 106

A 29-year-old man with a history of schizophrenia is brought to the emergency department in an ambulance for high fevers and altered mental status. According to previous records, the patient was recently started on haloperidol. The emergency medical technicians confirm that the patient said he takes haloperidol and is due for another dose. The patient then became unresponsive and could no longer answer questions. The technicians have the patient's haloperidol pill bottle and have not given him the dose that is now overdue. The patient's vital signs are as follows:

Temperature	105.2°F
Blood pressure	182/102 mmHg
Pulse rate	102 beats/min
Respirations	22/min

On examination, the patient is difficult to rouse and unable to answer questions. He is markedly diaphoretic and has markedly increased muscle tone in all extremities. The patient is drooling. His chest is clear to auscultation, the heart is tachycardic but with a regular rhythm, and the rest of the examination is unremarkable. Laboratory tests reveal the following:

Hemoglobin	16 gm/dL
Mean corpuscular volume	88 µm/cell
Sodium	137 mEq/L
Potassium	5.5 mEq/L
Chloride	104 mEq/L
CO_2 26 mEq/L	
Creatine kinase	8460 U/L
	(normal = 17–148)
Creatine kinase MB fraction	< 4% of total

What is the appropriate first intervention?

(A) Stop the haloperidol.
(B) Administer a bolus of haloperidol.
(C) Administer diphenhydramine.
(D) Give nitroglycerin.
(E) Perform an MRI of the brain.

Question 107

Which of the following is true regarding thermal injury or burns?

(A) Infection usually is secondary to *Corynebacterium diphtheriae* species.
(B) Third-degree burns are extremely painful, and liberal pain medication should be used.
(C) Skin with second-degree burns normally has blisters and open, weeping surfaces.
(D) Prophylactic intravenous antibiotics should be given for severe second-degree and all third-degree burns.
(E) Tetanus boosters are not required unless extensive third-degree burns are present.

Question 108

Which of the following is most likely to be associated with oligohydramnios?

(A) Renal agenesis
(B) Anencephaly
(C) Duodenal atresia
(D) Fetal hydrops
(E) Multiple gestation

Question 109

A 46-year-old man with renal failure secondary to adult polycystic kidney disease undergoes a kidney transplant using a cadaver kidney. The final vascular anastomosis is completed, and the vascular clamps are released. The transplanted kidney starts to turn a bluish black color within minutes. Which of the following is true?

(A) High-dose cyclosporine should be administered.
(B) The kidney should be removed.
(C) This is a form of rejection mediated by macrophages.
(D) This is an example of acute rejection.
(E) Large amounts of intravenous hydration should correct the process.

Question 110

A 32-year-old man is brought to the emergency department after an automobile accident in which he was an unrestrained passenger in the front seat. He is conscious, alert, and oriented but has abdominal pain. Vital signs are as follows:

Temperature	98.9°F
Blood pressure	136/88 mmHg
Pulse rate	96 beats/min
Respirations	16/min

On examination, the patient is in mild distress from pain. Intravenous access has been obtained, and lactated Ringer's solution is being infused. Pupils are equally round and reactive to light; chest and cardiac examinations are within normal limits; the abdomen is mildly tender to palpation with normal, active bowel sounds; and some ecchymosis of the skin is seen in the midline of the lower abdomen. There is no rebound or guarding. Rectal examination reveals a high-riding, boggy, tender prostate; stool is negative for occult blood. Genitalia examination reveals minimal blood at the urethral meatus. Extremity examination is within normal limits with no tenderness or pain to palpation and full range of active and passive motion. The nurse comes by to place a Foley catheter. What is the next appropriate step in the management of this patient?

(A) Order a retrograde urethrogram and cancel the Foley catheter.
(B) Write an order requesting strict urine output monitoring after the Foley catheter is placed.
(C) Order a CT scan of the abdomen without contrast enhancement.
(D) Administer broad-spectrum antibiotics.
(E) Obtain a urinalysis specimen from a catheterized urine specimen.

Question 111

A 66-year-old man presents to the emergency department with a chief complaint of abdominal pain. He describes a dull, crampy lower abdominal pain over the last 12 hours that is fairly constant. He mentions that he has not urinated in the last two days. Medical history is significant for hypertension, gout, hypercholesterolemia, and benign prostatic hypertrophy. Medications include terazosin, allopurinol, atorvastatin, and aspirin. Vital signs are within normal limits except for blood pressure of 158/94 mmHg. On physical examination, the patient has moderate suprapubic abdominal tenderness with a palpable, significantly distended bladder. Bowel sounds are normal and active. There is no rebound tenderness or guarding. Ultrasound exam reveals bilateral hydronephrosis and the serum creatinine is 2.2 mg/dL, though the patient has no history of renal insufficiency. You are unable to pass a Foley catheter into the bladder after multiple attempts. What is the next appropriate step in the management of this patient?

(A) Schedule a prostatectomy.
(B) Order an abdominal MR angiogram to exclude renal artery stenosis.
(C) Order an α-fetoprotein level.
(D) Perform suprapubic catheterization.
(E) Start the patient on heparin.

Question 112

A 65-year-old woman complains of sudden onset of severe right foot pain that began 2 hours ago at rest. There is no history of trauma. The pain is severe, constant, and throbbing. The woman said her right foot feels cold, and she is starting to feel some tingling in it. She felt completely healthy before these symptoms. She does not smoke, drink alcohol, or abuse drugs. Her medical history is significant for hypertension, arthritis, and rheumatic heart disease as a child. She takes ramipril, felodipine, and an aspirin for an "irregular heart beat."

On examination, vital signs are within normal limits. The heart rate and pulse are irregularly irregular. On extremity examination, the right foot is cold and tender compared with the left. The skin is slightly edematous around the right foot but is otherwise normal on both legs, as are the toenails. The dorsalis pedis pulse is not palpable on the right foot, whereas the left dorsalis pedis and both posterior tibial pulses are normal. As you are talking to the woman, she mentions that her left arm is feeling heavy. You note decreased strength in the left arm and a left facial droop that were not present 5 minutes ago. Which of the following conditions is most likely to account for this woman's presentation?

(A) Temporal arteritis with polymyalgia rheumatica
(B) Deep venous thrombosis with embolization
(C) Cardiac thrombus with embolization
(D) Severe peripheral vascular disease
(E) Thromboangiitis obliterans (Buerger's disease)

Question 113

A 63-year-old man presents to the office with a chief complaint of pain in the calf when walking. He claims that the further he walks, the more likely he is to get pain in his left calf, and the worse the pain is likely to get. When he stops to rest, the pain goes away. The pattern had been stable over a few months because the patient just avoided walking long distances, but he says it is now slowly getting worse, and shorter distances are bringing on the pain. Medical history is significant for a myocardial infarction 4 years ago, hypertension, hypercholesterolemia, gout, and tobacco use of 2 packs per day for the last 20 years. Medications include carvedilol, enalapril, pravastatin, aspirin, and allopurinol.

Vital signs are within normal limits. Extremity examination reveals shiny skin without hair on both legs below the knee and thickened, somewhat distorted toenails. Temperature is decreased on the surface of both feet compared with the rest of the body. Pedal and popliteal pulses are not palpable bilaterally, whereas femoral pulses are normal bilaterally. Which of the following should be the next step in the management of this patient?

(A) Encourage the patient to quit smoking.
(B) Start heparin.
(C) Refer for urgent revascularization procedure.
(D) Increase the dose of carvedilol.
(E) Stop the aspirin.

Question 114

A 69-year-old woman complains of the sudden onset of right arm weakness and heaviness that began 2 hours ago, associated with "clumsiness" in her right hand. She came immediately to the emergency department, but after sitting in the waiting room for 30 minutes, the arm felt back to normal and is no longer weak or clumsy. The patient has never experienced anything similar to this phenomenon before. Medical history is significant for diabetes, hypertension, congestive heart failure, and tobacco use since the age of 12. Medications include metformin, glipizide, pioglitazone, captopril, and furosemide. Examination is within normal limits except for the presence of a cardiac S3 sound and a bruit heard in the left carotid artery. A carotid duplex is ordered and reveals findings compatible with 85% stenosis in the left carotid artery and 40% stenosis in the right carotid artery. Which of the following interventions is most likely to result in the best long-term survival in relation to the patient's carotid artery disease?

(A) Left carotid endarterectomy
(B) Left and right carotid endarterectomies
(C) Aspirin
(D) Warfarin
(E) Simvastatin

Question 115

A 24-year-old woman comes to the office with the chief complaint of a headache. She says the headache started about 4 days ago and is getting worse. She has a hard time localizing the headache but says she feels pressure behind her face and gestures toward either side of her nose. She also admits to a "cold" involving greenish nasal discharge when she blows her nose, dry cough, and mild sore throat. She has not checked her temperature at home but has felt somewhat warm. She denies night sweats. Medical history is significant for dysmenorrhea and iron-deficiency anemia. The patient takes daily iron tablets and multivitamins. On examination, the area to the left of the nose is somewhat tender to palpation and the nasal mucosa is slightly congested. The pharynx is mildly erythematous, and the tympanic membranes are clear with a good light reflex. Which of the following is most likely to be true?

(A) The patient's current complaints are related to her dysmenorrhea.
(B) The patient has an immunodeficiency.
(C) The patient has cluster headaches.
(D) The patient has migraine headaches.
(E) The patient has sinusitis.

Question 116

An 18-month-old girl is brought in by her parents for fever and a runny nose. The child has a history of otitis media three times in the past year, and the parents note the child has been tugging on her left ear, which she had done with previous bouts of ear infection. The child has no other health problems and is developmentally normal. Height, weight, and head circumference are at the 60th percentile. On examination, you note an erythematous and bulging left tympanic membrane and what appears to be clear fluid with an air-fluid level behind the right tympanic membrane, where the child had a bout of otitis 2 months ago. There also is mild pharyngeal erythema, and the child has a temperature of 100.9°F. For which of the following is the child particularly at risk?

(A) Child abuse
(B) Lymphoma
(C) Leukemia
(D) Severe combined immunodeficiency
(E) Developmental cognitive or speech problems

Question 117

Which of the following organisms is most likely to cause otitis externa?

(A) *Staphylococcus epidermidis*
(B) *Streptococcus pneumoniae*
(C) *Pseudomonas aeruginosa*
(D) *Mycoplasma hominis*
(E) Coxsackievirus

Question 118

Which of the following is the most likely side effect of heparin?

(A) Thrombocytosis
(B) Teratogenicity
(C) Neutropenia
(D) Cardiomyopathy
(E) Thrombosis

Question 119

What is the best treatment for mumps orchitis?

(A) Intravenous corticosteroids
(B) Selective ablation of testicular veins
(C) Surgical drainage
(D) Acyclovir
(E) Prevention through immunization

Question 120

A 52-year-old obese man complains of progressive symptoms including increased thirst, excessive urination, weight loss, and fatigue over the past 3 weeks. The patient wakes up several times during the night to urinate and has been drinking several gallons of fluid a day. Past medical history is significant for hypertension and high cholesterol. Medications include valsartan and niacin. There is a strong family history of hypertension and diabetes. Vital signs are as follows:

Temperature	99.1°F
Blood pressure	142/92 mmHg
Pulse rate	110 beats/min
Respirations	20/min

Physical examination reveals dry mucous membranes, obesity, mild tachypnea, and tachycardia without murmurs; the rest of the examination is within normal limits. Laboratory tests reveal the following:

Hemoglobin	17 gm/dL
Mean corpuscular volume	87 mm/cell
Sodium	125 mEq/L
Potassium	4.0 mEq/L
Chloride	94 mEq/L
CO_2	24 mEq/L
BUN	22 mg/dL
Creatinine	1.0 mg/dL
Glucose	785 mg/dL

Which of the following is true regarding this patient?

(A) Hyperglycemia is most likely related to diabetic ketoacidosis.
(B) Decreased sodium level requires urgent hypertonic saline to prevent seizures.
(C) Decreased sodium level probably will correct itself with correction of the glucose.
(D) The patient is likely to have an elevated total body potassium even though the level is normal.
(E) The patient should receive a trial of vasopressin to determine if an appropriate renal response occurs.

Question 121

Which of the following antibiotics is the best choice for uncomplicated cases of otitis media?

(A) Vancomycin
(B) Nitrofurantoin
(C) Fluconazole
(D) Gentamicin
(E) Cefaclor

Question 122

Which of the following is **false** concerning a neck mass in a child?

(A) It may be due to thyroid abnormalities.
(B) If the mass elevates with tongue protrusion, it may represent a thyroglossal duct cyst.
(C) If in the midline, it is unlikely to represent a branchial cleft cyst.
(D) It may be due to lymphadenitis.
(E) It is more likely to be malignant than a neck mass in an adult.

Question 123

Which of the following is the most common cause of a nosebleed in a child?

(A) Angiofibroma
(B) Leukemia
(C) Idiopathic thrombocytopenic purpura
(D) Trauma
(E) Vascular ectasia

Question 124

Which of the following causes of rhinitis is most likely to have nasal secretions containing high numbers of eosinophils?

(A) Bacterial
(B) Allergic
(C) Viral
(D) Cancerous
(E) Fungal

Question 125

What is the most likely cause of vertigo in an elderly woman with no hearing loss or tinnitus who has dizzy spells and nystagmus only when she lies on her left side?

(A) Benign positional vertigo
(B) Bacterial labyrinthitis
(C) Ménière's disease
(D) Viral labyrinthitis
(E) Acoustic neuroma

Question 126

Which of the following is most important to perform after a child has a bout of bacterial meningitis?

(A) Formal objective developmental assessment using a standard battery of tests
(B) Objective auditory testing
(C) Objective vision screening by an ophthalmologist
(D) Repeat blood cultures
(E) Human immunodeficiency virus (HIV) testing

Question 127

Which of the following drugs is **least** likely to cause auditory disturbances?

(A) Amikacin
(B) Thioridazine
(C) Aspirin
(D) Loop diuretics
(E) Quinine

Question 128

Which of the following is **not** thought to improve long-term survival after a myocardial infarction?

(A) Atenolol
(B) Nitroglycerin
(C) Ramipril
(D) Aspirin
(E) Smoking cessation

Question 129

Which of the following is **not** thought to improve long-term survival in patients with stable congestive heart failure?

(A) Spironolactone
(B) Digoxin
(C) Carvedilol
(D) Enalapril
(E) Smoking cessation

Question 130

Which of the following is the most common cause of unilateral facial nerve paralysis that involves the entire left side of the face?

(A) Brain stem infarction
(B) Bell's palsy
(C) Acoustic neuroma
(D) Multiple sclerosis
(E) Middle ear infection

Question 131

A lesion of which of the following cranial nerves may result in hyperacusis?

(A) Trochlear nerve
(B) Facial nerve
(C) Vestibular branch of the vestibulocochlear nerve
(D) Glossopharyngeal nerve
(E) Vagus nerve

Question 132

Ignoring cost, which of the following would be the most effective measure to reduce the incidence of neural tube defects?

(A) Folate supplements given to all women of reproductive age
(B) Folate supplements given to all pregnant women starting at the first prenatal visit
(C) Regular prenatal care
(D) Control of maternal hypertension
(E) Smoking cessation

Question 133

A 36-year-old man who is a regular hiker and camper develops crampy abdominal pain and excessive foul-smelling, nonbloody diarrhea that floats to the top of the toilet bowl, which began 4 weeks ago. He denies fever. He does not take any medications. Physical examination is normal. Which of the following is likely to be true regarding the most likely cause of his diarrhea?

(A) It is caused by a bacteria susceptible to several different antibiotics.
(B) His stool is likely to have a decreased fat content.
(C) The cause is a virus.
(D) The stool may contain unique-appearing cysts.
(E) The site of involvement is the sigmoid colon.

Question 134

In a patient with increased intracranial pressure and moderate hypertension, which of the following should be **avoided**?

(A) Placing the patient in reverse Trendelenburg position
(B) Intubation
(C) Lowering of the blood pressure
(D) Mannitol
(E) Furosemide

Question 135

Which of the following is true concerning head trauma?

(A) Permanent neurologic deficits may occur in the setting of a normal CT scan.
(B) Heparin infusion should be started before head CT scan in the setting of a closed head injury.
(C) Lumbar puncture is the initial test of choice to look for intracranial hemorrhage.
(D) A fixed, dilated pupil in the setting of head trauma normally means there has been a shear injury to the ipsilateral third cranial nerve.
(E) Almost all skull fractures involving the calvaria require surgical intervention.

Question 136

A 58-year-old man complains of a sore big toe on the right foot with no history of trauma that woke him up in the middle of the night. The pain has gotten progressively worse since that time. He feels fine otherwise and has no other complaints. Medical history includes obesity, hypertension, and tobacco and alcohol use. The patient is divorced, is not currently sexually active, and denies any history of illicit drug use. The patient was started on hydrochlorothiazide 2 weeks ago for hypertension and has taken propranolol for several years. On examination, the patient is obese and in no apparent distress. Vital signs are within normal limits. The skin overlying the metatarsophalangeal joint of the right great (i.e., first) toe is swollen, hot, and erythematous. The joint is exquisitely tender to palpation. Laboratory tests reveal the following:

Hemoglobin	17 gm/dL
White blood cell count	10,000/μL
Sodium	140 mEq/L
Potassium	4.2 mEq/L
Chloride	102 mEq/L
CO_2	30 mEq/L
BUN	21 mg/dL
Creatinine	1.1 mg/dL
Uric acid	12.8 mg/dL (normal = 3–7)
Calcium	9.9 mg/dL (normal = 8.5–10.5)
Creatine kinase	70 U/L (normal = 17–148)
Total bilirubin:	0.6 mg/dL (normal = 0.1–1.0)

Which of the following is true concerning the patient's most likely condition?

(A) The symptoms may have been precipitated by hydrochlorothiazide.
(B) The patient currently needs allopurinol.
(C) The patient currently needs antibiotics.
(D) The patient currently requires admission to the hospital.
(E) Aspiration of the joint should be avoided in this setting.

Question 137

A 48-year-old man comes to the office asking for sleeping pills. On questioning, the patient, a Vietnam veteran, relates a history of terrible nightmares and insomnia. He admits to daytime flashbacks and recurrent dreams about the war and memory difficulties. He is divorced, lives alone, and has no friends that he is close to currently. When asked to elaborate on his combat experience, the patient becomes angry and asks you to "keep quiet about things you don't know." The patient seems quite anxious and distracted by the smallest stimulus. What is the best course of action for this patient?

(A) Diphenhydramine at bedtime
(B) Lorazepam during waking hours and at bedtime for several months
(C) Haloperidol every morning
(D) Referral to a psychotherapist doing group work with other Vietnam veterans
(E) Referral for electroconvulsive therapy, followed by daily fluoxetine indefinitely

Question 138

A 45-year-old man with a long smoking history presents with dyspnea. Vital signs are as follows:

Temperature	99.9°F
Blood pressure	168/92 mmHg
Pulse rate	90 beats/min
Respirations	22/min

Pulse oximetry reveals an oxygen saturation of 94%. Physical examination reveals decreased breath sounds and dull percussion note in the lower right chest. Chest radiograph reveals a large pleural effusion on the right with no other abnormalities. The patient denies exposure to anyone who has been sick or any change in his smoker's cough. Complete blood count and electrolytes are unremarkable. What is the best next step?

(A) Empirical coverage of tuberculosis and respiratory isolation
(B) PET scan
(C) Thoracentesis
(D) Pleural biopsy
(E) Insertion of a thoracostomy tube

Question 139

Which of the following is true concerning slipped capital femoral epiphysis?

(A) Treatment generally involves surgical pinning.
(B) It rarely affects obese children for unknown reasons.
(C) It usually occurs in children between the ages of 4 and 7.
(D) Patients usually complain of contralateral knee pain.
(E) Plain radiographs are not helpful in making the diagnosis.

Question 140

In the setting of acute trauma, fracture of which bone has the highest associated mortality?

(A) Lumbar vertebra
(B) Femur
(C) Rib
(D) Pelvis
(E) Humerus

Question 141

In a 50-year-old patient who complains of gradual onset of difficulty in reading the newspaper but no problem with vision when he or she is driving, what is the most likely diagnosis?

(A) Retinal detachment
(B) Macular degeneration
(C) Presbyopia
(D) New-onset diabetes mellitus with swelling of the lens resulting from hyperglycemia
(E) Cataract

Question 142

In a 6 month-old infant with a *lazy* eye (i.e., strabismus), with medial deviation of the right eye in the resting position, which of the following is most likely true?

(A) The condition usually resolves on its own and requires only routine follow-up.
(B) The infant has a right esotropia.
(C) If the condition persists, blindness is uncommon because of the early formation of visual neural connections.
(D) If the condition persists beyond age 8, glasses may be required for the affected eye.
(E) The infant most likely has a right oculomotor palsy.

Question 143

A 62-year-old woman presents for a routine examination and tells you she thinks that she may need antibiotics. When you ask her why, she mentions a rash on her left nipple that started 6 months ago and has not gone away. On physical examination, the left nipple demonstrates reddening, thickening and some crusting. You also palpate a 2 × 3 cm, irregular, solid left breast mass. The microscopic appearance of the woman's left nipple is shown below.

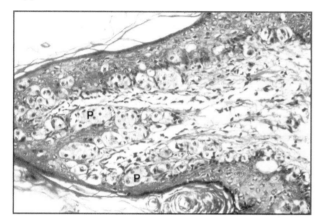

What is the most likely diagnosis?

(A) Paget's disease of the nipple
(B) Fibroadenoma
(C) Eczema of the nipple
(D) Cellulitis
(E) Chest wall sarcoma

Question 144

A 72-year-old woman comes to the office in a wheelchair, aided by her husband. Her husband hands you her medical records because you have never seen the woman before. In the woman's records is a CT scan of the brain:

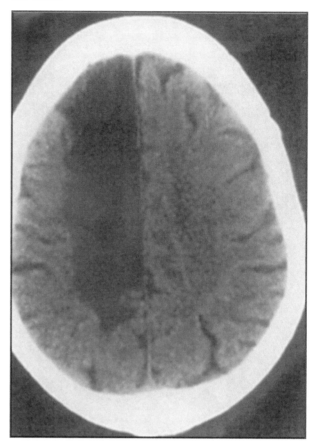

Which of the following is correct regarding the most likely cause of the lesion shown in the CT scan?

(A) It is due to interruption of blood supply from the right middle cerebral artery.
(B) Daily aspirin should be given to all those over 50 to lower the risk of this condition.
(C) The woman is likely to have weakness in her left leg.
(D) All of the above
(E) None of the above

Question 145

Which of the following causes hemorrhagic cystitis?
(A) Vincristine
(B) Vinblastine
(C) Cyclophosphamide
(D) Thioridazine
(E) Cyclosporine
(F) Isotretinoin
(G) Tetracycline
(H) Amiodarone
(I) Dihydroxycholecalciferol
(J) Verapamil
(K) None of the above

Question 146

Which of the following causes thyroid abnormalities?
(A) Vincristine
(B) Vinblastine
(C) Cyclophosphamide
(D) Thioridazine
(E) Cyclosporine
(F) Isotretinoin
(G) Tetracycline
(H) Amiodarone
(I) Dihydroxycholecalciferol
(J) Verapamil
(K) None of the above

Question 147

Which of the following can cause staining of the teeth when given to young children?
(A) Vincristine
(B) Vinblastine
(C) Cyclophosphamide
(D) Thioridazine
(E) Cyclosporine
(F) Isotretinoin
(G) Tetracycline
(H) Amiodarone
(I) Dihydroxycholecalciferol
(J) Verapamil
(K) None of the above

Question 148

Which of the following causes nephrotoxicity and immunosuppression?
(A) Vincristine
(B) Vinblastine
(C) Cyclophosphamide
(D) Thioridazine
(E) Cyclosporine
(F) Isotretinoin
(G) Tetracycline
(H) Amiodarone
(I) Dihydroxycholecalciferol
(J) Verapamil
(K) None of the above

Question 149

Which of the following is an antineoplastic agent that causes peripheral neuropathy?
(A) Vincristine
(B) Vinblastine
(C) Cyclophosphamide
(D) Thioridazine
(E) Cyclosporine
(F) Isotretinoin
(G) Tetracycline
(H) Amiodarone
(I) Dihydroxycholecalciferol
(J) Verapamil
(K) None of the above

Question 150

Which of the following is a vitamin A analog?
(A) Vincristine
(B) Vinblastine
(C) Cyclophosphamide
(D) Thioridazine
(E) Cyclosporine
(F) Isotretinoin
(G) Tetracycline
(H) Amiodarone
(I) Dihydroxycholecalciferol
(J) Verapamil
(K) None of the above

BLOCK 3 ANSWER KEY

101. C	111. D	121. E	131. B	141. C
102. C	112. C	122. E	132. A	142. B
103. B	113. A	123. D	133. D	143. A
104. E	114. A	124. B	134. C	144. C
105. C	115. E	125. A	135. A	145. C
106. A	116. E	126. B	136. A	146. H
107. C	117. C	127. B	137. D	147. G
108. A	118. E	128. B	138. C	148. E
109. B	119. E	129. B	139. A	149. A
110. A	120. C	130. B	140. D	150. F

Refer to Answers and Explanations Section for Block 3

Pages 221–229

Figure credits

Question 143: Stevens A, et al: Breast. From Stevens A, et al (eds): Wheater's Basic Histopathology, 4th ed. New York, Churchill Livingstone, 2002, pp 216–223.

Question 144: Rolak L (ed): Neurology Secrets, 2nd ed. Philadelphia, Hanley & Belfus, 1998, p 228.

BLOCK 4

50 QUESTIONS

TIME ALLOWED: 60 MINUTES

Question 151

What is the best measure to reduce the incidence of postoperative pulmonary complications?

(A) Cessation of smoking preoperatively
(B) Incentive spirometry preoperatively
(C) Refusal to give patients narcotics postoperatively
(D) Positive-pressure mechanical ventilation postoperatively
(E) Prophylactic antibiotics perioperatively

Question 152

A 42-year-old nonsmoking man with no medical history presents to the office with the chief complaint of hoarseness. He was at a basketball game the night before cheering loudly for his favorite team. When he woke up this morning, he noticed his voice was hoarse. Review of systems and physical examination are within normal limits. Which of the following is the next appropriate step?

(A) Laryngoscopy
(B) Empirical antibiotics
(C) Reassurance and repeat visit if symptoms fail to resolve
(D) Throat culture
(E) Full metabolic profile

Question 153

A 22-year-old woman is brought to the emergency department after an automobile accident and is unconscious, not breathing, and bleeding profusely with unstable vital signs. What is the first appropriate step in the management of this patient?

(A) Obtain a full medical history from family members.
(B) Perform a thorough physical examination.
(C) Establish an airway and institute mechanical ventilation.
(D) Blood type and crossmatch, then transfuse 2 units of packed red blood cells.
(E) Establish intravenous access, and administer a fluid challenge with Ringer's lactate.

Question 154

What is the most likely diagnosis in a previously healthy 14-year-old with periumbilical pain associated with nausea and vomiting whose pain subsequently shifts to the right lower quadrant and increases in severity?

(A) Cholecystitis
(B) Appendicitis
(C) Crohn disease
(D) Meckel's diverticulum
(E) Small bowel obstruction

Question 155

In a 45-year-old patient with epigastric pain that radiates through to the back and a markedly elevated amylase and lipase, which of the following is the **least** likely cause of the probable diagnosis?

(A) Corticosteroid treatment
(B) Hypocalcemia
(C) Alcohol abuse
(D) Gallstones
(E) Trauma

Question 156

In which of the following causes of peritonitis is laparotomy or laparoscopy **least** likely to be one of the appropriate treatment options?

(A) Appendicitis
(B) Cholecystitis
(C) Diverticulitis
(D) Spontaneous bacterial peritonitis
(E) Small bowel obstruction caused by adhesions

Question 157

Which of the following conditions does **not** have an increased incidence in the setting of a multiple-gestation pregnancy?

(A) Maternal preeclampsia
(B) Fetal macrosomia
(C) Postpartum uterine atony
(D) Vasa previa
(E) Perinatal morbidity

Question 158

Which of the following treatments is **least** likely to be helpful in a person with severe, acute liver failure?

(A) Intravenous fluids
(B) Glucose
(C) Fresh frozen plasma
(D) Vitamin K
(E) Addressing the underlying cause of the liver failure

Question 159

A G2P1 pregnant woman has a routine urinalysis that shows 4+ bacteria at 28 weeks. She is asymptomatic, afebrile, and has no abnormalities on physical examination. What is the best treatment?

(A) Nothing
(B) Amoxicillin
(C) Ciprofloxacin
(D) Repeat the urinalysis in 6 weeks
(E) Culture of the urine and treatment only if the culture reveals a gram-negative organism

Question 160

A pregnant woman has intractable nausea and vomiting in the first trimester that causes mild weight loss and requires hospitalization for electrolyte abnormalities and an inability to keep food down. Which of the following is most likely to be true?

(A) The woman is older than age 35.
(B) The woman has several children.
(C) The woman has multiple underlying social stressors.
(D) The woman does not meet the strict criteria for hyperemesis gravidarum.
(E) The woman has a malignant choriocarcinoma.

Question 161

A 42-year-old man comes to the office complaining of severe headaches, fatigue, and irritability. Withdrawal from which of the following substances is most likely?

(A) Barbiturates
(B) Marijuana
(C) LSD
(D) Benzodiazepines
(E) Caffeine

Question 162

A 17-year-old girl frequently has injected conjunctiva, locks herself in her room and listens to music for hours on end, and then comes into the family room looking for food and acting strange. Her parents complain that she has a total lack of motivation. Which of the following is true about the illegal drug she is most likely to be abusing?

(A) It is often used for its appetite-suppressing effects.
(B) It may be fatal in overdose.
(C) It has moderate to severe teratogenic effects.
(D) The physical withdrawal symptoms are severely uncomfortable but rarely fatal.
(E) It is the most commonly abused illicit drug.

Question 163

Which of the following is the most likely cause of death in a 16-year-old African American?

(A) Accident
(B) Homicide
(C) Suicide
(D) Cancer
(E) Congenital malformation

Question 164

A mother brings in her 2.5-year-old child complaining that the child wets her bed two to three times per week. This bedwetting has been going on since birth, although it has decreased in frequency, and it has not resolved with standard behavioral modification techniques that the mother read about. The child has no medical history. Physical examination and urinalysis are normal. Which of the following is true?

(A) Imipramine can be tried.
(B) Biofeedback is the next treatment of choice.
(C) The child should be spanked whenever bedwetting occurs.
(D) No further treatment for the bedwetting is required at this time.
(E) The child most likely has a congenital urinary tract abnormality.

Question 165

A 17-year-old girl comes to the office for a school physical. She is wearing baggy clothes and seems concerned about her appearance. Physical exam is essentially normal, but you notice some erosion of the skin over the knuckles of the right hand and erosion of some of the enamel on the back of the teeth. The patient has a weight appropriate for height. The patient has a normal mood and affect and says her only problem is that she is fat. Which of the following is most important to ask about?

(A) Arthritis
(B) Recurrent sore throats and fevers
(C) Familial bone disorders
(D) Purging behavior
(E) Regular brushing of the teeth with fluoridated toothpaste

Question 166

A 17-year-old girl broke up with her boyfriend three weeks ago and has been moping around the house, crying many times a day since the breakup. She is not interested in talking to her girlfriends when they call to console her. She has missed a day of school as well. Which of the following is the most likely diagnosis?

(A) Major depression
(B) Cyclothymia
(C) Adjustment disorder with depressed mood
(D) Bipolar I disorder, currently depressed
(E) Dysthymia

Question 167

Which of the following is the most likely source of error if an experimenter knows which subjects have been assigned into the treatment and placebo groups?

(A) Recall bias
(B) Unacceptability bias
(C) Interviewer bias
(D) Lead-time bias
(E) Nonresponse bias

Question 168

An experimenter does a prospective study after placing 50,000 subjects who are equally matched for demographic and lifestyle variables into one of two groups based on the number of pills they take each day (< 3 pills, > 3 pills). He measures only the number of pills subjects take and their mortality data over a 5-year period. He notes that subjects who take more pills are more likely to die and concludes that medications cause an unacceptable number of deaths. Which of the following is the most likely reason for his conclusion to be invalid?

(A) Nonrandom bias
(B) Lead-time bias
(C) Confounding variables
(D) Type II error
(E) Interviewer bias

Question 169

Which of the following is true regarding commonly used tests that screen for or confirm disease?

(A) Highly specific tests are preferred for screening.
(B) Increased specificity can be obtained by increasing sensitivity.
(C) Screening usually is not recommended for chronic, untreatable conditions.
(D) Positive predictive value increases when the disease is rare.
(E) The primary goal with screening tests is to have the lowest possible false-positive rate.

Question 170

Which of the following is true regarding indications for the measles-mumps-rubella vaccine in adults, assuming that they have not yet been vaccinated?

(A) All immunocompromised patients should be vaccinated.
(B) Pregnant women should be vaccinated.
(C) Health care workers should not be vaccinated because of the potential risk of giving the diseases to patients.
(D) Human immunodeficiency virus–positive patients should receive the vaccine.
(E) This vaccine is especially indicated in those with an anaphylactic reaction to eggs.

Question 171

Which of the following concerning vaccines is correct?

(A) Patient desire is not a valid indication for the hepatitis B vaccine.
(B) Influenza should be offered to all adults older than age 50, regardless of health status.
(C) The pneumococcal vaccine should not be given to any patients younger than age 20.
(D) Pediatric patients who take aspirin should avoid the influenza vaccine because of concerns over Reye's syndrome.
(E) A tetanus booster vaccine should not be given to adults, unless they sustain a nonclean or nonminor wound, owing to vaccine toxicity concerns.

Question 172

Which of the following is true concerning persons older than age 65?

(A) About 40% suffer from dementia.
(B) Only about 5% live in a nursing home.
(C) Approximately 2–3% of the population is older than age 65.
(D) *Sundowning* is a normal phenomenon in the elderly.
(E) Elderly people are less likely to commit suicide than younger people are.

Question 173

A 29-year-old man presents to the emergency department with shortness of breath, fatigue, and headache. Medical history is insignificant, although the patient has noted feeling tired with a nagging dry cough and diarrhea over the past few months. The man is a homosexual with multiple partners and denies alcohol, tobacco, or illicit drug use. He mentions that his pants seem a little loose on him lately, but he is not sure if he has lost weight. On examination, the man is thin and mildly tachypneic with a temperature of 101.2° F. His breath sounds are clear bilaterally, and the heart rate is mildly tachycardic but regular. A radiograph shows diffuse, bilateral interstitial infiltrates, and an arterial blood gas measurement reveals a PaO_2 of 58. Which of the following is most likely to be true?

(A) Pneumococcal pneumonia is likely.
(B) The white blood cell count is probably normal or low.
(C) A broad-spectrum cephalosporin or fluoroquinolone is the preferred treatment.
(D) The sexual history is not relevant.
(E) The clear breath sounds point toward a noninfectious cause.

Question 174

Which of the following is true regarding human immunodeficiency virus (HIV) infection?

(A) HIV infection is automatically called acquired immunodeficiency syndrome (AIDS) when the CD4 count drops to less than $400/mm^3$, even without symptoms.
(B) Initial infection with HIV often clinically resembles infectious mononucleosis.
(C) Initial testing for HIV is done with enzyme-linked immunosorbent assay (ELISA), which also is the confirmatory test.
(D) The HIV test is nearly universally positive within 2 weeks of initial infection.
(E) HIV patients should not receive any form of polio vaccine.

Question 175

Which of the following is **not** considered an example of a cytotoxic or type II hypersensitivity reaction?

(A) Goodpasture's syndrome
(B) Hyperacute transplant rejection
(C) Pemphigus
(D) Autoimmune hemolytic anemia caused by methyldopa
(E) The tuberculosis skin test (purified protein derivative [PPD])

Question 176

A 32-year-old man is given oral amoxicillin in the emergency department and 20 minutes later develops shortness of breath, wheezing, facial swelling, and decreased blood pressure. He rapidly begins to deteriorate with unstable vital signs, and you attempt intubation for respiratory failure. You are unable to pass the tube because of laryngeal edema, and the patient subsequently loses consciousness. What should you do next?

(A) Start intravenous fluids.
(B) Administer diphenhydramine.
(C) Perform cricothyroidotomy.
(D) Administer subcutaneous epinephrine.
(E) Administer corticosteroids.

Question 177

Which of the following is **not** true regarding muscular dystrophy?

(A) It is an X-linked recessive disorder.
(B) Creatine phosphokinase levels usually are low at the time of presentation.
(C) It normally affects children before age 7.
(D) Muscle biopsy can be used to confirm the diagnosis.
(E) The condition is thought to be due to a disorder of dystrophin.

Question 178

A 36-year-old female smoker comes to the office complaining of fatigue and vision problems. She notes intermittent double vision, usually toward the end of the day accompanied by muscular fatigue for the last 3 weeks. The fatigue has been gradually getting worse. The woman denies previous problems similar to this and denies any change in visual acuity. Physical examination reveals mild ptosis and global, mild muscular weakness that gets worse with continued testing. Reflexes and sensory examination are within normal limits, and there is no muscular tenderness to palpation. The creatine phosphokinase level is normal. Which of the following is true concerning the most likely diagnosis?

(A) Thymectomy usually is advised.
(B) The pathophysiology involves vasculitis as the primary event.
(C) The patient needs immediate corticosteroid administration.
(D) The histologic type is most likely to be small cell.
(E) Diagnosis is made by muscle biopsy.

Question 179

A 67-year-old man has gradual onset of slow movement, muscular rigidity, resting hand tremor, and an unstable, shuffling gait. His affect also seems quite flat. Which of the following is **not** likely to be true?

(A) He is at an increased risk of suicide.
(B) His symptoms could be caused by medication.
(C) He has an increased risk of developing dementia.
(D) He may need medications that block dopamine receptors to treat these symptoms.
(E) He may need medications that block anticholinergic receptors to treat these symptoms.

Question 180

Which of the following is true regarding cancer screening in adults?

(A) Annual stool testing for occult blood should be done starting at age 50, with a baseline sigmoidoscopy or barium enema around this time as well.
(B) In smokers, annual sputum cytology and chest radiograph should be done after age 50.
(C) Annual breast self-examinations for women should begin at the age of 30.
(D) Annual Pap smear for women should begin at the age of 30 whether or not women are sexually active.
(E) Annual prostate-specific antigen (PSA) levels for men should begin at age 35.

Question 181

A 32-year-old woman complains of excessive perspiration, palpitations, and fatigue. On questioning, she admits to anxiety, difficulty sleeping, and diarrhea. She was diagnosed with generalized anxiety disorder by her previous physician and given buspirone, which she is still taking. On examination, you note tachycardia with an irregular rate and shiny, red, indurated skin over both shins. Which of the following is true concerning the most likely diagnosis?

(A) It is mediated by a viral infection.
(B) Alprazolam is more effective for treatment.
(C) Thymectomy usually is indicated.
(D) Radioactive ablation is used commonly in treatment.
(E) Markedly elevated urinary catecholamine breakdown products are likely.

Question 182

A 24-year-old patient presents with a chief complaint of an itchy rash. On examination, the patient has vesicles, papules, and wheals on the extensor aspects of the elbows and knees with excoriations. The rest of the examination is within normal limits. The patient also mentions 6 months of diarrhea and some weight loss for which he had a colonoscopy 3 months ago, which was negative. The patient denies any history of abdominal pain. A biopsy of the skin lesions reveals IgA deposits. Stool testing reveals steatorrhea. Which of the following is most likely to be true?

(A) A jejunal biopsy would reveal fingerlike villi with a villus to crypt ratio of roughly 4:1.

(B) A gluten-free diet most likely would reduce symptoms.

(C) Antibiotics would cure the symptoms.

(D) Serum gastrin level is extremely high.

(E) You would expect to see a small bowel stricture with a barium study.

Question 183

A 32-year-old African American woman presents with shortness of breath that has been increasing gradually in severity over the past several months. On examination, the breath sounds are clear. The patient mentions a painful shin rash as well, and you notice a lesion on the anterior aspect of her left shin similar to the one shown in the figure below. A chest radiograph reveals hilar adenopathy and bilateral interstitial parenchymal lung infiltrates.

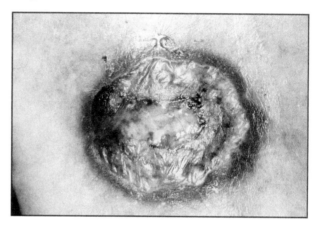

Which of the following is most likely?

(A) Leukemia
(B) Goodpasture's syndrome
(C) Paragonimiasis
(D) Tuberculosis
(E) Sarcoidosis

Question 184

Which of the following antibiotics is most likely to cause photosensitivity?

(A) Doxycycline
(B) Ciprofloxacin
(C) Amoxicillin
(D) Ceftriaxone
(E) Chloramphenicol

Question 185

A 10-year-old child is brought to the emergency department 2 days after playing with a neighbor's cat and being bitten on the hand by the cat. The bite appears deep. Which of the following is a correct part of the initial management of the wound?

(A) Suture any lacerations present.
(B) Give the rabies vaccine.
(C) Cauterize the wound.
(D) Avoid cleaning the wound with soap.
(E) Give prophylactic antibiotics.

Question 186

A 10-month-old infant is brought to the office in January because of "the flu." The infant had a runny nose and low-grade fever 2 days ago and now is breathing faster than normal. On examination, you hear expiratory wheezing and note some intercostal retractions. Which is true of the most likely diagnosis?

(A) You should not examine the throat because you may precipitate airway obstruction.
(B) Ampicillin and erythromycin are good choices for treatment.
(C) Chest radiograph is most likely to show bilateral, diffuse infiltrates.
(D) The best treatment is supportive (e.g. oxygen, intravenous fluids, bronchodilators).
(E) The most likely cause is *Staphylococcus aureus*.

Question 187

A 27-year-old man presents to the emergency department 2 weeks after a hiking trip in Virginia, complaining of severe headache, fever, and fatigue. He says the symptoms started 3 days ago and have been getting worse. He mentions a rash on his arms and legs that started this morning and is starting to spread. On examination, the patient is ill appearing and has an erythematous macular rash on the distal aspects of all four extremities ranging from the wrist and ankle to the mid-forearm and shin. His temperature is 104°F. Which of the following is most likely true?

(A) The patient was bitten by a tick.
(B) The patient was exposed recently to someone with a severe sore throat.
(C) The patient was exposed recently to a sexually transmitted disease.
(D) The patient has not received standard childhood immunizations.
(E) The patient has been exposed recently to *Borrelia burgdorferi*.

Question 188

A 22-year-old woman presents to the office complaining of sore throat, headache, fever, severe fatigue, and "feeling lousy" for the past 6 days. On examination, you note prominent cervical adenopathy, pharyngeal erythema, mild splenomegaly, and a temperature of 99.9° F. The patient has not been sick or had sexual intercourse in more than 2 years. She reports no abnormal weight loss or other symptoms. Which of the following would be **inconsistent** with the most likely diagnosis on the complete blood count and peripheral blood smear?

(A) Large numbers of atypical, toxic-appearing lymphocytes
(B) Lymphocytosis
(C) Mild anemia
(D) Auer rods
(E) Thrombocytopenia

Question 189

A 42-year-old woman presents for a routine Pap smear. She is single and sexually active with multiple partners, but has no history of sexually transmitted diseases and uses condoms regularly. She has no complaints. A Pap smear is performed and reveals the appearance shown below.

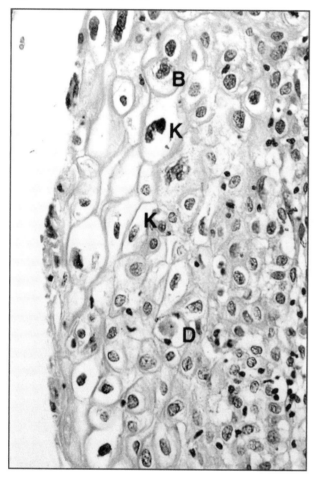

Which of the following is true regarding this patient's Pap smear?

(A) It demonstrates no abnormalities.

(B) It demonstrates invasive cervical carcinoma.

(C) It demonstrates cervical carcinoma in situ with severe dysplasia

(D) It demonstrates mild changes of human papillomavirus infection.

(E) It indicates the presence of pelvic inflammatory disease (PID), probably due to *Chlamydia* infection.

Question 190

A 6-year-old child is brought in by her mother due to a growth on her ear that developed gradually in the months following attempted ear piercing in the upper portion of the child's ear. The appearance of the child's ear is shown below.

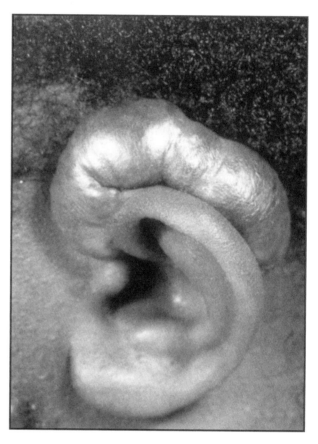

Which of the following is true regarding the most likely diagnosis?

(A) Metastases have likely already occurred.

(B) The lesion will probably regress spontaneously within a year or two.

(C) It is an unusual lesion in those of African American descent.

(D) It is of primarily cosmetic concern.

(E) Prompt excision should be recommended.

Question 191

Which personality disorder is characterized by the following statement: "The rules are more important than the objectives"

(A) Paranoid
(B) Schizoid
(C) Schizotypal
(D) Avoidant
(E) Histrionic
(F) Narcissistic
(G) Antisocial
(H) Borderline
(I) Dependent
(J) Obsessive-compulsive

Question 192

Which personality disorder could be described as a pervasive *inferiority complex*?

(A) Paranoid
(B) Schizoid
(C) Schizotypal
(D) Avoidant
(E) Histrionic
(F) Narcissistic
(G) Antisocial
(H) Borderline
(I) Dependent
(J) Obsessive-compulsive

Question 193

A wife who continuously stays with an abusive husband would be most likely to have which personality disorder?

(A) Paranoid
(B) Schizoid
(C) Schizotypal
(D) Avoidant
(E) Histrionic
(F) Narcissistic
(G) Antisocial
(H) Borderline
(I) Dependent
(J) Obsessive-compulsive

Question 194

The classic loner who does not desire company describes which personality disorder?

(A) Paranoid
(B) Schizoid
(C) Schizotypal
(D) Avoidant
(E) Histrionic
(F) Narcissistic
(G) Antisocial
(H) Borderline
(I) Dependent
(J) Obsessive-compulsive

Question 195

Splitting and constant crises are common in which personality disorder?

(A) Paranoid
(B) Schizoid
(C) Schizotypal
(D) Avoidant
(E) Histrionic
(F) Narcissistic
(G) Antisocial
(H) Borderline
(I) Dependent
(J) Obsessive-compulsive

Question 196

Which personality disorder requires that a pediatric disorder have been present to make a formal diagnosis?

(A) Paranoid
(B) Schizoid
(C) Schizotypal
(D) Avoidant
(E) Histrionic
(F) Narcissistic
(G) Antisocial
(H) Borderline
(I) Dependent
(J) Obsessive-compulsive

Question 197

In a 28-year-old obese woman with papilledema, normal blood pressure, and negative head CT scan, which of the following cerebrospinal fluid analysis profiles is most likely?

	Cells/μL	Main cell type	Glucose (mg/dL)	Protein (mg/dL)	Pressure (mmHg)
Normal CSF	0–3	Lymphocytes	50–100	20–45	50–200
A.	1200	Neutrophils	25	100	220
B.	50	Lymphocytes	60	60	130
C.	1	Lymphocytes	60	35	300
D.	1000	Red blood cells	65	54	224
E.	500	Lymphocytes	30	120	230

Question 198

In a 29-year-old man with normal temperature and leukocyte count with sudden onset of the worst headache of his life who then becomes unconscious, which of the following cerebrospinal fluid analysis profiles is most likely?

	Cells/μL	Main cell type	Glucose (mg/dL)	Protein (mg/dL)	Pressure (mmHg)
Normal CSF	0–3	Lymphocytes	50–100	20–45	50–200
A.	1200	Neutrophils	25	100	220
B.	50	Lymphocytes	60	60	130
C.	1	Lymphocytes	60	35	300
D.	1000	Red blood cells	65	54	224
E.	500	Lymphocytes	30	120	230

Question 199

In a 2-year-old with high fevers, high white count, altered level of consciousness and lethargy with vomiting, which of the following cerebrospinal fluid analysis profiles is most likely?

	Cells/μL	Main cell type	Glucose (mg/dL)	Protein (mg/dL)	Pressure (mmHg)
Normal CSF	0–3	Lymphocytes	50–100	20–45	50–200
A.	1200	Neutrophils	25	100	220
B.	50	Lymphocytes	60	60	130
C.	1	Lymphocytes	60	35	300
D.	1000	Red blood cells	65	54	224
E.	500	Lymphocytes	30	120	230

Question 200

In a 28-year-old woman with waxing and waning neurologic symptoms in different areas of the body over the last year and a history of optic neuritis, which of the following cerebrospinal fluid analysis profiles is most likely?

	Cells/μL	Main cell type	Glucose (mg/dL)	Protein (mg/dL)	Pressure (mmHg)
Normal CSF	0–3	Lymphocytes	50–100	20–45	50–200
A.	1200	Neutrophils	25	100	220
B.	50	Lymphocytes	60	60	130
C.	1	Lymphocytes	60	35	300
D.	1000	Red blood cells	65	54	224
E.	500	Lymphocytes	30	120	230

BLOCK 4 ANSWER KEY

151. A	161. E	171. B	181. D	191. J
152. C	162. E	172. B	182. B	192. D
153. C	163. B	173. B	183. E	193. I
154. B	164. D	174. B	184. A	194. B
155. B	165. D	175. E	185. E	195. H
156. D	166. C	176. C	186. D	196. G
157. B	167. C	177. B	187. A	197. C
158. D	168. C	178. A	188. D	198. D
159. B	169. C	179. D	189. D	199. A
160. C	170. D	180. A	190. D	200. B

Refer to Answers and Explanations Section for Block 4

Pages 231–238

Figure credits

Question 183: du Vivier A: The skin and systemic disease. In du Vivier A (ed): Atlas of Clinical Dermatology, 3rd ed. New York, Churchill Livingstone, 2002, pp. 509–561.

Question 189: Stevens A, et al: Infections of histologic importance. In Stevens A, et al (eds): Wheater's Basic Histopathology, 4th ed. New York, Churchill Livingstone, 2002, pp. 35–55.

Question 190: du Vivier A: Benign tumours of the skin. In du Vivier A (ed): Atlas of Clinical Dermatology, 3rd ed. New York, Churchill Livingstone, 2002, pp. 125–161.

50 QUESTIONS

TIME ALLOWED: 60 MINUTES

Question 201

Which of the following is related most closely to neurologic prognosis after spinal cord compression, as from an injury, tumor, or abscess?

(A) Sex of the patient
(B) Pretreatment function
(C) Antibiotic selection
(D) Skill of the neurosurgeon
(E) Age of the patient

Question 202

A woman was stuck with a rose thorn while gardening and a week later developed a pustule on the skin, which ulcerated, and lymphadenopathy in the arm. She has little pain and no fever. Which of the following is the most likely causative organism?

(A) *Trichophyton rubrum*
(B) *Streptococcus*
(C) *Staphylococcus*
(D) *Vibrio parahaemolyticus*
(E) *Sporothrix schenckii*

Question 203

Which of the following organisms would become a more likely cause of sepsis after splenectomy?

(A) *Staphylococcus aureus*
(B) *Candida albicans*
(C) *Sporothrix schenckii*
(D) *Haemophilus influenzae*
(E) *Pseudomonas aeruginosa*

Question 204

A pulmonary infection with which of the following organisms is most likely to cause a "typical" type of pneumonia?

(A) *Chlamydia pneumoniae*
(B) *Mycoplasma pneumoniae*
(C) *Haemophilus influenzae*
(D) *Chlamydia psittaci*
(E) *Francisella tularensis*

Question 205

Which of the following tumors is matched properly with its most commonly used tumor marker?

(A) Liver cancer—CA 19-9
(B) Ovarian cancer—carcinoembryonic antigen (CEA)
(C) Choriocarcinoma—human chorionic gonadotropin (HCG)
(D) Pancreatic cancer—acid phosphatase
(E) Breast cancer—S-100

Question 206

A 49-year-old male accountant in the hospital for recently diagnosed pancreatic cancer is refusing surgery or chemotherapy for his condition. You have discussed the risks and benefits of treatment, and the patient understands but says he just wants to go home. He is not clinically depressed and denies it when you ask him. What should you do next?

(A) Give a trial of antidepressants, then ask the patient again if he wants therapy.
(B) Discharge the patient to home.
(C) Get a court order allowing treatment.
(D) Have the courts determine the patient's competency.
(E) Get the patient's wife to persuade the patient to undergo therapy.

Question 207

Which of the following is **least** likely to be associated with oral cancer?

(A) Erythroplakia
(B) Chewing tobacco
(C) Smoking
(D) Alcohol abuse
(E) Hairy leukoplakia

Question 208

A 72-year-old, retired, outdoor construction worker presents to the office at his wife's request because of a "bump" near his eye. On examination, the patient has a 1-cm, pearly, umbilicated lesion with peripheral telangiectasias lateral to the left eyelid. He says it has been growing slowly for the last 6 months. What is the next best step?

(A) Provide reassurance.
(B) Provide careful observation with a follow-up visit in 2 weeks.
(C) Obtain a biopsy specimen of a small piece of the lesion for pathology.
(D) Perform an excisional biopsy.
(E) Prescribe tetracycline and see the patient again in 2 weeks.

Question 209

Which of the following would **not** be expected as a result of a carcinoid tumor that began in the bowel and has metastasized to the liver?

(A) Aortic valve fibrosis
(B) Flushing
(C) Elevated urinary 5-hydroxyindoleacetic acid
(D) Diarrhea
(E) Pulmonary valve fibrosis

Question 210

Which of the following genetic syndromes does **not** increase the tendency toward developing thrombosis?

(A) Factor V Leiden mutation
(B) Protein C deficiency
(C) Factor XI deficiency
(D) Antithrombin III deficiency
(E) Factor S deficiency

Question 211

A 27-year old G2P0 woman with a history of two miscarriages comes into the office with pain and swelling in her right leg. She denies other symptoms on thorough review of systems. An ultrasound reveals a blood clot in the right femoral vein. She is otherwise healthy, thin, and active; has no recent trauma or prolonged immobilization; and is not taking any medications or pills. Laboratory tests reveal the following:

Prothrombin time	Normal
Partial thromboplastin time	Slightly prolonged
Bleeding time	Normal
Hemoglobin	14 gm/dL
Mean corpuscular volume	90 μm/cell
Platelet count	250,000/μL
VDRL syphilis test	Positive
HIV test	Negative

What is the most likely cause of this woman's blood clot?

(A) Syphilis-induced phlebitis
(B) Protein S deficiency
(C) Underlying malignancy
(D) Lupus anticoagulant
(E) Protein C deficiency

Question 212

A 58-year-old smoker comes to the emergency department with a chief complaint of bleeding when he shaves. He also mentions a 40-lb weight loss and decreased appetite. He is visibly jaundiced and cachectic. You insert an intravenous catheter, and the site continues to ooze blood after holding pressure for 1 minute. Laboratory tests reveal the following:

Hemoglobin	12 gm/dL
Mean corpuscular volume	88 μm/cell
White blood cell count	7200/μL
Platelet count	33,000/μL
Prothrombin time	Prolonged
Partial thromboplastin time	Prolonged
Bleeding time	Prolonged
Fibrin level	Decreased
Total bilirubin	8.0 mg/dL (normal = 0.1–1.0)

What is the likely cause for the patient's bleeding tendency?

(A) Acute hepatic necrosis
(B) Fibrin deficiency
(C) Disseminated intravascular coagulation
(D) Surreptitious warfarin ingestion
(E) von Willebrand disease

Question 213

A 31-year-old woman presents with nearly continuous muscle pain for the last 2 months. She is quite upset over her pain and claims she is unable to sleep well because of it. She also relates a high-degree of stress at work, which requires her to be pain-free to perform her job activities well. Review of systems is positive for frequent bilateral headaches. Examination reveals anterior cervical, fore-arm, trapezius and knee tenderness to palpation. Laboratory tests reveal the following:

Hemoglobin	14 g/dL
Mean corpuscular volume	87 μm/cell
Erythrocyte sedimentation rate	5 mm/h (normal = 0–150)
Creatine phosphokinase	24 U/L (normal = 10–79)

What is the most likely diagnosis?

(A) Polymyositis
(B) Fibromyalgia
(C) Polymyalgia rheumatica
(D) Polyarteritis nodosa
(E) Dermatomyositis

Question 214

A 32-year-old man who is a heavy smoker comes to the office with a complaint of pain and tingling in the fingers and toes bilaterally. The patient says the problem began about 2 months ago but is starting to get much worse. Review of systems is otherwise negative. On examina-tion, the fingertips are cold in both hands with a mottled appearance, both dorsalis pedis pulses are slightly decreased, and some of the toes are cold and mildly cyan-otic. A small ulcer is also noted over one of the patient's fingertips. The vital signs and the rest of the physical examination are within normal limits. A complete blood count and basic metabolic profile are within normal limits. Antinuclear, anticentromere, and antitopoiso-merase antibodies as well as rheumatoid factor are all negative. What is the treatment most likely to relieve this patient's current symptoms?

(A) Cessation of smoking
(B) Corticosteroids
(C) Plasmapheresis
(D) Hydroxychloroquine
(E) Broad-spectrum antibiotics

Question 215

A 28-year-old woman comes to the office complaining of a headache and joint pains. On questioning, she mentions that she went on a camping trip to Wisconsin 1 month ago and developed a strange skin rash on her thigh when she got home. The rash started out as a "small, red bump" and got larger over the next few days until it was roughly the diameter "of a grapefruit, but the center cleared up while the outside red part kept getting bigger." The rash subse-quently went away, and the patient forgot about it until today. Her left knee is swollen and hot but not erythema-tous, and she has a temperature of 100° F. Her eyes are irritated by the light in the room, and she constantly shields them with her hand during the interview and examination. What is the treatment of choice for the most likely underlying disorder?

(A) Corticosteroids
(B) Hydroxychloroquine
(C) Doxycycline
(D) Aspirin
(E) Intravenous immunoglobulins

Question 216

A middle-aged patient presents with a hot, swollen knee, and aspiration of the joint is performed. Joint fluid analy-sis reveals the following:

White blood cell count	4000/μL (normal < 200)
Percentage of neutrophils	16% (normal < 25%)
Viscosity	Lower than normal
Gram stain	Negative
Crystals present	Yes
Crystal description	Rhomboid-shaped crystals with weakly positive birefringence
Serum uric acid level	9.2 mg/dL (normal = 3.0–7.0)

What is the most likely cause of the inflamed knee joint?

(A) Gout
(B) Pseudogout
(C) Podagra
(D) Septic arthritis
(E) Rheumatoid arthritis

Question 217

A 42-year-old obese woman had an uncomplicated laparoscopic cholecystectomy yesterday afternoon, and the nurse calls you this morning because the patient has a fever. When you go to see the patient, she is sleeping. You wake her up, and she clearly is disappointed about being woken up. She has not gotten out of bed or sat up since the surgery. Her medication list includes meperidine every 4 hours and acetaminophen with codeine on request. Vital signs are as follows:

Temperature	100.1°F
Blood pressure	128/86 mmHg
Pulse rate	88 beats/min
Respirations	12/min

On examination, the surgical incisions are clean, dry, and intact. The lungs are clear to auscultation with an occasional crackle heard in the lower left lung field. The rest of the examination is within normal limits. Which of the following is true about the most likely cause of the patient's fever?

(A) Incentive spirometry and early ambulation can help prevent this condition.

(B) Narcotics generally improve this condition by suppressing the cough reflex.

(C) Broad-spectrum antibiotics are indicated because the patient had recent abdominal surgery.

(D) A first-generation penicillin or cephalosporin is appropriate in this situation.

(E) Obesity is unrelated to this condition.

Question 218

An obese, otherwise healthy 24-year-old woman comes to the office complaining of headaches that have developed over the last 2 weeks and are getting worse, especially in the morning. Vital signs are as follows:

Temperature	98.6°F
Blood pressure	130/84 mmHg
Pulse rate	72 beats/min
Respirations	14/min

On vision testing, the patient's vision is 20/20 in the right eye and 20/25 in the left eye. The patient does not wear glasses and has never had trouble seeing distant objects. Funduscopic examination reveals swollen-appearing disks with indistinct disk margins. The physical examination is within normal limits. Neurologic examination is unremarkable, and a CT scan of the brain and electroencephalogram reveal no abnormalities. Which of the following is the most likely cause of the patient's headaches?

(A) Posterior fossa brain tumor, which often is poorly seen with CT scan

(B) Pseudotumor cerebri

(C) Optic neuritis

(D) Subarachnoid hemorrhage

(E) Leukemia

Question 219

A 32-year-old asymptomatic woman and her husband, both of Italian descent, come to see you for the first time. They have three healthy children without medical problems. The woman's medical history is significant for a miscarriage between her first and second child and for recently discovered anemia. The patient was recently put on iron tablets by another physician, who has since retired from practice. The woman complains that the iron pills are making her constipated, and she wants to know if she still needs them. Vital signs are within normal limits. A blood workup reveals the following:

Hemoglobin	12 gm/dL
Mean corpuscular volume	72 µm/cell
Reticulocyte count	4% (normal = 0.5–2.5)
Hemoglobin A$_2$	4.9% (normal = < 3.5)
Peripheral smear	Mild hypochromia, 1+ target cells

Which of the following is true regarding the likely cause of this woman's anemia?

(A) She needs at least another 3 months of iron therapy because the reticulocytosis shows the bone marrow has responded to the iron supplements.

(B) She needs a work-up for her constipation to exclude colon cancer or other obstructive lesion.

(C) Iron therapy should be stopped.

(D) The miscarriage was most likely due to a genetic anemia in the fetus, and the woman and her husband should undergo genetic testing.

(E) Blood transfusion is indicated if the hemoglobin falls to less than 10 mg/dL.

Question 220

Which of the following does **not** increase the risk of forming calcium stones in the kidney?

(A) Hyperoxaluria
(B) Hypercalcemia
(C) Hyperparathyroidism
(D) Thiazide diuretics
(E) Hypercalciuria

Question 221

A 41-year-old man presents to the emergency department complaining of severe, intermittent right flank pain with radiation to the groin for the last 2 hours. Abdominal radiograph reveals a 4 mm, round calcified denisty in the area of the lower right ureter. Which of the following is **not** an appropriate part of the initial management?

(A) Encouraging high levels of fluid intake
(B) Giving narcotics for pain
(C) Checking a urinalysis
(D) Surgically removing the stone
(E) Checking a serum calcium level

Question 222

A 3-year-old child is brought in by her mother for a nosebleed 1 week after a bout of severe, bloody diarrhea. There is no history of trauma to the nose, and the child was under close supervision when the nosebleed started. The child's diarrhea resolved without incident 5 days ago, and the child had been doing fine. The child is noted to be lethargic, irritable, and pale and has mild tachycardia, but the nosebleed has stopped, and the rest of the examination is within normal limits. Laboratory tests reveal the following:

Hemoglobin	8 gm/dL (normal: 11–13)
Mean corpuscular volume	93 µm/cell
White blood cell count	8000/µL
Platelet count	34,000/µL
Peripheral smear	3+ schistocytes, 2+ helmet cells
Urinalysis	Red blood cell casts noted
Prothrombin time	Normal

What is the most likely diagnosis?

(A) Idiopathic thrombocytopenic purpura
(B) Thrombotic thrombocytopenic purpura
(C) Hemolytic uremic syndrome
(D) Henoch-Schönlein purpura
(E) Acute leukemia

Question 223

Which of the following is a retroperitoneal structure?

(A) Ileum
(B) Transverse colon
(C) Adrenal gland
(D) Gallbladder
(E) Anal canal

Question 224

A 24-year-old woman comes to the clinic with a chief complaint of urinary urgency and frequency. Pelvic examination reveals no cervical discharge or erythema, and a urinalysis of a clean-catch mid-stream urine sample reveals large numbers of bacteria, no epithelial cells, positive nitrite, and positive leukocyte esterase. Which of the following organisms is most likely the cause of the woman's symptoms?

(A) *Trichomonas vaginalis*
(B) *Chlamydia trachomatis*
(C) *Escherichia coli*
(D) *Streptococcus bovis*
(E) *Staphylococcus saprophyticus*

Question 225

A 36-year-old asymptomatic woman comes to the clinic requesting a pregnancy test. A pregnancy test is negative, and a urinalysis performed on the patient's urine reveals the following:

Specific gravity	1.011
Urobilinogen	Negative
Bacteria	1+
Epithelial cells	4+
Nitrite	Negative
Leukocyte esterase	Negative
Protein	Negative
Glucose	Negative
Hemoglobin	2+
Microscopic examination	2+ red blood cells; numerous normal epithelial cells, negative for white blood cells, casts or crystals

What is the most likely cause for the woman's hematuria?

(A) Urinary tract infection
(B) Menstrual bleeding
(C) Nephrolithiasis
(D) Glomerulonephritis
(E) Urinary tract neoplasm

Question 226

Which of the following choices is **not** generally prescribed to a patient with chronic renal failure?

(A) Water-soluble vitamin supplements
(B) Erythropoietin
(C) Calcium supplements
(D) Magnesium supplements
(E) Potassium restriction in the diet

Question 227

Which of the following is **false** concerning obesity?

(A) It increases the risk of osteoporosis.
(B) It increases the risk of type II diabetes mellitus.
(C) It increases the risk of endometrial cancer.
(D) It increases the risk of overall mortality.
(E) It is commonly associated with sleep apnea.

Question 228

A 48-year-old woman with small cell lung cancer is admitted to the hospital in severe pain and given morphine and continuous normal saline through an intravenous catheter. Electrolytes are normal on admission, but 4 days later the patient has a sodium level of 123 mEq/L. She does not appear to have any signs of fluid overload. What is the best way to attempt to correct the hyponatremia?

(A) Switch the intravenous fluid to hypertonic saline.
(B) Increase the intravenous fluid rate but leave it as normal saline.
(C) Give demeclocycline.
(D) Stop the intravenous fluids and restrict free water intake.
(E) Resect the lung cancer.

Question 229

Which of the following derangements in the corticosteroid hormone axis would you expect to see after surgical pituitary gland removal? (CRH = corticotropin-releasing hormone; ACTH = adrenocorticotropin hormone)

	CRH	ACTH	Cortisol
(A)	High	Low	Low
(B)	High	High	Low
(C)	Low	Low	Low
(D)	High	Low	Normal
(E)	Normal	Low	Low

Question 230

If a person took too much oral thyroxine hormone, how would you expect the following thyroid parameters to change? (TRH = thyroid-stimulating releasing hormone, TSH = thyroid stimulating hormone)

	TRH	TSH	Free thyroxine
(A)	Low	Low	High
(B)	Low	High	High
(C)	High	High	High
(D)	High	Low	High
(E)	Normal	Normal	High

Question 231

Which of the following is **false** regarding physiologic jaundice of the newborn?

(A) It often is present at birth in premature infants.

(B) It is more common in premature infants.

(C) It rarely causes kernicterus.

(D) It is thought to be due to immature liver function.

(E) Of normal term infants, up to 50% may develop physiologic jaundice.

Question 232

Three days after birth, a term newborn develops mild jaundice in the absence of other signs. The infant seems healthy and active, and there were no complications with the delivery. Total bilirubin is 3.5 mg/dL (normal = < 1.2 mg/dL in adults), and unconjugated bilirubin is 3.0 mg/dL. Complete blood count, peripheral smear, and liver function tests are all within normal limits. What is the next step in the management of the infant?

(A) No further treatment other than routine follow-up

(B) Observation and repeat of the bilirubin levels every 6 hours for 72 hours

(C) Phototherapy

(D) Exchange transfusion

(E) Elective intubation and hyperventilation

Question 233

A 2-year-old normally healthy child is brought to the emergency department with fever and diarrhea as well as one episode of vomiting this morning. On examination, the pharynx is erythematous, and the left tympanic membrane is erythematous and bulging outward, obscuring the normal anatomy. The mother reports that the child has been tugging on the ear for the past 24 hours. The child's temperature is 102° F, and the child's diapers contain liquid brown stool that is negative for occult blood. What is the most likely cause of the child's gastrointestinal symptoms?

(A) Otitis media

(B) Viral gastroenteritis

(C) Bacterial gastroenteritis

(D) Child abuse

(E) Ulcerative colitis

Question 234

Which of the following is a potential complication of severe reflux esophagitis?

(A) Pancreatitis

(B) Gastric cancer

(C) Esophageal cancer

(D) Duodenal ulcer

(E) Pernicious anemia

Question 235

Which of the following is **not** usually indicated in a case of acute pancreatitis?

(A) Preventing the patient from eating initially

(B) Intravenous fluids

(C) Antibiotics

(D) Nasogastric tube if nausea and vomiting are present

(E) Narcotics for pain

Question 236

Which of the following is **least** helpful in the management of typical chronic calcific pancreatitis?

(A) Alcohol abstinence

(B) Corticosteroids

(C) Oral pancreatic enzyme replacement

(D) Fat-soluble vitamin supplements

(E) None of the above

Question 237

A 31-year-old woman with repeated bouts of intermittent, severe, substernal chest pain has had a negative cardiac workup. A barium swallow reveals a distal narrowing of the esophagus with a *bird's beak* appearance and esophageal dilation proximal to the narrowing. The patient also reports dysphagia but denies heartburn. What is the most likely diagnosis?

(A) Scleroderma

(B) Barrett's esophagus

(C) Esophageal carcinoma

(D) Gastric carcinoma

(E) Achalasia

Question 238

What is the usual cause of a conjugated hyperbilirubine-mia with jaundice, darkening of the urine, and clay-col-ored stools?

(A) Parenchymal liver disease
(B) Obstruction in the biliary system
(C) Liver malignancy
(D) Hepatitis
(E) Pancreatitis

Question 239

An infant is born prematurely at 30 weeks to a diabetic mother. After delivery, the child has labored, rapid respi-rations, substernal retractions, cyanosis, grunting, nasal flaring, and diffuse microatelectasis with diffuse ground-glass type infiltrates seen on chest radiograph. What is the most likely cause of the child's respiratory difficulty?

(A) Carbon monoxide poisoning
(B) Chlamydial pneumonia
(C) Cystic fibrosis
(D) Deficiency of surfactant
(E) Pulmonary hypoplasia

Question 240

A 19-year-old woman presents with a chief complaint of "zits." She has no medical history and takes no medications.

Which of the following is true regarding acne vulgaris?

(A) It is generally considered to be an autoimmune phe-nomenon.
(B) The patient's diet is likely to be the cause.
(C) Oral isotretinoin is the preferred first-line agent.
(D) A biopsy of one of the more inflamed-appearing lesions is required to confirm the diagnosis.
(E) None of the above

Question 241

A 24-year-old white man comes into the office complain-ing of "white spots" on his skin that he noticed after tan-ning at the beach. The patient has no other complaints, and the physical examination is unremarkable other than the skin (shown below), which does not itch.

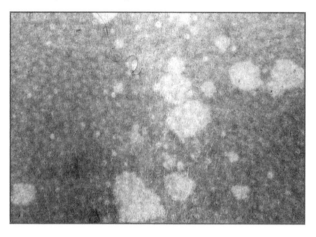

Which of the following is the most likely condition?

(A) Pityriasis rosea
(B) Tinea versicolor
(C) Kaposi's sarcoma
(D) Contact dermatitis
(E) Lichen planus

Question 242

An otherwise healthy 3-year-old girl presents with a third episode of pneumonia in the right middle lobe over the past 4 months. The child never had pneumonia before 4 months ago. What is the most likely reason for the recur-rent pneumonias?

(A) Cystic fibrosis
(B) Congenital lung anomaly
(C) Bruton's X-linked agammaglobulinemia
(D) Foreign body aspiration
(E) HIV infection

Question 243

What is the most likely method of inheritance for schizo-phrenia?
(A) Autosomal dominant
(B) Autosomal recessive
(C) X-linked recessive
(D) Polygenic disorder

Question 244

What is the most likely method of inheritance for Duchenne muscular dystrophy?
(A) Autosomal dominant
(B) Autosomal recessive
(C) X-linked recessive
(D) Polygenic disorder

Question 245

What is the most likely method of inheritance for bipolar disorder?
(A) Autosomal dominant
(B) Autosomal recessive
(C) X-linked recessive
(D) Polygenic disorder

Question 246

What is the most likely method of inheritance for Wilson's disease?
(A) Autosomal dominant
(B) Autosomal recessive
(C) X-linked recessive
(D) Polygenic disorder

Question 247

What is the most likely method of inheritance for neurofibromatosis?
(A) Autosomal dominant
(B) Autosomal recessive
(C) X-linked recessive
(D) Polygenic disorder

Question 248

What is the most likely method of inheritance for multiple endocrine neoplasia I syndrome?
(A) Autosomal dominant
(B) Autosomal recessive
(C) X-linked recessive
(D) Polygenic disorder

Question 249

What is the most likely method of inheritance for the condition depicted below:

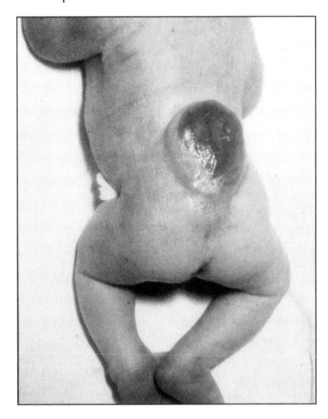

(A) Autosomal dominant
(B) Autosomal recessive
(C) X-linked recessive
(D) Polygenic disorder

Question 250

What is the most likely method of inheritance for familial polyposis coli?
(A) Autosomal dominant
(B) Autosomal recessive
(C) X-linked recessive
(D) Polygenic disorder

BLOCK 5 ANSWER KEY

201. B	211. D	221. D	231. A	241. B
202. E	212. C	222. C	232. A	242. D
203. D	213. B	223. C	233. A	243. D
204. C	214. A	224. C	234. C	244. C
205. C	215. C	225. B	235. C	245. D
206. B	216. B	226. D	236. B	246. B
207. E	217. A	227. A	237. E	247. A
208. D	218. B	228. D	238. B	248. A
209. A	219. C	229. A	239. D	249. D
210. C	220. D	230. A	240. E	250. A

Refer to Answers and Explanations Section for Block 5

Pages 239–246

Figure credits

Question 241: du Vivier A: The dermatologic diagnosis. In du Vivier A (ed): Atlas of Clinical Dermatology, 3rd ed. New York, Churchill Livingstone, 2002, pp 1–21.

Question 249: Hoffbrand AV, Pettit JE: Megaloblastic anemias. In Hoffbrand AV, Pettit JE (eds): Color Atlas of Clinical Hematology, 3rd ed. St. Louis, Mosby, 2000, pp 57–70.

BLOCK 6

50 QUESTIONS

TIME ALLOWED: 60 MINUTES

Question 251

A 64-year-old man with home oxygen–requiring emphysema presents with shortness of breath and fever as well as an increase in chronic cough. Chest radiograph reveals no acute changes compared with old films, and a good sputum sample reveals large numbers of gram-negative diplococci. What is the most likely organism?

(A) *Neisseria gonorrhoeae*
(B) *Neisseria meningitidis*
(C) *Moraxella catarrhalis*
(D) *Streptococcus pneumoniae*
(E) *Mycoplasma pneumoniae*

Question 252

What cause of potentially severe atypical pneumonia is classically associated with exposure to a contaminated environmental water source?

(A) *Mycoplasma pneumoniae*
(B) *Chlamydia pneumoniae*
(C) *Chlamydia psittaci*
(D) *Legionella pneumophila*
(E) *Coxiella burnetii*

Question 253

Which of the following is more likely to be present in an atypical pneumonia than a pneumonia caused by *Streptococcus pneumoniae*?

(A) Fever greater than 102°F
(B) Age greater than 40
(C) Single-lobe involvement on chest radiograph
(D) Prodromal symptoms for more than 3 days
(E) Positive blood cultures

Question 254

Which of the following descriptions of the circulation during the perinatal period is **not** accurate?

(A) The first breaths after birth decrease pulmonary vascular resistance.
(B) After birth, higher blood oxygen concentration stimulates prostaglandin production, causing gradual closure of the ductus arteriosus.
(C) After birth, clamping of the cord and increased pulmonary venous return cause increased left-sided heart pressures, which results in functional closure of the foramen ovale.
(D) The highest oxygen content in the fetus during intrauterine life is in the umbilical veins.
(E) During intrauterine life, blood going to the upper extremities is higher in oxygen content than blood going to the lower extremities.

Question 255

Which of the following agents is useful in the setting of diastolic cardiac dysfunction?

(A) Digoxin
(B) Metoprolol
(C) Isosorbide dinitrate
(D) Furosemide
(E) Hydralazine

Question 256

Which of the following has **not** been associated with ventricular septal defects?

(A) Fetal alcohol syndrome
(B) Maternal smoking
(C) Intrauterine TORCH infections
(D) Down syndrome
(E) Tetralogy of Fallot

Question 257

What is the treatment for most ventricular septal defects present at birth?

(A) Observation
(B) Primary surgical closure
(C) Indomethacin to induce closure
(D) Prostaglandins to induce closure
(E) Intracardiac administration of growth factors to allow stimulation of cardiac muscle growth over the defect

Question 258

A 1-year-old boy is brought to the office because his mother is concerned over his marked bleeding tendency and easy bruising. You measure the following parameters:

Prothrombin time	Normal
Partial thromboplastin time	Prolonged
Bleeding time	Normal
Peripheral smear	Normal
Hemoglobin	11 gm/dL

What is the most likely cause of the child's problem?

(A) Idiopathic thrombocytopenia
(B) Henoch-Schönlein purpura
(C) Hemophilia A
(D) Hemophilia B
(E) von Willebrand's disease

Question 259

A 22-year-old man is brought to the emergency department after an automobile accident. His femur is clearly broken because the proximal portion of the bone has penetrated through the skin. He is alert and oriented but in excruciating pain. Pulses are absent distal to the fracture. Which of the following is the appropriate management?

(A) Observation and stabilization
(B) Immediate closed reduction in the emergency department
(C) Immediate closed reduction under general anesthesia
(D) Immediate open reduction and internal fixation under general anesthesia
(E) Elective open reduction and internal fixation the next day with intravenous fluids, antibiotics, and traction overnight

Question 260

A 62-year-old woman with a history of rheumatic fever as a child presents with shortness of breath. On examination, she has a loud, late diastolic blowing murmur best heard in the apex. Which of the following areas is **not** likely to have increased pressure within it because of the valvular dysfunction most likely present?

(A) Pulmonary artery
(B) Right ventricle
(C) Left atrium
(D) Left ventricle
(E) Pulmonary veins

Question 261

A 62-year-old woman with hypertension, diabetes, hypercholesterolemia, and a long smoking history comes to the emergency department with altered mental status. She is started on supplemental oxygen, and an intravenous catheter is inserted. Oxygen saturation is 95% on 3 L nasal cannula, pulse is 102 beats/min, temperature is 96.2° F, and the blood pressure is 78/42 mmHg. The chest has scattered rhonchi, but the patient is unable to cooperate enough to take a deep breath.

She is given 2 L of normal saline, and her blood pressure remains unchanged while her pulse increases. The patient is noted to have moderate jugular venous distention. A chest radiograph shows patchy infiltrates bilaterally that resemble a combination of infiltrate and pulmonary edema. Laboratory studies are pending. The patient is tachypneic but appears to be in only mild distress. She does seem to be confused, however, and is unable to give a good history. What is the next best step in the management of this patient?

(A) Provide intubation and mechanical ventilation.
(B) Provide anticoagulation with heparin.
(C) Give 2 more liters of normal saline.
(D) Begin invasive hemodynamic monitoring (Swan-Ganz catheterization).
(E) Discuss the patient's wishes regarding intubation and cardiopulmonary resuscitation.

Question 262

A 25-year-old man is brought to the emergency department after being assaulted. He is awake but mildly disoriented. Physical examination reveals a bleeding leg with a fairly deep laceration from a sharp object and a bruise over the abdomen. He is able to talk and does not appear markedly short of breath, although respiratory rate is 20/min. Blood pressure is 70/30 mmHg, and pulse rate is 140 beats/min. Oxygen saturation is 97% on room air. Physical exam reveals mild abdominal tenderness but no rebound or guarding. An intravenous catheter is inserted, and the patient is given 1 L of Ringer's lactate. Blood pressure is remeasured at 82/50 mmHg, and pulse rate now is 122 beats/min. Lab tests are pending. What is the best next step?

(A) Administer another liter of Ringer's lactate.
(B) Administer 5% dextrose in water.
(C) Administer 10% dextrose in water.
(D) Perform immediate CT scan of the head.
(E) Proceed to the operating room for exploratory laparotomy.

Question 263

A mother brings her 4-year-old girl with Down syndrome to the office because the child has a fever and a skin rash. The child takes no medications and has no significant medical history other than repair of a ventricular septal defect shortly after birth. The child is pale and somewhat lethargic compared with normal. The child's temperature is 102° F, pulse is 138 beats/min, and respiratory rate is 22/min. Blood pressure is normal. The child has severe, exudative pharyngitis and widespread petechiae. A complete blood count reveals the following:

Hemoglobin	5 gm/dL
White blood cell count	1200/μL
Platelets	28,000/μL

Which of the following is the most likely cause of the child's symptoms?

(A) Child abuse
(B) Parvovirus B19 infection
(C) Aplastic anemia from toxin exposure
(D) Acute lymphocytic leukemia
(E) Non-Hodgkin's lymphoma

Question 264

Which of the following is true regarding epidural hematomas?

(A) They classically cause a gradual onset of symptoms.
(B) They often are associated with temporal bone fracture.
(C) They usually are due to trauma involving cerebral veins or a dural sinus.
(D) They usually appear crescent shaped on CT scan.
(E) Loss of consciousness is rare in the setting of an epidural hematoma, although neurologic deficits may be present.

Question 265

Which of the following would be **least** expected in fluid removed from a pleural effusion if the effusion is due to an early empyema?

(A) Positive Gram stain
(B) High neutrophil count
(C) Low glucose level
(D) Pleural fluid to serum protein ratio less than 0.5
(E) Pleural fluid to serum lactate dehydrogenase ratio of 0.76

Question 266

Which of the following agents is **not** thought to increase cardiac contractility at the doses typically used?

(A) Phenylephrine
(B) Isoproterenol
(C) Dobutamine
(D) Dopamine
(E) Milrinone

Question 267

Which of the following complications of type II or adult-onset diabetes is **not** seen in patients with type I or juvenile-onset diabetes?

(A) Retinopathy
(B) Kidney disease
(C) Accelerated atherosclerosis
(D) Autonomic neuropathy
(E) None of the above

Question 268

In which of the following patients would enalapril be the best first-line agent for high blood pressure control?

(A) A 62-year-old man with renal artery stenosis
(B) A 32-year-old pregnant woman
(C) A 41-year-old woman with hyperkalemia
(D) A 58-year-old man prone to go into atrial fibrillation with a rapid ventricular rate
(E) A 56-year-old diabetic woman

Question 269

Which of the following is **false** concerning coarctation of the aorta?

(A) It commonly is associated with Turner syndrome.
(B) Rib notching may be present and is seen on the inferior aspects of the ribs.
(C) In adults with uncorrected coarctation, a ruptured cerebral aneurysm is a fairly common cause of death.
(D) The stenotic area usually is just proximal to the right subclavian artery.
(E) Upper extremity-only hypertension is commonly present.

Question 270

Which of the following antibiotic/infection combinations is most likely to result in effective treatment of the infection?

(A) Tetracycline for streptococcal pharyngitis
(B) Piperacillin and tazobactam for *Chlamydia* urethritis
(C) Azithromycin for *Legionella* pneumonia
(D) Aztreonam for a positive blood culture containing *Enterococcus faecalis*
(E) Gentamicin for *Clostridium difficile* colitis

Question 271

Which of the following symptoms is **not** likely to be related directly or indirectly to diabetes in a patient with long-standing, poorly controlled diabetes?

(A) Sudden onset of double vision
(B) Shortness of breath
(C) Orthostatic hypotension
(D) Nausea and vomiting shortly after eating
(E) None of the above

Question 272

Which of the following patients with hypertension and a recent myocardial infarction should **not** be put on beta blocker therapy?

(A) A 59-year-old man with stable congestive heart failure
(B) A 45-year-old diabetic man with angina
(C) A 69-year-old woman with severe asthma
(D) A 52-year-old man with intermittent claudication
(E) All of the above

Question 273

A 41-year-old obese woman with no other medical history is in the hospital and status-post cholecystectomy, having had surgery 4 days ago. She still is not eating and has been on 5% dextrose and half-normal saline for maintenance intravenous fluid at 175 mL/h since surgery. She has remained afebrile, and a chest radiograph taken yesterday showed clear lungs. The patient has not had flatus or a bowel movement since surgery. The patient requires only acetaminophen for pain control but has complained of severe, worsening weakness and increasing abdominal distention over the last 2 days. An abdominal radiograph showed an ileus pattern with no obstruction seen. Chart review reveals a basic chemistry profile, performed 2 days ago:

Sodium	137 mEq/L
Potassium	3.2 mEq/L
Chloride	108 mmol/L
CO_2	26 mEq/L
BUN	8 mg/dL
Creatinine	0.8 mg/dL

The patient has had no changes in therapy or medication since that time. The nurse calls because the patient is starting to have some trouble breathing secondary to "weakness." What is the most likely physical finding in this patient?

(A) Increased, high-pitched bowel sounds that come in waves
(B) High fever
(C) Pulmonary rales
(D) Abnormal tendon reflexes
(E) Distended neck veins

Question 274

Assuming the person has no other medical problems and takes no medications, which of the following symptoms or signs would be **least** expected in a 36-year-old patient who presents with new-onset, uncontrolled diabetes mellitus type II?

(A) Blurry vision
(B) Orthostatic hypotension
(C) Loss of sensation below the knee bilaterally
(D) Excessive hunger with recent history of frequent eating
(E) Nocturia

Question 275

A 29-year-old woman has a chief complaint of severe muscle pain and weakness, primarily in the shoulders and back. She has no other medical problems, although she admits to trouble sleeping recently. Her muscles are extremely tender to palpation, but strength is normal in the affected muscles. Laboratory tests show a normal erythrocyte sedimentation rate, complete blood count, and creatine phosphokinase level. What is the next best step in the workup of this patient?

(A) Electromyography

(B) Nerve conduction studies

(C) Muscle biopsy

(D) Inquiry about the patient's mood and stress level

(E) High-dose corticosteroids

Question 276

A 39-year-old man who smokes presents for health maintenance. You have never seen him before because he is new in town. He takes metoprolol for hypertension and glipizide for diabetes. Although the man has no known heart disease, his father died of a heart attack at the age of 40. A screening lipid profile is performed after an overnight fast because the patient did not know any information about his cholesterol levels. The test reveals the following:

Total cholesterol	238 mg/dL
LDL cholesterol	148 mg/dL
HDL cholesterol	30 mg/dL
Triglycerides	300 mg/dL

Which of the following actions is most appropriate regarding the patient's laboratory values?

(A) The patient should have the test repeated in 1 week to ensure there has not been a laboratory error.

(B) The patient should begin lifestyle modifications, including exercise and a low-calorie, low-fat diet.

(C) The patient needs only routine follow-up because he meets current recommended cholesterol goals.

(D) The patient should be started on niacin.

(E) The patient should be started on atorvastatin.

Question 277

Which cancer is currently the number one cause of cancer death in women?

(A) Breast

(B) Lung

(C) Colon

(D) Uterine

(E) Leukemia

Question 278

Which of the following is usually inherited in an autosomal-recessive manner and results in an increased risk of cancer?

(A) Familial polyposis coli

(B) Multiple endocrine syndrome, type I

(C) Neurofibromatosis

(D) Xeroderma pigmentosa

(E) Down syndrome

Question 279

A 24-year-old man presents to the office with complaints of stomachaches. He brings with him a thick stack of papers that he says is his medical record. He demands that you read the "file" because all his other physicians have been unable to figure out what is wrong with him. What is the best thing to say to the patient?

(A) "I'll read the files as soon as our appointment is over."

(B) "I'll read the files if I have time."

(C) "Why don't you tell me a little more about your stomachaches?"

(D) "Why don't we go over the file together?"

(E) "Are you feeling depressed or sad?"

Question 280

Which of the following would be **unexpected** in a patient with chronic end-stage renal failure who missed her last two dialysis sessions?

(A) Hypertension

(B) Respiratory acidosis

(C) Hypocalcemia

(D) Hyperkalemia

(E) None of the above

Question 281

Which of the following is **least** likely to cause acute renal failure or insufficiency, assuming no pre-existing renal disease?

(A) Right nephrectomy
(B) Dehydration
(C) Benign prostatic hypertrophy
(D) Rhabdomyolysis
(E) Congestive heart failure

Question 282

A 33-year-old woman complains of fatigue that started about 2 or 3 weeks ago. She is a nurse who just began working a second full-time job 3 weeks ago but claims to get enough sleep. She reports no other symptoms and reports being "happy." Her affect and mood seem normal. She takes birth control pills but no other medications. She is sexually active with her boyfriend but denies being promiscuous. Physical examination and vital signs are within normal limits. Baseline laboratory tests reveal the following:

Hemoglobin	13.8 gm/dL
Hematocrit	41%
Mean corpuscular volume	93 µm/cell
White blood cell count	8100/mL
Platelet count	184,000/µL
Thyroid-stimulating hormone	2.5 µU/mL (normal = 0.5–5.0)
Total thyroxine level (T4)	14 µg/dL (normal= 4–12)

What is the most likely cause of this patient's fatigue?

(A) Graves' disease
(B) Surreptitious ingestion of thyroxine
(C) HIV infection
(D) Major depression
(E) None of the above

Question 283

A 32-year-old restaurant manager has a nerve conduction study done for symptoms of carpal tunnel syndrome that confirms the diagnosis of carpal tunnel syndrome. The patient also has fatigue and constipation. Which of the following is most important in the management of this patient?

(A) Check for Tinel's sign.
(B) Check for Phalen's sign.
(C) Check a thyroid-stimulating hormone (TSH) level.
(D) Check the stool for occult blood.
(E) Order a blood test for anti–acetylcholine receptor antibodies.

Question 284

A 28-year-old woman presents with a fever and neck pain that started 2 days ago. She said she had a "cold" a week ago that went away just before the neck pain started. The neck pain is made worse by swallowing and turning of the head. On physical examination, the pharynx is minimally erythematous without exudate. There is no palpable lymphadenopathy, and the tympanic membranes are clear. The thyroid gland is enlarged, tender, and firm. Which of the following is likely to be true?

(A) The patient has several first-degree relatives with hypothyroidism.
(B) Fine-needle aspiration of the gland is needed in the firm area to rule out a neoplasm.
(C) The patient most likely has an elevated thyroid-stimulating immunoglobulin titer.
(D) The patient has a fungal thyroid infection.
(E) None of the above

Question 285

A 46-year-old man complains of increasing abdominal girth and fatigue that has developed gradually over the past few months. Past medical history is significant for alcoholism and a vague history of hepatitis C. The man takes no medications and family history is remarkable only for alcoholism. Physical examination reveals a firm, nodular liver that is not enlarged and mild splenomegaly. Shifting dullness to percussion and a fluid wave are elicited on abdominal exam as well. A liver biopsy is performed and a sample slide shown below.

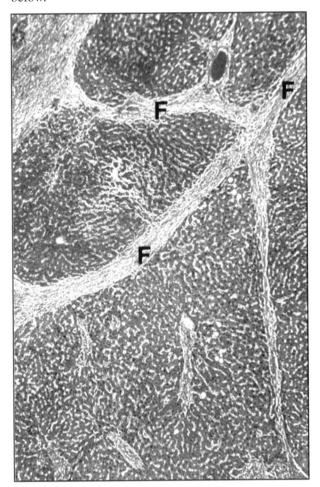

What diagnosis is confirmed by the figure?

(A) Cirrhosis
(B) Chronic active hepatitis, mild
(C) Chronic active hepatitis, severe
(D) Hepatic adenoma
(E) Hepatocellular carcinoma

Question 286

Which of the following causes of hyperbilirubinemia is **least** likely to result in elevated levels of bilirubin in the urine?

(A) Crigler-Najjar syndrome
(B) Biliary atresia
(C) Acute viral hepatitis
(D) Hemolysis
(E) Neonatal cholestasis

Question 287

A 22-year-old man presents with cervical lymphadenopathy, night sweats, malaise, and weight loss over the past 8 weeks. A lymph node biopsy is performed and reveals distinct-looking binucleated cells. What is the most likely diagnosis?

(A) Cat-scratch disease
(B) Burkitt lymphoma
(C) Hodgkin lymphoma
(D) Acute lymphoblastic leukemia
(E) Infectious mononucleosis

Question 288

A 41-year-old man presents with severe odynophagia that developed over the past few weeks. Endoscopy is performed and reveals whitish patches and plaques on the esophageal mucosa, which are also noted in the man's pharynx. A sample taken during the endoscopy procedure revealed the presence of numerous organisms whose appearance is shown below.

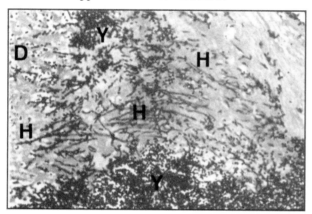

Which of the following is true regarding the most likely cause of the man's symptoms?

(A) Penicillin is the treatment of choice.
(B) Chronic esophageal reflux likely led to this infection.
(C) 6-12 months of anti-tuberculous therapy will be needed, preferably using directly observed therapy (DOT).
(D) The man needs a work-up for immunodeficiency.
(E) Infection typically occurs via hematogenous spread from distal sites.

Question 289

You are called to do a routine newborn examination on a female infant who is status-post a vaginal breech delivery without complications. You notice that the left leg is slightly shorter than the right leg. On abduction of the thighs with the hips and knees flexed, there is an audible click coming from the left side. The rest of your examination is normal. Which of the following is **false** regarding the most likely condition?

(A) Hip ultrasound often is more useful than hip radiograph to confirm the diagnosis.
(B) The child may be at an increased risk for arthritis of the hip as an adult.
(C) Surgical pinning done under local anesthesia is the treatment of choice.
(D) The fact that the patient is female and was born breech is significant in the history.
(E) The earlier treatment is instituted, the better the outcome generally is.

Question 290

An obese 41-year-old woman presents to the emergency department with a chief complaint of abdominal pain. The pain started 3 hours earlier, is constant, is located in the right upper portion of the abdomen, and is accompanied by severe nausea. The patient admits to having similar pains in the past that went away on their own after several minutes, which she attributed to "gas." The patient's past medical history is significant for high blood pressure and a right knee arthroscopy for arthritis. She takes hydrochlorothiazide daily and as-needed acetaminophen when her knee "acts up." Vital signs are as follows:

Temperature	99.8°F
Blood pressure	158/90 mmHg
Pulse rate	92 beats/min
Respirations	14/min

On examination, the only abnormalities are obesity and right upper quadrant tenderness to palpation, especially under the rib cage. There are no palpable abdominal masses or organs; however, the patient is fairly obese, making the examination somewhat difficult. Laboratory tests reveal the following:

Hemoglobin	14 gm/dL
Mean corpuscular volume	88 µm/cell
White blood cell count	10,000/µg with 90% neutrophils
ALT	15 (normal = 1–21)
Alkaline phosphatase	95 U/L (normal = 13–39)
Total bilirubin	0.7 mg/dL (normal = 0.1–1.0)
Sodium	142 mEq/L
Creatinine	1.0 mg/dL

What should you do next?

(A) Order an ultrasound of the right upper quadrant.

(B) Order a CT scan of the abdomen with contrast enhancement.

(C) Order acute hepatitis A, B, C, and D panels.

(D) Order a 5'-nucleotidase level.

(E) Delay any planned surgical intervention until the blood pressure is better controlled.

Question 291

An 18-year-old man presents to the emergency department with headache, malaise and fever. A sore throat and dry cough started 5 days ago and progressed to a severe headache several hours ago accompanied by sweating alternating with chills. He has no history of trauma, recent travel, or hiking and lives in a dormitory at the local college where he is a student. He is sexually active with two different girls. He says he is starting to feel "a little weird, like cloudy in my brain" and is slightly confused. Vital signs are as follows:

Temperature	102.8°F
Blood pressure	100/58 mmHg
Pulse rate	118 beats/min
Respirations	18/min

On examination, the skin is flushed and warm. There are several petechiae bilaterally on the lower extremities below the knee. When examining the hands, you notice similar petechiae on the tips of two different fingers of the left hand. Funduscopic examination is within normal limits, and pupils are equal and reactive, although the patient says the light hurts his eyes. The patient has severe neck pain when he tries to touch his chin to his chest and resists your attempts to assist him. He begins to have shaking chills as you are examining him and pushes you away, curling up into the fetal position and moaning softly. What is the next best course of action?

(A) Administer prophylactic anticonvulsants.

(B) Perform a lumbar puncture and start empiric antibiotics based on the gram stain results.

(C) Order an MRI of the brain, then do a lumbar puncture.

(D) Start intravenous fluids and broad-spectrum antibiotics while preparing to perform lumbar puncture.

(E) Order a complete metabolic profile.

Question 292

A 62-year-old man comes to see you for the first time because he has just moved to the area. His medical history is significant for hypertension, high cholesterol, and diabetes. He freely admits that he is a "pretty lousy" patient who often fails to take his medicines, smokes, and has especially poor blood pressure control. His medications include nifedipine, captopril, metformin, insulin, simvastatin, and aspirin. Physical examination reveals obesity and an S4 heart sound. When you stroke the plantar aspect of the feet, the toes of the right foot react by flexing downward, whereas the great toe of the left foot extends and the other toes extend upward in a fanlike pattern. Sensation is intact, and reflexes are symmetric, other than a left ankle jerk reflex that is more brisk than the right. Which of the following is most likely to be **false** regarding this patient?

(A) He has a left lower motor neuron lesion by physical examination.
(B) He is a type II diabetic.
(C) He has left ventricular hypertrophy.
(D) He has atherosclerosis.
(E) He has had at least one small stroke.

Question 293

A 32-year-old man presents to your office complaining of infertility. He and his wife have tried for more than 2 years to conceive without success. The patient is tall and thin with little facial hair. On examination, he has mild gynecomastia and small, firm testes. There are no other stigmata of liver disease. The patient has not noticed any recent change in body habitus. Which of the following is most likely to be **false** regarding this patient?

(A) A buccal smear would reveal the presence of Barr bodies.
(B) He is infertile.
(C) He is mentally retarded.
(D) He is heterosexual.
(E) His testicles are likely to have little or no functional capacity.

Question 294

A 21-year-old woman comes to see you for primary amenorrhea. She has no significant medical history. She is short and on examination has widely spaced nipples with no breast development and juvenile-appearing external genitalia. You also note mild ptosis and a low hairline on the back of the neck. Which of the following is most likely to be true regarding this patient?

(A) She has a pituitary neoplasm.
(B) She has functional ovaries with end-organ unresponsiveness to hormone stimulation.
(C) She is likely to be mentally retarded with a low verbal IQ.
(D) Her genotype is most likely 47 XXX.
(E) A buccal smear would reveal an absence of Barr bodies.

Question 295

Which of the following can worsen hypercalcemia?

(A) Sulfonamides
(B) Beta blockers
(C) HMG-CoA reductase inhibitors
(D) Angiotensin-converting enzyme inhibitors
(E) Aminoglycosides
(F) Loop diuretics
(G) Thiazide diuretics
(H) Calcium channel blockers
(I) Tricyclic antidepressants
(J) Fluoroquinolones

Question 296

Which of these agents requires monitoring of liver function tests?

(A) Sulfonamides
(B) Beta blockers
(C) HMG-CoA reductase inhibitors
(D) Angiotensin-converting enzyme inhibitors
(E) Aminoglycosides
(F) Loop diuretics
(G) Thiazide diuretics
(H) Calcium channel blockers
(I) Tricyclic antidepressants
(J) Fluoroquinolones

Question 297

Which class of agentss is one of the most common causes of Stevens-Johnson syndrome?

(A) Sulfonamides
(B) Beta blockers
(C) HMG-CoA reductase inhibitors
(D) Angiotensin-converting enzyme inhibitors
(E) Aminoglycosides
(F) Loop diuretics
(G) Thiazide diuretics
(H) Calcium channel blockers
(I) Tricyclic antidepressants
(J) Fluoroquinolones

Question 298

Which class of agents can prolong neuromuscular blockade in the setting of general anesthesia?

(A) Sulfonamides
(B) Beta blockers
(C) HMG-CoA reductase inhibitors
(D) Angiotensin-converting enzyme inhibitors
(E) Aminoglycosides
(F) Loop diuretics
(G) Thiazide diuretics
(H) Calcium channel blockers
(I) Tricyclic antidepressants
(J) Fluoroquinolones

Question 299

Which class of agents can cause dangerous cardiac side effects in overdose?

(A) Sulfonamides
(B) Beta blockers
(C) HMG-CoA reductase inhibitors
(D) Angiotensin-converting enzyme inhibitors
(E) Aminoglycosides
(F) Loop diuretics
(G) Thiazide diuretics
(H) Calcium channel blockers
(I) Tricyclic antidepressants
(J) Fluoroquinolones

Question 300

Which class of agents hould be used with caution in patients with gout or a sulfa allergy?

(A) Sulfonamides
(B) Beta blockers
(C) HMG-CoA reductase inhibitors
(D) Angiotensin-converting enzyme inhibitors
(E) Aminoglycosides
(F) Loop diuretics
(G) Thiazide diuretics
(H) Calcium channel blockers
(I) Tricyclic antidepressants
(J) Fluoroquinolones

BLOCK 6 ANSWER KEY

251. C	261. D	271. E	281. A	291. D
252. D	262. A	272. C	282. E	292. A
253. D	263. D	273. D	283. C	293. C
254. B	264. B	274. C	284. E	294. E
255. B	265. D	275. D	285. A	295. G
256. B	266. A	276. B	286. A	296. C
257. A	267. E	277. B	287. C	297. A
258. C	268. E	278. D	288. D	298. E
259. D	269. D	279. C	289. C	299. I
260. D	270. C	280. B	290. A	300. G

Refer to Answers and Explanations Section for Block 6

Pages 247–255

Figure credits

Question 285: Stevens A, et al: Hepatobiliry system and pancreas. In Stevens A, et al (eds): Wheater's Basic Histopathology, 4th ed. New York, Churchill Livingstone, 2002, pp 154–164.

Question 288: Stevens A, et al: Infections of histologic importance. In Wheater's Basic Histopathology, 4th ed. New York, Churchill Livingstone, 2002, pp 35–55.

BLOCK 7

USMLE Step 2 Mock Exam, 2e

50 QUESTIONS

**TIME ALLOWED:
60 MINUTES**

Question 301

In the fetal circulation, which of the following lists, from highest to lowest, the blood oxygen saturation levels inside the named vessels (highest oxygen saturation first, lowest last)?

(A) Umbilical artery, carotid artery, femoral vein, umbilical vein

(B) Carotid artery, femoral vein, umbilical artery, umbilical vein

(C) Carotid artery, umbilical artery, femoral vein, umbilical vein

(D) Umbilical vein, carotid artery, umbilical artery, femoral vein

(E) Umbilical vein, carotid artery, femoral vein, umbilical artery

Question 302

A 57-year-old female alcoholic presents to the emergency department with increasingly severe epigastric pain radiating through to the back, nausea, and vomiting. The vital signs are as follows:

Temperature	98.9°F
Blood pressure	172/92 mmHg
Pulse rate	96 beats/min
Respirations	18/min

Physical examination reveals epigastric tenderness with voluntary guarding but no rebound tenderness or involuntary guarding. Abdominal radiograph is unremarkable. Laboratory tests reveal the following:

Hemoglobin	9.5 gm/dL
Hematocrit	32%
Mean corpuscular volume	102 μm/cell
White blood cell count	11,100/μL
Platelet count	90,000/μL
Sodium	140 mEq/L
Potassium	4.2 mEq/L
Chloride	108 mEq/L
CO_2	24 mEq/L
BUN	26 mg/dL
Creatinine	1.4 mg/dL
Amylase	764 U/L (normal = 53–123 u/L)

What is the best way to manage this patient?

(A) Send patient home after making a follow up appointment with her physician and prescribing a nonsteroidal analgesic for pain.

(B) Admit to the hospital for a blood transfusion.

(C) Admit to the hospital for medical management.

(D) Admit to the hospital for surgery.

(E) Perform esophagogastroduodenoscopy.

Question 303

Which of the following is **least** likely as an explanation for a patient's anemia?

(A) Pregnancy

(B) Prematurity

(C) Peptic ulcer disease

(D) Emphysema

(E) Dietary habits

Question 304

A 24-year-old woman with lupus nephritis progresses to renal failure despite treatment. Which of the following electrolyte disturbances is she most likely to develop?

(A) Hypokalemia
(B) Hyperkalemia
(C) Hypercalcemia
(D) Hypomagnesemia
(E) Alkalosis

Question 305

Given his electrocardiogram findings, which antihypertensive is this 54-year-old male patient most likely taking, assuming the electrocardiogram was normal before drug therapy was started?

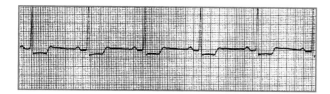

(A) Atenolol
(B) Nifedipine
(C) Captopril
(D) Terazosin
(E) Irbesartan

Question 306

A 53-year-old woman presents with significant weight loss and fatigue. Rectal exam reveals no masses, but melena is present. A barium enema is performed and reveals an abnormality in the ascending colon (arrow in figure). Which of the following is true regarding the most likely etiology?

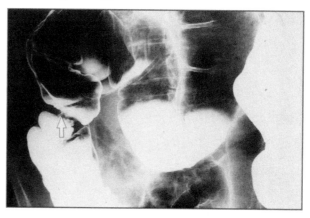

Which of the following is true regarding the most likely etiology?

(A) The cause is likely to be adhesions from prior surgery.
(B) Surgical resection is the initial treatment of choice.
(C) The 5-year survival is typically less than 5%.
(D) It is an uncommon cause of lower GI bleeding.
(E) It is more common in adolescents and young adults.

Question 307

Flight of ideas is seen most commonly in which of the following disorders?

(A) Mania
(B) Schizoid personality disorder
(C) Borderline personality disorder
(D) Depression
(E) Obsessive-compulsive disorder

Question 308

A 29-year-old gravida 3 para 2 (G3P2) woman with a 13-week intrauterine pregnancy develops a deep venous thrombosis of the left lower extremity. What is the most appropriate treatment?

(A) Heparin or low-molecular weight heparin
(B) Heparin acutely, then gradually switch the patient to warfarin for the remainder of the pregnancy
(C) Warfarin
(D) Aspirin
(E) No treatment should be advised

Question 309

Which of the following is **least** correct regarding Huntington's disease?

(A) It can cause dementia.
(B) It can cause psychosis.
(C) It is inherited in an autosomal dominant fashion.
(D) Early diagnosis is crucial for prognosis.
(E) CT scan or MRI often reveals changes in the basal ganglia.

Question 310

Which of the following represents the **least** appropriate single agent for treatment of bipolar disorder?

(A) Venlafaxine
(B) Lithium
(C) Valproic acid
(D) Carbamazepine
(E) Lamotrigine

Question 311

Which of the following is **not** an expected finding in patients due to untreated systemic lupus erythematosus?

(A) Malar rash
(B) Hirsutism
(C) Serositis
(D) Arthritis
(E) Oral ulcers

Question 312

Which of the following is an expected part of Felty's syndrome?

(A) Hepatomegaly
(B) Glossitis
(C) Neutropenia
(D) Diffuse lymphadenopathy
(E) Skeletal dysplasia

Question 313

Assuming detection occurs only after a patient presents with symptoms from cancer, which of the following cancers is most likely to be curable?

(A) Esophageal carcinoma
(B) Pancreatic carcinoma
(C) Ovarian carcinoma
(D) Gestational choriocarcinoma
(E) Hepatocellular carcinoma

Question 314

A woman is found to have a 4 cm invasive ductal carcinoma in her right breast that is noted to be positive for both estrogen and progesterone receptors. Which of the following cancer therapies would be **least** likely to improve her long-term prognosis?

(A) Infliximab
(B) Anastrozole
(C) Tamoxifen
(D) Goserelin
(E) Fulvestrant

Question 315

In which type of bacterial infection would aztreonam most likely be an effective monotherapy?

(A) Pyelonephritis
(B) Community-acquired typical pneumonia
(C) Community-acquired atypical pneumonia
(D) Pharyngitis
(E) Osteomyelitis

Question 316

Which of the following is the best agent to treat confirmed *Chlamydia* pneumonia?

(A) Azithromycin
(B) Piperacillin
(C) Amikacin
(D) Clindamycin
(E) Imipenem

Question 317

Which of the following is **not** one of the potential or regular functions of the spleen?

(A) To remove senescent red blood cells
(B) To store red blood cells
(C) To produce red blood cells
(D) To act as a lymphoid organ
(E) None of the above

Question 318

Which of the following is the most common form of cancer affecting the skin?

(A) Basal cell carcinoma
(B) Squamous cell carcinoma
(C) Malignant melanoma
(D) Cutaneous T cell lymphoma
(E) Metastatic lung cancer

Question 319

A city being studied has a population of 100,000. Using culture as the gold standard test, 5000 people in the city are found to have chlamydial infection. A new DNA probe chlamydial test is positive in 4000 people in the city, of whom only 3000 tested positive by culture. What is the sensitivity of the new DNA probe test?

(A) 50%
(B) 60%
(C) 75%
(D) 80%
(E) >95%

Question 320

What is the most likely cause of death in a 67-year-old black male?

(A) Homicide
(B) An accident
(C) Suicide
(D) Cancer
(E) AIDS

Question 321

What is the most likely cause of death in a 17-year-old white male?

(A) Homicide
(B) An accident
(C) Suicide
(D) Cancer
(E) AIDS

Question 322

When is a fetus most susceptible to teratogenic agents?

(A) The first 3 weeks after conception
(B) The 4th through the 9th weeks after conception
(C) The 10th through 15th weeks after conception
(D) The 16th through 21st weeks after conception
(E) The 22nd through 27th weeks after conception

Question 323

A 64-year-old woman presents with a large, ulcerating breast mass that is highly suspicious for cancer. She tells you that she is not interested in knowing the diagnosis. What is the best initial approach to this patient?

(A) Ask her why she does not want to know the diagnosis.
(B) Tell her that you think it is best that she know the diagnosis.
(C) Respect the patient's wishes and do not tell her the diagnosis.
(D) Call the patient's relatives and discuss the option with them.
(E) Refuse to withhold the diagnosis from the patient and urge her to consider immediate treatment.

Question 324

Which of the following agents acts by direct binding to the luminal aspect of the gastric mucosa?

(A) Sucralfate
(B) Magnesium hydroxide
(C) Omeprazole
(D) Ranitidine
(E) Metoclopramide

Question 325

What is the treatment of choice for a β-blocker overdose?

(A) Isoproterenol
(B) Epinephrine
(C) Glucagon
(D) Growth hormone
(E) Cortisol

Question 326

Which of the following statements regarding gestational trophoblastic disease is **incorrect**?

(A) A human chorionic gonadotropin level that fails to return to zero after an abortion or delivery often is helpful in making the diagnosis.
(B) An ultrasound can help establish the diagnosis and may reveal a "snowstorm" pattern.
(C) A choriocarcinoma can be excluded if the symptoms occur after a term delivery.
(D) A dilation and curettage is adequate treatment for most cases.
(E) If metastases occur, the disease often still responds to chemotherapy.

Question 327

A 33-year-old sexually active woman presents with a complaint of vaginal lesions. On examination, the woman has exophytic, pedunculated, soft, moist, discrete lesions on the external genitalia. The lesions are nontender and do not appear ulcerated. What is the most likely diagnosis?

(A) Condyloma acuminatum
(B) Condyloma latum
(C) Vaginal squamous cell cancer
(D) Chancroid
(E) Herpes genitalis

Question 328

In which of the following conditions would a pulmonary artery wedge pressure of 26 mmHg (normal = 8–12 mmHg) be **unexpected**?

(A) Severe mitral regurgitation
(B) Cardiogenic shock
(C) Untreated renal failure
(D) Septic shock
(E) Severe mitral stenosis

Question 329

Which of the following is **unlikely** in significant hypovolemia?

(A) Lower than normal skin temperature
(B) Low pulmonary capillary wedge pressure
(C) Low systemic vascular resistance
(D) Low urine output
(E) Low blood pressure

Question 330

Which of the following would be **least** likely to result purely from cor pulmonale?

(A) Distended neck veins
(B) Pulsus alternans
(C) Hepatomegaly
(D) Nocturia
(E) Lower extremity edema

Question 331

A 64-year-old woman with a family history of breast cancer presents with a new self-detected right breast mass. On physical examination, the mass is hard and slightly mobile, and it is difficult to feel distinct margins of the lesion. You estimate that the lesion is 3-4 cm in diameter. The left breast is unremarkable on examination, and no axillary lymph nodes are palpable. What is the most appropriate management of the mass?

(A) MRI
(B) Stereotactic biopsy
(C) CT scan of the chest to look for metastatic disease
(D) Repeat clinical exam in 1-2 months
(E) Excisional biopsy

Question 332

Which of the following complications is **unlikely** in a person with bulimia nervosa, assuming that no other psychiatric disturbances are present?

(A) Weight less than 75% of ideal body weight
(B) Laxative abuse
(C) Heavy, prolonged exercise
(D) Periods of binge eating during which the person feels no control
(E) Female sex

Question 333

An 18-month-old boy is brought in with a fever, and a urinalysis reveals that the infant is having his third urinary tract infection since birth. Physical examination is within normal limits, and the infant has no other notable history. Which of the following is most likely to be the underlying cause of the infections?

(A) Vesicoureteral reflux
(B) Exstrophy of the bladder
(C) Hypospadias
(D) Ureterocolic fistula
(E) Prune-belly syndrome (Eagle-Barrett syndrome)

Question 334

Which of the following is **least** likely to be a result of hemolytic-uremic syndrome?

(A) Acute renal failure requiring dialysis
(B) History of recent gastroenteritis
(C) Microangiopathic hemolytic anemia
(D) Thrombocytopenia
(E) Antiplatelet antibodies

Question 335

Which neoplasm is **least** likely in a 3-year-old child?

(A) Wilms' tumor (nephroblastoma)
(B) Neuroblastoma
(C) Leukemia
(D) Posterior fossa brain tumor
(E) Osteogenic sarcoma

Question 336

Which neoplasm is **least** likely in a 13-year-old child?

(A) Neuroblastoma
(B) Primary malignant bone tumor
(C) Leukemia
(D) Lymphoma
(E) Soft tissue sarcoma

Question 337

Which of the following would best describe a 7-month-old infant with thrombocytopenia, eczema, and immunodeficiency?

(A) Glanzmann's thrombasthenia
(B) Bernard-Soulier syndrome
(C) Idiopathic thrombocytopenic purpura
(D) Wiskott-Aldrich syndrome
(E) Kasabach-Merritt syndrome

Question 338

A 57-year-old man undergoes open cholecystectomy for gangrenous cholecystitis. On postoperative days 1 and 2, the man appears increasingly anxious and tremulous but denies pain and simply says "hospitals make him nervous." On postoperative day 3, the man becomes disoriented and agitated, calling out that he is being attacked when no one else is in the room. Other than the mental status changes, the physical examination is unremarkable. Vital signs are unremarkable other than a blood pressure of 168/88 mmHg, and the patient has been afebrile since surgery. Complete blood count and electrolytes are within normal limits. The patient is on no pain medications and oxygen saturation measured by pulse oximetry is 97%. What is the most likely cause of the patient's symptoms?

(A) Delirium tremens
(B) Pulmonary embolus
(C) Sepsis
(D) Acute hypoadrenalism
(E) Occult hyponatremia

Question 339

A 36-year-old term gravida 6, para 5, woman with two prior cesarean sections using "classic" or vertical incisions has sudden onset of severe abdominal pain and hypotension during oxytocin infusion. Which of the following causes of third trimester bleeding best fits this description?

(A) Placenta previa
(B) Abruptio placentae
(C) Uterine rupture
(D) Vasa previa
(E) Cervical lesions (e.g., herpes, gonorrhea, *Chlamydia*, *Candida*)
(F) Bleeding disorder in the mother
(G) Cervical cancer
(H) Bloody show

Question 340

A 26-year-old gravida 1, para 0, woman with triplets has painless vaginal bleeding and stable vital signs, and one of the fetuses shows marked tachycardia and decreased spontaneous movements. Which of the following causes of third trimester bleeding best fits this description?

(A) Placenta previa
(B) Abruptio placentae
(C) Uterine rupture
(D) Vasa previa
(E) Cervical lesions (e.g., herpes, gonorrhea, *Chlamydia*, *Candida*)
(F) Bleeding disorder in the mother
(G) Cervical cancer
(H) Bloody show

Question 341

A 22-year-old gravida 1, para 0, woman has a blood-tinged, mucouslike discharge that resolved immediately (before she got to the hospital) and subsequently went into labor. The woman is anxious, and the cervix is dilated to 4 cm. The fetus seems stable by external fetal monitoring. Which of the following causes of third trimester bleeding best fits this description?

(A) Placenta previa
(B) Abruptio placentae
(C) Uterine rupture
(D) Vasa previa
(E) Cervical lesions (e.g., herpes, gonorrhea, *Chlamydia*, *Candida*)
(F) Bleeding disorder in the mother
(G) Cervical cancer
(H) Bloody show

Question 342

A 34-year-old gravida 5, para 4, woman with multiple uterine fibroids and a history of a normal Pap smear at her first prenatal visit presents with profuse, painless bleeding at 40 weeks. She said the bleeding became bright red and more diffuse as she got nearer to the hospital. Which of the following causes of third trimester bleeding best fits this description?

(A) Placenta previa
(B) Abruptio placentae
(C) Uterine rupture
(D) Vasa previa
(E) Cervical lesions (e.g., herpes, gonorrhea, *Chlamydia*, *Candida*)
(F) Bleeding disorder in the mother
(G) Cervical cancer
(H) Bloody show

Question 343

A 19-year-old gravida 3, para 0, woman presents with bleeding, a tender uterus, and fetal distress. Urine toxicology screen is positive for cocaine. Which of the following causes of third trimester bleeding best fits this description?

(A) Placenta previa
(B) Abruptio placentae
(C) Uterine rupture
(D) Vasa previa
(E) Cervical lesions (e.g., herpes, gonorrhea, *Chlamydia*, *Candida*)
(F) Bleeding disorder in the mother
(G) Cervical cancer
(H) Bloody show

Question 344

A 37-year-old promiscuous gravida 4, para 3, woman with an extensive smoking history and no routine medical care over the last 10 years presents with vaginal bleeding and a friable, eroded cervix. Cervical cultures are negative. Which of the following causes of third trimester bleeding best fits this description?

(A) Placenta previa
(B) Abruptio placentae
(C) Uterine rupture
(D) Vasa previa
(E) Cervical lesions (e.g., herpes, gonorrhea, *Chlamydia*, *Candida*)
(F) Bleeding disorder in the mother
(G) Cervical cancer
(H) Bloody show

Queston 345

Persons with this condition are most likely to have been sexually abused as children.

(A) Somatization disorder
(B) Conversion disorder
(C) Agoraphobia
(D) Body dysmorphic disorder
(E) Factitious disorder
(F) Malingering
(G) Dissociative fugue
(H) Dissociative identity disorder
(I) Social phobia

Question 346

The patient's only secondary gain is to assume the sick role.

(A) Somatization disorder
(B) Conversion disorder
(C) Agoraphobia
(D) Body dysmorphic disorder
(E) Factitious disorder
(F) Malingering
(G) Dissociative fugue
(H) Dissociative identity disorder
(I) Social phobia

Question 347

The patient focuss on symptoms but with no overt secondary gain

(A) Somatization disorder
(B) Conversion disorder
(C) Agoraphobia
(D) Body dysmorphic disorder
(E) Factitious disorder
(F) Malingering
(G) Dissociative fugue
(H) Dissociative identity disorder
(I) Social phobia

Question 348

A woman has a fight with her boyfriend, then soon after is unable to move her arm.

(A) Somatization disorder
(B) Conversion disorder
(C) Agoraphobia
(D) Body dysmorphic disorder
(E) Factitious disorder
(F) Malingering
(G) Dissociative fugue
(H) Dissociative identity disorder
(I) Social phobia

Question 349

Patients with this condition often desire cosmetic plastic surgery.

(A) Somatization disorder
(B) Conversion disorder
(C) Agoraphobia
(D) Body dysmorphic disorder
(E) Factitious disorder
(F) Malingering
(G) Dissociative fugue
(H) Dissociative identity disorder
(I) Social phobia

Question 350

The appearance of the angle of the mouth/lips shown in the figure below is associated with a deficiency of which substance?

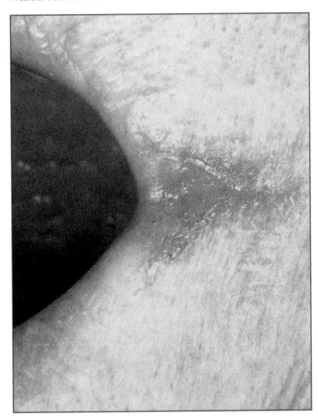

(A) Vitamin D
(B) Thiamine
(C) Riboflavin
(D) Calcium
(E) Magnesium

BLOCK 7 ANSWER KEY

301. D	311. B	321. B	331. E	341. H
302. C	312. C	322. B	332. A	342. A
303. D	313. D	323. A	333. A	343. B
304. B	314. A	324. A	334. E	344. G
305. A	315. A	325. C	335. E	345. H
306. B	316. A	326. C	336. A	346. E
307. A	317. E	327. A	337. D	347. A
308. A	318. A	328. D	338. A	348. B
309. D	319. B	329. C	339. C	349. D
310. A	320. D	330. B	340. D	350. C

Refer to Answers and Explanations Section for Block 7

Pages 258–265

Figure credits

Question 305: Seelig CB: Simplified EKG Analysis. Philadelphia, Hanley & Belfus, 1992.

Question 306: Hoffbrand AV, Pettit JE: Hypochromic anaemias and iron overload. In Hoffbrand AV, Pettit JE (eds): Color Atlas of Clinical Hematology, 3rd ed. St. Louis, Mosby, 2000, pp. 41–56.

Question 350: Hoffbrand AV, Pettit JE: Megaloblastic anaemias. In Hoffbrand AV, Pettit JE (eds): Color Atlas of Clinical Hematology, 3rd ed. St. Louis, Mosby, 2000, pp 57–70.

50 QUESTIONS

**TIME ALLOWED:
60 MINUTES**

Question 351

Which of the following is **least** consistent with Marfan's syndrome?

(A) X-linked recessive inheritance
(B) Arachnodactyly
(C) Ectopia lentis
(D) Aortic dissection at an early age
(E) Greater than average height

Question 352

A mother brings in her 5-month-old infant because the infant is bowlegged. The mother is interested in finding out surgical treatment options. Examination reveals minimal bowlegs without other abnormalities. Radiograph shows only a mild bowleg deformity without other bony abnormalities. What is the best therapeutic option for the infant?

(A) Observation
(B) Leg splints
(C) High-dose oral calcium
(D) Open surgical fixation
(E) Cast application

Question 353

Which of the following correctly characterizes a difference between marasmus and kwashiorkor?

(A) Children with kwashiorkor are usually alert and aggressive, whereas children with marasmus are generally apathetic.
(B) Children with kwashiorkor may take in enough calories, whereas children with marasmus always have a deficit in total calories.
(C) Children with kwashiorkor usually have subcutaneous wasting, whereas children with marasmus usually have diffuse edema.
(D) Children with kwashiorkor usually have a normal liver, whereas children with marasmus usually have an enlarged, fatty liver.
(E) Children with kwashiorkor rarely develop anemia, whereas children with marasmus almost always have significant anemia.

Question 354

Which of the following is **least** likely to occur in starvation?

(A) Weight loss
(B) Reduced basal metabolic rate
(C) Amenorrhea in a female
(D) Decreased glucagon levels
(E) Diarrhea

Question 355

Which vitamin deficiency is most likely in a vegan (one who eats no animal products whatsoever)?

(A) Vitamin B_1
(B) Vitamin B_3
(C) Vitamin B_6
(D) Vitamin B_{12}
(E) Vitamin D

Question 356

In which condition is a nontender, palpable gallbladder most likely?

(A) Pancreatic cancer
(B) Chronic cholecystitis
(C) Cholelithiasis
(D) Acute cholecystitis
(E) Cholangitis

Question 357

Which of the following is thought to be the most potent risk factor for pancreatic cancer?

(A) Smoking
(B) Alcohol
(C) Diabetes
(D) White race
(E) Cholelithiasis

Question 358

Which of the following is **least** likely to cause pancreatitis?

(A) Hypocalcemia
(B) Coxsackievirus infection
(C) Dideoxyinosine
(D) Sulfonamides
(E) Familial hypertriglyceridemia

Question 359

Which of the following is **least** likely to cause high amylase levels?

(A) Mumps
(B) Perforated peptic ulcer
(C) Intestinal infarction
(D) Renal failure
(E) Hypoglycemia

Question 360

What is the most likely presenting sign or symptom of renal cell carcinoma?

(A) Hematuria
(B) Palpable flank mass
(C) Cough secondary to lung metastasis
(D) Hypertension
(E) Renal failure

Question 361

Which of the following is **least** likely to increase the risk of transitional cell carcinoma of the bladder?

(A) Smoking
(B) Chronic *Schistosoma haematobium* infestation
(C) Long-term exposure to cyclophosphamide
(D) Chronic ingestion of phenacetin
(E) Industrial exposure to aromatic amines

Question 362

Which of the following is **false** regarding priapism?

(A) It may be caused by trazodone.
(B) It may be caused by sickle cell disease.
(C) Prolonged cases (i.e. those that last more than several hours) commonly result in impotence.
(D) Surgical decompression is ineffective and has many complications that preclude its use.
(E) Estrogen therapy sometimes is effective as prophylaxis in individuals with repeated episodes.

Question 363

A 59-year-old woman with four children reports involuntary loss of urine when coughing, sneezing, or lifting. What is the most likely mechanism for the woman's incontinence?

(A) Stress incontinence
(B) Urge incontinence
(C) Overflow incontinence
(D) Neurogenic bladder dysfunction
(E) Psychogenic incontinence

Question 364

A 31-year-old man presents with acute pain in the right testicle. He says the pain came on gradually over the last several hours. The patient denies any history of sexually transmitted disease but admits to being promiscuous. Physical examination reveals a temperature of 100.1°F, a tender right testicle, and mild erythema of the scrotal skin overlying the testicle. The testicular pain is relieved by elevation of the testicle. An ultrasound study reveals increased blood flow into the right testicle. What is likely to be the most effective treatment for the most likely condition?

(A) Immediate surgical exploration and orchiopexy of the affected testicle
(B) Immediate surgical exploration and orchiopexy of both testicles
(C) Unilateral orchiectomy
(D) Doxycycline
(E) Penicillin

Question 365

A 56-year-old woman with schizophrenia and on haloperidol for the last 10 years gradually develops involuntary darting movements of the tongue. She also intermittently and frequently grimaces involuntarily. Which of the following is true of the most likely condition?

(A) Immediately stopping the haloperidol would reverse the condition.
(B) The dose of haloperidol should be increased.
(C) An anticholinergic, such as diphenhydramine or benztropine, would stop the symptoms.
(D) Switching to clozapine would reverse the symptoms promptly.
(E) None of the above

Question 366

A 64-year-old man with a long smoking history is found to have a 2-cm lung nodule on chest radiograph. A CT scan of the chest shows a suspicious-looking lung nodule as well as multiple enlarged mediastinal lymph nodes. A biopsy of the lung nodule reveals a small cell lung carcinoma. What is the best current single therapeutic option in terms of improving survival?

(A) Surgical pneumonectomy of the affected lung
(B) Surgical lobectomy of the affected lobe
(C) Radiation therapy
(D) Chemotherapy
(E) Hormonal therapy with an estrogen-containing compound

Question 367

A 42-year-old obese man complains of excessive day-time sleepiness. He says he sleeps a lot but never feels rested when he wakes up, often feeling more tired after waking up than when he went to bed. He frequently wakes during the night and often has a headache in the morning on waking. He mentions that his wife complains about his snoring, especially after he "goes out drinking with the boys," which he says happens about once a week. Which of the following is **incorrect** regarding the most likely condition?

(A) It places him at a much higher risk of having a car accident.
(B) Obesity increases the risk of this condition.
(C) It has been associated with hypertension and heart disease.
(D) The primary treatment is surgical in obese patients.
(E) It may cause depression and memory problems.

Question 368

A 29-year-old black woman presents for a routine checkup. She has a medical history significant only for asthma during childhood, which she claims to have "outgrown." She does not smoke, drink alcohol, or use drugs. She is sexually active and has not seen a physician in 6 years. She is 4, feet 11 inches (150 cm) tall and weighs 247.5 lb (112.5 kg). Physical examination is unremarkable other than obesity. Which of the following is true?

(A) The patient has a body mass index of 50 kg/m^2.
(B) The patient, given her age, has no outstanding health maintenance issues other than anticipatory guidance.
(C) Given her race and sex, the patient's obesity is of little concern at this age.
(D) The patient should be referred promptly for gastric bypass surgery.
(E) The patient should be prescribed a β_2-agonist because people do not "outgrow" asthma.

Question 369

Which of the following scenarios would be considered a coronary disease risk factor when deciding treatment goals for cholesterol-lowering therapy?

(A) A 44-year-old woman on hormone replacement therapy
(B) A male patient with an aunt who had a myocardial infarction at age 42
(C) A female patient who used to smoke but successfully quit a few months ago
(D) A female patient taking a calcium channel blocker for high blood pressure
(E) A male patient whose father died of a myocardial infarction at the age of 62

Question 370

In the United States, which form of acute hepatitis is most likely in an adult who is not sexually active, has never received a blood transfusion, and has never used intravenous drugs?

(A) Hepatitis A
(B) Hepatitis B
(C) Hepatitis C
(D) Hepatitis D
(E) Hepatitis E

Question 371

Which of the following donor-recipient combinations would be **least** likely to produce a transfusion reaction?

	Donor blood type	Recipient blood type
(A)	B–	A–
(B)	A+	AB–
(C)	AB+	B–
(D)	O+	A–
(E)	B–	AB+

Question 372

A 19-year-old woman comes to the office requesting birth control. She says she is not sure which method would be best for her but says that her previous and current boyfriends did not like to use condoms. She has no plans of having children "anytime soon" but wants them eventually. She admits to being promiscuous and is not currently looking for a monogamous relationship. Other than "occasional" smoking, drinking, and marijuana use, her health history is unremarkable. Which of the following methods of contraception would be **least** appropriate for her?

(A) Intrauterine device
(B) Birth control pills
(C) Long-acting medroxyprogesterone depot injections
(D) Long-acting levonorgestrel implant
(E) Diaphragm with spermicide

Question 373

A 27-year-old female attorney presents with a chief complaint of severe "cramps" around the time of menstruation each month. She describes colicky, midline lower abdominal pain that begins just before her menstrual flow begins and lasts for 2 days "like clockwork" every month. She takes acetaminophen, which she says is not helping. Physical examination, including a full pelvic examination, is unremarkable. Which of the following is the most appropriate empirical therapy for the most likely condition?

(A) A cyclooxygenase inhibitor
(B) A gonadotropin-releasing hormone analogue
(C) A corticosteroid
(D) A synthetic testosterone analogue
(E) A cephalosporin

Question 374

A mother brings in her 7-month-old infant because she is concerned that the baby cries frequently for no apparent reason. You have never seen the infant before because the family has just moved here from another town. The infant last saw a physician 3 months ago for routine vaccinations. The infant, the woman's first, cries at least twice a day, sometimes for 15 minutes at a time. The woman says she tries to soothe the infant, but the infant often continues crying for several minutes. The woman admits that the crying has gotten better since the infant was a newborn. Physical examination is unremarkable, and the infant seems alert and responsive. What is the best way to proceed in the management of the infant?

(A) Perform ultrasound of the abdomen.
(B) Order an MRI of the brain.
(C) Take routine blood tests including complete blood count and chemistries.
(D) Ask the woman if she ever strikes the child.
(E) Give anticipatory guidance and administer routine immunizations.

Question 375

Which demographic group has the highest risk of being involved in a fatal car accident?

(A) Women age 15 to 24
(B) Men age 15 to 24
(C) Men age 35 to 55
(D) Women older than 65
(E) Men older than 65

Question 376

Which of the following is true regarding teen pregnancy?

(A) Approximately 1 in 10 adolescent girls age 15 to 19 years old gets pregnant each year.
(B) Black teens have a similar pregnancy rate compared with white teens but are less likely to have an abortion and so have a higher birth rate.
(C) Pregnancy rates among U.S. teens are lower than in most other developed countries for which data exist.
(D) Roughly 5% to 10% of teenage pregnancies are terminated via an elective abortion.
(E) Roughly 55% of teen pregnancies are intentional.

Question 377

Which of the following is **incorrect** regarding sex, sexually transmitted diseases (STDs), and adolescents?

(A) Approximately half of teen pregnancies occur during the first 6 months of sexual activity.
(B) An intrauterine device offers moderate protection against STDs, although it cannot protect against viral diseases.
(C) Blacks have a higher rate of STDs than whites.
(D) *Chlamydia trachomatis* is the most common bacterial STD.
(E) Sexually active adolescents have a higher incidence of STDs than middle-aged adults.

Question 378

Which of the following is the most widely recommended annual screening procedure in adolescents?

(A) Fasting lipid profile in teens with a positive family history of cardiovascular disease
(B) Prostate examination in black males
(C) Tuberculosis skin test
(D) Complete blood count or hemoglobin and hematocrit levels in males
(E) Gonorrhea and chlamydia cultures in females who are sexually active

Question 379

Which of the following is **incorrect** concerning autistic disorder?

(A) It is more common in males than females.
(B) By definition, onset of symptoms begins before 3 years of age.
(C) Affected children may have stereotypic motor behavior, such as flapping hands or rocking.
(D) Most affected children are mentally retarded.
(E) The congenital rubella syndrome is thought to cause most cases.

Question 380

Which of the following is correct regarding the newborn period?

(A) The infant's umbilical cord should be inspected to ensure that there is only one artery and one vein.
(B) A milky white vaginal discharge in girls often is normal shortly after birth.
(C) Gastroschisis can be recognized because it occurs in the midline, and the herniated sac usually contains liver and bowel.
(D) A heart rate of 56 beats/min is reassuring in a sleeping newborn.
(E) The pupillary light reflex should start to be present roughly 10 to 14 days after birth in a term newborn.

Question 381

Which of the following can cause apnea in a preterm newborn?

(A) Lung disease
(B) Hypoglycemia
(C) Intraventricular hemorrhage
(D) Infection
(E) All of the above

Question 382

A woman gives birth to an infant who is found to have a subarachnoid hemorrhage shortly after birth. Which of the following is **least** likely to cause this scenario?

(A) Prematurity
(B) Very low birth weight
(C) Breech presentation
(D) Fetal-maternal disproportion
(E) Cesarean section

Question 383

Which of the following is **false** concerning the fragile X syndrome?

(A) It is a common cause of diagnosable mental retardation.
(B) The chromosomal defect can be diagnosed in the prenatal period.
(C) The syndrome is due to amplification of a trinucleotide sequence with a threshold effect that determines the condition's severity.
(D) Males are affected more commonly, but carrier females may develop aspects of the syndrome.
(E) Genetic counseling is not needed because almost all individuals with the syndrome are sterile.

Question 384

Which of the following would be **unexpected** in a 27-year-old man going through heroin withdrawal?

(A) Heightened sensitivity to pain
(B) Excessive somnolence and sleep
(C) Diarrhea
(D) Piloerection (*gooseflesh*)
(E) Mydriasis

Question 385

Which of the following statements is **least** true regarding specific personality disorders?

(A) Antisocial persons are generally incapable of charm.
(B) Borderline persons often perform acts of self-mutilation.
(C) Histrionic persons often consider their relationships more intimate than they are.
(D) Narcissistic persons tolerate criticism poorly and may react to it with rage.
(E) Schizoid persons are "loners," preferring solitary activities.

Question 386

A 61-year-old man presents with abdominal pain that began the prior night. He has a history of hypertension, high cholesterol, and benign prostatic hypertrophy. He is a smoker and a "social" drinker, and his medications include terazosin and simvastatin. On examination, the patient is noted to have a heart rate of 104 beats/min and a blood pressure of 162/88 mmHg. Abdominal examination reveals a slightly tender mass in the hypogastrium. Abdominal ultrasound reveals the mass to be a massively distended bladder filled with urine without other bladder abnormality. Bilateral hydronephrosis with normal-appearing kidneys is noted in the study. Laboratory examination reveals a creatinine of 3.1 mg/dL and blood urea nitrogen of 39. The patient relates no history of kidney disease. Which of the following is true?

(A) Terazosin is a good first-line drug for hypertension.
(B) The symptoms likely are due to occult renal disease that has progressed slowly.
(C) The patient most likely has nephrolithiasis.
(D) The patient most likely has acute renal insufficiency secondary to prostatism.
(E) A bladder (Foley) catheter should not be placed until a normal retrograde urethrogram is obtained.

Question 387

A mother comes in worrying that her 1-year-old infant's development may be delayed because the infant seems "slower" than his siblings were at this age. The infant was born at term and has had normal growth and development noted on previous studies, but you have not seen the infant for 3 months. Which of the following would be most reassuring for normal age-appropriate development?

(A) The infant crawls without difficulty.
(B) The infant babbles incoherently frequently.
(C) The infant can build a tower of 2 blocks.
(D) The infant reaches for familiar objects.
(E) The infant can feed himself with a bottle.

Question 388

A mother brings in her 8-month-old daughter for trouble breathing. She says the infant has not had a fever but seems "sleepy." Examination reveals a lethargic, apathetic infant with a respiratory rate of 30/min. Bilateral retinal hemorrhages and a full anterior fontanel are noted on examination. The mouth and pharynx are clear without evidence of inflammation, and the lungs are clear to auscultation. The infant has no evidence of bruises. A CT scan is ordered and reveals a subdural hematoma. Which of the following is **least** appropriate?

(A) Ordering neurosurgical consultation
(B) Calling the local child protective services agency to report suspected child abuse
(C) Ordering a skeletal survey to look for old fractures
(D) Checking oxygenation with pulse oximetry
(E) Ordering lateral neck films to look for a foreign body in the trachea

Question 389

An 18-year-old gravida 1, para 0, woman comes in for a routine prenatal visit at 30 weeks. She complains of mild ankle edema and some heartburn. You hear what sound like normal fetal heart sounds on examination, and the distance from the symphysis pubis to the top of the fundus is roughly 24 cm. Routine urinalysis and vital signs are within normal limits. What should you do next?

(A) Tell the woman she is to remain on strict bed rest for the rest of the pregnancy.
(B) Perform fetal ultrasound.
(C) Give assurance and schedule next routine prenatal visit.
(D) Perform esophagogastroduodenoscopy.
(E) Admit the woman to the hospital for further testing and observation.

Question 390

Which of the following is **not** a sign that suggests a diagnosis of current pregnancy?

(A) Amenorrhea
(B) Chadwick's sign
(C) Hegar's sign
(D) Transverse-appearing cervical os
(E) Linea nigra

Question 391

What is the most common cause of secondary amenorrhea?

(A) Pregnancy
(B) Diabetes mellitus
(C) Anorexia nervosa
(D) Ovarian failure
(E) Chemotherapy

Question 392

A mother brings in her 3-year-old daughter because she has something protruding from her vagina that resembles a "bunch of grapes." What is the most likely diagnosis based on this history?

(A) Choriocarcinoma
(B) Hydatiform mole
(C) Normal physiologic discharge of childhood
(D) Nonspecific vaginitis
(E) Sarcoma botryoides

Question 393

What is the appropriate treatment for an 11-year-old boy who has recently developed secondary sexual characteristics and received a diagnosis of idiopathic precocious puberty from his primary care physician?

(A) No treatment
(B) MRI of the brain to rule out intracranial neoplasm
(C) Administration of gonadotropin-releasing hormone analogue to prevent premature epiphyseal closure
(D) Administration of growth hormone
(E) CT scan of the abdomen to rule out an adrenal neoplasm

Question 394

A 3-year-old boy has a sore throat and nosebleeds. What is the most likely blood dyscrasia?

(A) Acute lymphocytic leukemia
(B) Acute myelocytic leukemia
(C) Chronic lymphocytic leukemia
(D) Chronic myelocytic leukemia
(E) Multiple myeloma
(F) Waldenström's macroglobulinemia
(G) Hairy cell leukemia
(H) Mycosis fungoides
(I) Hodgkin's lymphoma
(J) Polycythemia vera

Question 395

A 62-year-old man has a skin rash that has not responded to multiple treatments. What is the most likely blood dyscrasia?

(A) Acute lymphocytic leukemia
(B) Acute myelocytic leukemia
(C) Chronic lymphocytic leukemia
(D) Chronic myelocytic leukemia
(E) Multiple myeloma
(F) Waldenström's macroglobulinemia
(G) Hairy cell leukemia
(H) Mycosis fungoides
(I) Hodgkin's lymphoma
(J) Polycythemia vera

Question 396

A 65-year-old man complains of painful fingers in the cold weather, and a recent history of worsening headaches and visual disturbances. He has a low-normal hemoglobin level. What is the most likely blood dyscrasia?

(A) Acute lymphocytic leukemia
(B) Acute myelocytic leukemia
(C) Chronic lymphocytic leukemia
(D) Chronic myelocytic leukemia
(E) Multiple myeloma
(F) Waldenström's macroglobulinemia
(G) Hairy cell leukemia
(H) Mycosis fungoides
(I) Hodgkin's lymphoma
(J) Polycythemia vera

Question 397

A 53-year-old woman with worsening back pain and fatigue presents with pneumonia, high serum protein level, and severe renal insufficiency that fails to resolve with rehydration. What is the most likely blood dyscrasia?

(A) Acute lymphocytic leukemia
(B) Acute myelocytic leukemia
(C) Chronic lymphocytic leukemia
(D) Chronic myelocytic leukemia
(E) Multiple myeloma
(F) Waldenström's macroglobulinemia
(G) Hairy cell leukemia
(H) Mycosis fungoides
(I) Hodgkin's lymphoma
(J) Polycythemia vera

Question 398

A 64-year-old man with a white blood cell count of 88,000/µL lives 16 years after refusing any type of treatment. What is the most likely blood dyscrasia?

(A) Acute lymphocytic leukemia
(B) Acute myelocytic leukemia
(C) Chronic lymphocytic leukemia
(D) Chronic myelocytic leukemia
(E) Multiple myeloma
(F) Waldenström's macroglobulinemia
(G) Hairy cell leukemia
(H) Mycosis fungoides
(I) Hodgkin's lymphoma
(J) Polycythemia vera

Question 399

An infant born after 36 weeks gestation to a healthy mother with no pregnancy complications has severe respiratory distress immediately after delivery. Examination demonstrates tachypnea and gurgling, tinkling noises heard in the left hemithorax. The child is intubated, and a chest x-ray is obtained:

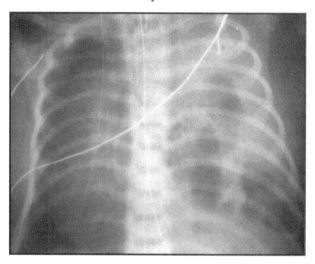

Which of the following is true regarding the most likely diagnosis?

(A) Prognosis is most closely related to pulmonary function
(B) Prognosis is most closely related to the technical success of surgical repair
(C) It more commonly occurs on the right side
(D) Prognosis is most closely related to the underlying chromosomal aneuploidy
(E) A nasogastric tube is contraindicated in this setting

Question 400

A 28-year-old man complains of gradual onset of a painless, nonpruritic rash on his chest and hands over the past several months. Examination reveals confluent, non-palpable areas of depigmentation with the appearance shown below. A scraping for fungi is negative.

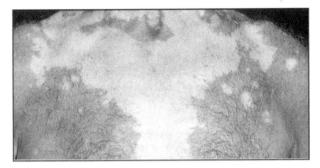

Which of the following is **false** regarding the most likely condition?

(A) A biopsy would likely reveal an absence of melanocytes in affected areas

(B) The patient has an increased risk for other autoimmune disorders

(C) Corticosteroids should be started promptly

(D) The erythrocyte sedimentation rate is likely to be within normal limits

(E) The affected skin is unlikely to return to its normal level of pigmentation in the absence of treatment

BLOCK 8 ANSWER KEY

351. A	361. B	371. E	381. E	391. A
352. A	362. D	372. A	382. E	392. E
353. B	363. A	373. A	383. E	393. A
354. D	364. D	374. E	384. B	394. A
355. D	365. E	375. B	385. A	395. H
356. A	366. D	376. A	386. D	396. F
357. A	367. D	377. B	387. C	397. E
358. A	368. A	378. E	388. E	398. C
359. E	369. D	379. E	389. B	399. A
360. A	370. A	380. B	390. D	400. C

Refer to Answers and Explanations Section for Block 8

Pages 267–276

Figure credits

Question 399: Katz DS, Math KR, Groskin SA (eds): Radiology Secrets. Philadelphia, Hanley & Belfus, 1998, p 381.

Question 400: Hoffbrand AV, Pettit JE: Megaloblastic anaemias. In Hoffbrand AV, Pettit JE (eds): Color Atlas of Clinical Hematology, 3rd ed. St. Louis, Mosby, 2000, pp 57-70.

50 QUESTIONS

**TIME ALLOWED:
60 MINUTES**

Question 401

Which of the following is true regarding drowning and near-drowning?

(A) Infants less than 1 year old commonly drown in a bathtub.
(B) Children age 2 to 6 are most likely to drown in a swimming pool.
(C) At least half of drowning accidents in adolescents and adults are related to alcohol consumption.
(D) Given a similar duration of submersion, cold-water submersion is associated with a higher likelihood of survival than warm-water submersion.
(E) All of the above
(F) None of the above

Question 402

Which of the following is true regarding an acutely psychotic and violent patient?

(A) An antipsychotic should not be given at the same time as a sedative.
(B) Pupillary miosis suggests possible cocaine intoxication.
(C) Violent behavior makes mania extremely unlikely.
(D) Restraints are indicated if the well-being of the staff is at risk.
(E) Diphenhydramine should be avoided in young men given antipsychotic medication because of the risk of hyperpyrexia.

Question 403

Which of the following descriptions of the multiaxial system used in psychiatry is **incorrect**?

(A) Axis I: clinical psychiatric syndromes
(B) Axis II: developmental disorders and personality disorders
(C) Axis III: nonpsychiatric medical conditions, whether related or not
(D) Axis IV: current or recent psychosocial stressors, given as a number value between 1 and 6, with 6 representing the highest stress level
(E) Axis V: global assessment of current functioning, given as a number value between 1 and 5, with 5 representing the highest level

Question 404

Which of the following is a correct example of an ego defense mechanism?

(A) Projection—A man with strong homosexual impulses believes most of his colleagues are homosexual.
(B) Sublimation—A woman claims all people can be only either good or bad.
(C) Intellectualization—A former drug addict becomes a drug counselor.
(D) Dissociation—A person who cheats on tests claims he has to cheat because the tests are unfairly written.
(E) Denial—A man diagnosed with lung cancer begins to act childish and asks the staff to help him with activities he is capable of performing himself.

Question 405

Which of the following statements regarding preventive medicine is correct?

(A) An example of primary prevention is screening of asymptomatic men for prostate cancer with an annual digital rectal examination.
(B) An antismoking campaign is an example of secondary prevention.
(C) A subsidized work and supervised independent-living program for schizophrenics is an example of tertiary prevention.
(D) All of the above
(E) None of the above

Question 406

Which of the following is true regarding behavioral conditioning?

(A) A fixed schedule of reinforcement is more likely to produce behavior that resists extinction than a variable schedule of reinforcement.
(B) Positive and negative reinforcement can be equally effective in producing desired behavior.
(C) Shaping occurs when a person performs a behavior to avoid a noxious stimuli.
(D) If the stimulus and reward or punishment are separated by a longer time period, the response often is learned more quickly.
(E) Scolding a child immediately after an undesirable behavior ensures that the child performs the undesired activity less frequently.

Question 407

A 65-year-old man presents with subacute onset of confusion and is found to have a positive rapid plasmin reagin (RPR) syphilis test. The man's wife thinks he may have had a sexually transmitted disease while in the army 40 years ago but does not know if he was treated for it. The man has not been sexually active for 3 years, according to his wife. Which of the following is true?

(A) A more specific serologic test for syphilis is not needed in this setting.

(B) Treatment for syphilis often causes the RPR test to become negative.

(C) A Venereal Disease Research Laboratory (VDRL) test for syphilis can be used to confirm the diagnosis of syphilis.

(D) The man needs a urethral swab to check for spirochetes.

(E) None of the above

Question 408

Which of the following is **incorrect** regarding therapy for hyperlipidemia?

(A) Niacin usually is effective at raising high-density lipoproteins but often is poorly tolerated.

(B) Liver function tests must be monitored when simvastatin is used.

(C) Cholestyramine works at least partly by binding bile acids in the gut.

(D) Gemfibrozil is a useful agent to reduce low-density lipoproteins.

(E) None of the above

Question 409

A 31-year-old gravida 1, para 0, woman is 23 weeks pregnant. An ultrasound was done secondary to maternal concern over the status of the pregnancy. The otherwise normal-appearing fetus is noted to be in a breech presentation. Which of the following is **least** correct?

(A) The fetus probably will change spontaneously to a vertex presentation before delivery.

(B) Congenital anomalies have an increased incidence in fetuses with a persistent breech presentation.

(C) The incidence of breech presentation at delivery is inversely proportional to the length of gestation.

(D) In a frank breech, the thighs are flexed while the knees are extended, causing the feet to be close to the head.

(E) Complete breech is the most common type of malpresentation and often can be delivered vaginally.

Question 410

Which of the following is true regarding uterine fibroids?

(A) They can cause menorrhagia and dysmenorrhea.

(B) They often grow rapidly once menopause occurs.

(C) Fibroids have no malignant potential but can cause serious symptoms secondary to local effects.

(D) They are an uncommon indication for a cesarean section.

(E) Gonadotropin-releasing hormone analogues often cause a paradoxic enlargement of fibroids and should not be used.

Question 411

The incidence of which of the following conditions becomes more common after menopause?

(A) Fibroid tumors

(B) Adenomyosis

(C) Endometriosis

(D) Pelvic relaxation

(E) Corpus luteum cysts

Question 412

A 24-year-old gravida 1, para 1, woman is 4 days postpartum, having delivered a healthy infant, and comes to the office complaining of emotional lability and trouble concentrating. A physical examination is unremarkable. What is the most likely cause of these symptoms?

(A) Postpartum blues

(B) Postpartum depression

(C) Postpartum psychosis

(D) Endomyometritis

(E) None of the above

Question 413

A 48-year-old man is brought to the emergency department unconscious with extremely labored breathing. The patient's identity is unknown and no known family members are available. You are unaware of any advanced directives or living wills and believe that the patient requires urgent intubation and mechanical ventilation. One of the staff is worried about getting sued for giving treatment to someone who potentially does not want it. Which of the following is true?

(A) You should treat the patient as you see fit.
(B) You should call the courts to give you permission to treat the patient.
(C) You should give only supportive care (i.e., fluids and nutrition).
(D) You should call an emergency meeting of the hospital's ethics committee to help you make a decision.
(E) You should withhold treatment until a family member can be located.

Question 414

A bluish discoloration of the flanks resulting from retroperitoneal hemorrhage

(A) Beck's triad   (K) Kehr's sign
(B) Charcot's triad   (L) Courvoisier's sign
(C) Brudzinski's sign   (M) Murphy's sign
(D) Homan's sign   (N) Prehn's sign
(E) Leriche's syndrome   (O) Grey Turner's sign
(F) Rovsing's sign   (P) Trousseau's syndrome
(G) Trousseau's sign   (Q) Barlow's sign
(H) Ortolani's sign   (R) Chvostek's sign
(I) Tinel's sign   (S) None of the above
(J) Cullen's sign

Question 415

Buttock claudication and atrophy secondary to aortoiliac occlusive disease

(A) Beck's triad   (K) Kehr's sign
(B) Charcot's triad   (L) Courvoisier's sign
(C) Brudzinski's sign   (M) Murphy's sign
(D) Homan's sign   (N) Prehn's sign
(E) Leriche's syndrome   (O) Grey Turner's sign
(F) Rovsing's sign   (P) Trousseau's syndrome
(G) Trousseau's sign   (Q) Barlow's sign
(H) Ortolani's sign   (R) Chvostek's sign
(I) Tinel's sign   (S) None of the above
(J) Cullen's sign

Question 416

The sign of appendicitis elicited by deep palpation in the right lower quadrant

(A) Beck's triad   (K) Kehr's sign
(B) Charcot's triad   (L) Courvoisier's sign
(C) Brudzinski's sign   (M) Murphy's sign
(D) Homan's sign   (N) Prehn's sign
(E) Leriche's syndrome   (O) Grey Turner's sign
(F) Rovsing's sign   (P) Trousseau's syndrome
(G) Trousseau's sign   (Q) Barlow's sign
(H) Ortolani's sign   (R) Chvostek's sign
(I) Tinel's sign   (S) None of the above
(J) Cullen's sign

Question 417

Forced dorsiflexion of the foot causing calf pain in the setting of a deep venous thrombosis

(A) Beck's triad   (K) Kehr's sign
(B) Charcot's triad   (L) Courvoisier's sign
(C) Brudzinski's sign   (M) Murphy's sign
(D) Homan's sign   (N) Prehn's sign
(E) Leriche's syndrome   (O) Grey Turner's sign
(F) Rovsing's sign   (P) Trousseau's syndrome
(G) Trousseau's sign   (Q) Barlow's sign
(H) Ortolani's sign   (R) Chvostek's sign
(I) Tinel's sign   (S) None of the above
(J) Cullen's sign

Question 418

Carpopedal spasm provoked in hypocalcemic patient by pumping up a blood pressure cuff or applying a tourniquet

(A) Beck's triad   (K) Kehr's sign
(B) Charcot's triad   (L) Courvoisier's sign
(C) Brudzinski's sign   (M) Murphy's sign
(D) Homan's sign   (N) Prehn's sign
(E) Leriche's syndrome   (O) Grey Turner's sign
(F) Rovsing's sign   (P) Trousseau's syndrome
(G) Trousseau's sign   (Q) Barlow's sign
(H) Ortolani's sign   (R) Chvostek's sign
(I) Tinel's sign   (S) None of the above
(J) Cullen's sign

Question 419

Migratory thrombophlebitis in the setting of a visceral malignancy

(A) Beck's triad
(B) Charcot's triad
(C) Brudzinski's sign
(D) Homan's sign
(E) Leriche's syndrome
(F) Rovsing's sign
(G) Trousseau's sign
(H) Ortolani's sign
(I) Tinel's sign
(J) Cullen's sign
(K) Kehr's sign
(L) Courvoisier's sign
(M) Murphy's sign
(N) Prehn's sign
(O) Grey Turner's sign
(P) Trousseau's syndrome
(Q) Barlow's sign
(R) Chvostek's sign
(S) None of the above

Question 420

The click heard or felt while abducting the hips when a newborn's hips and knees are flexed, which often indicates developmental dysplasia of the hip

(A) Beck's triad
(B) Charcot's triad
(C) Brudzinski's sign
(D) Homan's sign
(E) Leriche's syndrome
(F) Rovsing's sign
(G) Trousseau's sign
(H) Ortolani's sign
(I) Tinel's sign
(J) Cullen's sign
(K) Kehr's sign
(L) Courvoisier's sign
(M) Murphy's sign
(N) Prehn's sign
(O) Grey Turner's sign
(P) Trousseau's syndrome
(Q) Barlow's sign
(R) Chvostek's sign
(S) None of the above

Question 421

Referred left shoulder pain from splenic rupture

(A) Beck's triad
(B) Charcot's triad
(C) Brudzinski's sign
(D) Homan's sign
(E) Leriche's syndrome
(F) Rovsing's sign
(G) Trousseau's sign
(H) Ortolani's sign
(I) Tinel's sign
(J) Cullen's sign
(K) Kehr's sign
(L) Courvoisier's sign
(M) Murphy's sign
(N) Prehn's sign
(O) Grey Turner's sign
(P) Trousseau's syndrome
(Q) Barlow's sign
(R) Chvostek's sign
(S) None of the above

Question 422

Seen in cardiac tamponade

(A) Beck's triad
(B) Charcot's triad
(C) Brudzinski's sign
(D) Homan's sign
(E) Leriche's syndrome
(F) Rovsing's sign
(G) Trousseau's sign
(H) Ortolani's sign
(I) Tinel's sign
(J) Cullen's sign
(K) Kehr's sign
(L) Courvoisier's sign
(M) Murphy's sign
(N) Prehn's sign
(O) Grey Turner's sign
(P) Trousseau's syndrome
(Q) Barlow's sign
(R) Chvostek's sign
(S) None of the above

Question 423

Painful neck flexion with meningitis

(A) Beck's triad
(B) Charcot's triad
(C) Brudzinski's sign
(D) Homan's sign
(E) Leriche's syndrome
(F) Rovsing's sign
(G) Trousseau's sign
(H) Ortolani's sign
(I) Tinel's sign
(J) Cullen's sign
(K) Kehr's sign
(L) Courvoisier's sign
(M) Murphy's sign
(N) Prehn's sign
(O) Grey Turner's sign
(P) Trousseau's syndrome
(Q) Barlow's sign
(R) Chvostek's sign
(S) None of the above

Question 424

A male infant presents with vomiting, poor feeding, and progressive abdominal distention at 3 weeks of age. The parents note that the infant has not passed stool or flatus since birth. Rectal examination reveals absent stool in the vault, and the infant has what feels like stool-filled bowel loops throughout the abdomen. Which of the following is the most likely cause of this presentation?

(A) Duodenal atresia
(B) Anal atresia
(C) Hirschsprung's disease
(D) Strangulated hernia
(E) Necrotizing enterocolitis

Question 425

What is the most likely cause of a pathologic fracture in adults?

(A) Primary bone tumor
(B) Osteoporosis
(C) Paget's disease
(D) Metastatic cancer
(E) Osteomyelitis

Question 426

What is the most likely cause of neonatal conjunctivitis that begins in the first 24 hours of life?

(A) Chemical
(B) *Chlamydia*
(C) Gonorrhea
(D) Allergic
(E) *Streptococcus viridans*

Question 427

Which of the following is **least** consistent with cardiac tamponade in the setting of trauma?

(A) Clear breath sounds
(B) Hypertension
(C) Muffled heart sounds
(D) Penetrating trauma to the left chest
(E) Distended neck veins

Question 428

Which of the following has been associated with prolonged gestation (> 42 weeks)?

(A) Maternal chlamydial pelvic infection
(B) Premature rupture of the membranes
(C) Anencephaly
(D) Multiple gestation
(E) Maternal smoking

Question 429

What method is most often employed to monitor high-risk pregnancies as women approach 40 weeks' gestation?

(A) Serial amniocentesis with amniotic fluid examination
(B) Automatic labor induction at 36 weeks
(C) Biophysical profile once or twice a week
(D) Serial pelvic examinations three times a week
(E) Outpatient fetal heart monitoring

Question 430

A 34-year-old man is brought to the emergency department unconscious. His respiratory rate is 5/min, and he is intubated promptly. There is no evidence of trauma, and the man has multiple scabs on both forearms. He was found on the floor of a known drug house with an empty needle and a piece of thin, rubber tubing on the floor next to him. He has pinpoint pupils. Which of the following is true regarding the drug that most likely caused this man's symptoms?

(A) Administration of naloxone can reverse respiratory depression caused by this drug
(B) It is potentially fatal in withdrawal
(C) Users of this drug have a low risk of HIV because of impotence
(D) Withdrawal symptoms include hypersomnolence and constipation
(E) Violent behavior is typical with intoxication

Question 431

A mother complains that her 6-year-old boy does not want to go to school. She says he has many friends in the neighborhood who come over to play almost daily, and the child denies a problem with the teacher or other children. The child often resorts to complaining of headaches or stomachaches but sometimes flat out refuses to go. The mother claims she and the child otherwise have a good relationship. The boy's father died 4 years ago, but the child's history is otherwise unremarkable. Physical examination reveals no abnormalities. Which of the following is the most likely diagnosis?

(A) Conduct disorder
(B) Oppositional-defiant disorder
(C) Separation anxiety disorder
(D) Child abuse
(E) Attention-deficit hyperactivity disorder

Question 432

An 8-year-old child comes to the office with his mother with a chief complaint of abdominal pain and anorexia. Medical history is significant only for attention-deficit hyperactivity syndrome, for which the child takes dextroamphetamine. Physical examination is within normal limits other than a minimally tender abdomen with deep palpation. Which of the following is true?

(A) Insomnia and growth suppression also may occur.
(B) The child most likely has Henoch-Schönlein purpura.
(C) The child is malingering.
(D) The child most likely has a somatization disorder.
(E) Immediate psychiatric referral is needed.

Question 433

A woman develops what appears to be preeclampsia at 16 weeks' gestation with proteinuria and hypertension. An ultrasound reveals a grainy image that looks almost like a snowstorm with no evidence of a fetus. Which of the following is likely to be true?

(A) The fetus is small for gestational age.
(B) The woman has a teratoma.
(C) The β-human chorionic gonadotropin level is abnormally elevated.
(D) The woman cannot have preeclampsia because she is only in the second trimester.
(E) Fetal heart tones would be markedly tachycardic.

Question 434

Which of the following methods of birth control is considered the most effective in reducing pregnancy rates?

(A) Levonorgestrol subcutaneous implants
(B) Oral contraceptive pills
(C) Condoms
(D) Intrauterine device
(E) Withdrawal method in conjunction with natural family planning (rhythm method)

Question 435

A 48-year-old otherwise healthy gravida 7, para 7, woman comes into the office complaining of gradually worsening urinary incontinence. On examination, a small bulge is noted in the lower anterior vaginal wall. What is the most likely diagnosis?

(A) Rectocele
(B) Enterocele
(C) Ectopic ureterocele
(D) Urethrocele/urethral displacement
(E) Bladder cancer with extension into the vagina

Question 436

A new article is published comparing the efficacy of immediate surgery versus preoperative adjuvant chemotherapy plus surgery in the treatment of colon cancer. The outcome measured is death. The author concludes that immediate surgery is significantly better at improving survival compared with adjuvant chemotherapy plus surgery ($p < 0.05$). What does the p-value mean in this instance?

(A) The study has a low power.
(B) There is less than a 5% chance that the difference in mortality was due to random chance.
(C) The difference in survival between the groups was less than 5%, making both treatments equal in efficacy.
(D) There is a 5% chance of making a type II error.
(E) Surgery improves mortality in colon cancer more than surgery plus chemotherapy.

Question 437

A student compiles data on two medical schools regarding specialty choice after graduation. She decides to group the graduates of the schools into one of two groups: primary care or specialization. What test might help her compare the schools in terms of the number of graduates that go into primary care from each school?

(A) T-test
(B) Paired T-test
(C) Analysis of variance (ANOVA)
(D) Chi-squared test
(E) P-value

Question 438

A 67-year old thin smoker develops rapid onset of areas of skin thickening and increased pigmentation with a velvety feel. The lesions, which are most prominent in the axillae (see figure), are extensive, nonpruritic and painless. The man also relates an unintentional 30 pound weight loss over the last 2 months.

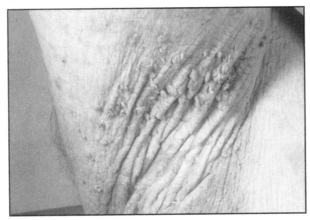

Which of the following is the patient's most likely skin condition?

(A) Acathosis nigricans
(B) Hidradenitis suppurativa
(C) Pemphigus vulgaris
(D) Pemphigoid
(E) Dermatitis herpetiformis

Question 439

A 34-year-old woman presents with a blood-stained right nipple discharge. Ultrasound reveals a subcentimeter, smooth, solid nodule within a dilated major duct close to the nipple that can be appreciated on galactography (a contrast study of the interior of the milk ducts) as a filling defect. Biopsy reveals a papillary lesion within the excised portion of duct with no cellular atypia that has a histologic appearance identical to the figure shown below:

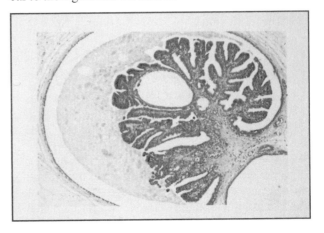

Which of the following is the most likely diagnosis?

(A) Invasive ductal carcinoma
(B) Invasive lobular carcinoma
(C) Intraductal papilloma
(D) Fibroadenoma
(E) Phyllodes tumor

Question 440

Which of the following would be **least** likely as an explanation for large bowel obstruction in an adult?

(A) Neoplasm
(B) Fecal impaction
(C) Sigmoid volvulus
(D) Intussusception
(E) Diverticulitis

Question 441

What is the most common type of hernia in women?

(A) Incisional
(B) Femoral
(C) Direct
(D) Indirect
(E) Strangulated

Question 442

Which of the following is **least** appropriate in the initial management of atrial fibrillation?

(A) Anticoagulation with heparin
(B) Controlling the ventricular rate with digoxin
(C) Controlling the ventricular rate with propranolol
(D) Unsynchronized cardioversion
(E) Chemical cardioversion with amiodarone

Question 443

Which of the following is **least** likely to cause a dilated cardiomyopathy?

(A) Alcohol
(B) Amyloidosis
(C) Coronary artery disease
(D) Myocarditis
(E) Doxorubicin

Question 444

A 14-year-old girl who had her ears pierced 10 days ago presents with bilateral earlobe rashes around the area of the piercings. The rash is well circumscribed, nontender, erythematous, and pruritic and contains several vesicles. Which of the following is most likely to be true?

(A) A type IV hypersensitivity reaction has occured
(B) The child has not been vaccinated against chickenpox
(C) An oral first-generation penicillin should be prescribed
(D) Cultures of an affected area are likely to yield the causative gram positive cocci
(E) The child has asthma

Question 445

Which of the following organisms, if untreated, would be the most likely to cause scarlet fever?

(A) *Corynebacterium diphtheriae*
(B) Group A streptococcus
(C) Epstein-Barr virus
(D) *Staphylococcus epidermidis*
(E) *Streptococcus bovis*

Question 446

A 10-year-old girl is brought into the clinic by her mother secondary to abrupt onset of "smoke"-colored urine and puffy eyes. A urinalysis reveals red blood cell casts and mild proteinuria. The child has hypertension and elevated creatinine. Physical examination is normal except for mild periorbital and ankle edema. Which of the following is most likely true?

(A) The child has a family history of polycystic kidney disease.
(B) The child had a sore throat roughly 1 to 2 weeks ago.
(C) Electron microscopy of a renal biopsy specimen would show loss of podocyte foot processes.
(D) The child has pancreatic insufficiency.
(E) The child's serum is lipemic appearing.

Question 447

A 6-year-old boy is brought in by his mother for a facial rash and fever. The child has bilateral erythematous cheeks, almost looking as if he had been slapped, and a temperature of 99.9° F. The rest of the examination is normal. Which of the following is most likely to be **false** concerning the most likely diagnosis?

(A) The child will develop a maculopapular rash on the torso.
(B) The causative organism can cause transient bone marrow suppression.
(C) Outbreaks of this condition most commonly occur in the spring.
(D) The child needs only supportive measures for treatment.
(E) Oral erythromycin would shorten the duration of symptoms.

Question 448

Which of the following is **least** correct concerning osteosarcoma?

(A) Peak incidence is in individuals older than age 50.
(B) It may be associated with long-standing Paget's disease.
(C) It may be associated with chronic osteomyelitis lesions.
(D) It may produce a "sunburst" appearance in the affected bone.
(E) It is most common in the distal femur and proximal tibia.

Question 449

Which of the following is **not** generally associated with an increased risk of stomach cancer?

(A) Japanese race
(B) Chronic aspirin use
(C) Increasing age
(D) Smoking
(E) *Helicobacter pylori* infection

Question 450

Which of the following tumors is most likely to arise from the adrenal gland?

(A) Wilms' tumor
(B) Paraganglioma
(C) Neuroblastoma
(D) Carcinoid
(E) Nephroblastoma

BLOCK 9 ANSWER KEY

401. E	411. D	421. K	431. C	441. D
402. D	412. A	422. A	432. A	442. D
403. E	413. A	423. C	433. C	443. B
404. A	414. O	424. C	434. A	444. A
405. C	415. E	425. B	435. D	445. B
406. B	416. S	426. A	436. B	446. B
407. B	417. D	427. B	437. D	447. E
408. D	418. G	428. C	438. A	448. A
409. E	419. P	429. C	439. C	449. B
410. A	420. H	430. A	440. D	450. C

Refer to Answers and Explanations Section for Block 9

Pages 277–285

Figure credits

Question 438: du Vivier A: The skin and systemic disease. In du Vivier A: Original Atlas of Clinical Dermatology, 3rd ed. New York, Churchill Livingstone, 2002, pp. 509–561.

Question 439: Stevens A, et al: Breast. In Stevens A, et al (eds): Wheater's Basic Histopathology, 4th ed. New York, Churchill Livingstone, 2002, pp 216–223.

BLOCK 10

50 QUESTIONS

TIME ALLOWED: 60 MINUTES

Question 451

A 16-month-old infant is brought to the emergency department with hypotonia and seizures by a neighbor who was babysitting. A lumbar puncture reveals gram-positive cocci in pairs and a cerebrospinal fluid profile consistent with acute bacterial meningitis. You order antibiotics to be given. The parents arrive in the emergency department and refuse all treatment on religious grounds. They refuse to listen to your arguments and threaten to sue if you treat the child. You feel the child will die without antibiotics. What is the appropriate next step?

(A) Do not treat the child.
(B) Call the staff psychiatrist to evaluate the parents' level of competence.
(C) Ignore the parents and treat the child as you see fit.
(D) Attempt to obtain a court order allowing you to treat the child.
(E) Discharge the child to the parents' care.

Question 452

A woman brings in her 4-year-old son after his second urinary tract infection that was treated with ampicillin 1 week ago by an emergency department physician who recommended follow-up. You have never seen the child before. According to the mother, all immunizations are up to date, and the boy has no other health problems. The woman just moved to the area and agrees to have old records forwarded to your office. The child seems to have normal cognitive development for his age. He is quite active, and height and weight are at the 50th percentile for age. Physical examination is unremarkable. Urinalysis reveals the following:

pH	6.0
Specific gravity	1.010
Protein	Negative
Glucose	Negative
Ketones	Negative
Nitrite	Negative
Leukocyte esterase	Negative
White blood cells	None detected
Red blood cells	None detected
Gram stain	No organisms seen, few epithelial cells

What is the next appropriate step?

(A) Nothing
(B) Follow-up appointment in 6 months for routine health maintenance
(C) CT scan of the abdomen and pelvis
(D) Repeat urinalysis in 2 months
(E) Renal ultrasound and voiding cystourethrogram

Question 453

A 3-week-old boy is brought to the emergency department for vomiting and lethargy. The infant has had nonbilious-appearing vomitus shortly after feedings that has gotten progressively worse over the past week. The child has a palpable olive-shaped mass in the epigastrium without abdominal distention. What is the most likely diagnosis?

(A) Esophageal atresia
(B) Duodenal atresia
(C) Splenic hematoma
(D) Hypertrophic pyloric stenosis
(E) Hirschsprung's disease

Question 454

What is the most likely cause of a bone tumor in an adult?

(A) Metastases
(B) Osteosarcoma
(C) Unicameral bone cyst
(D) Chondroma
(E) Chondrosarcoma

Question 455

Which of the following is true regarding the most common form of glaucoma?

(A) Attacks often are painful.
(B) A surgical procedure is performed promptly once the diagnosis is made.
(C) Affected patients often have an increased cup-to-disk ratio on funduscopy.
(D) An attack may be precipitated by the use of anticholinergic medications.
(E) Patients often describe seeing "halos" around lights or having blurred vision.

Question 456

Which of the following is **inaccurate** regarding conjunctivitis?

(A) Preauricular lymphadenopathy often indicates a viral cause
(B) Allergic conjunctivitis tends to be bilateral
(C) Conjunctivitis often causes a decrease in visual acuity that resolves gradually over weeks
(D) Neonates are at risk for bacterial conjunctivitis acquired from passage through an infected birth canal
(E) Viral conjunctivitis is often highly contagious

Question 457

Which of the following is **least** consistent with an isolated tension pneumothorax?

(A) Decreased breath sounds on the affected side
(B) Dull percussion note on the affected side
(C) Distended neck veins
(D) History of blunt trauma to the chest
(E) Dyspnea

Question 458

Which of the following drugs is considered safe in pregnancy?

(A) Lithium
(B) Warfarin
(C) Heparin
(D) Diphenylhydantoin
(E) Ciprofloxacin

Question 459

A 34-year-old healthy pregnant woman is found to have an elevated serum alpha fetoprotein level at 16 weeks' gestation. What is the next step in the workup?

(A) Repeat test in 1 week
(B) Fetal ultrasound
(C) Amniocentesis
(D) Chorionic villus sampling
(E) Intrauterine fetal transfusion

Question 460

A 42-year-old male immigrant from Southeast Asia presents with productive cough, night sweats and an unintentional 10 pound weight loss. The man is a non-smoker. Chest x-ray reveals a cavitary lesion in the right upper lobe.

What is the next best step in the management of this patient?

(A) Acquire bacterial sputum cultures
(B) PET scan of the chest
(C) Open surgical biopsy
(D) Respiratory isolation
(E) Chemotherapy

Question 461

Which of the following is **not** thought to represent a significant risk factor for suicide?

(A) Age less than 45 years
(B) Substance abuse
(C) Presence of a psychiatric disorder
(D) Male sex
(E) Single marital status

Question 462

A woman brings in her 34-year-old husband because he is "acting crazy." She says that he was completely normal 1 week ago but lost his job the next day and went "bonkers." The woman claims her husband has been talking to imaginary people, has incoherent speech, thinks people are out to get him, and acts "bizarre." Assuming that you confirm this information in an interview and physical examination is within normal limits, what is the diagnosis?

(A) Schizophreniform disorder
(B) Schizophrenia
(C) Schizoid personality
(D) Acute psychotic disorder
(E) Schizoaffective disorder

Question 463

What is the best way to increase the power of a study?

(A) Increase the number of people in the study
(B) Increase the number of variables
(C) Decrease the stratification of the sample groups
(D) Decrease the amount of matching of confounding variables
(E) Decrease the number of people in the study

Question 464

An experimenter tests a new hypertension drug on two groups of 10 people with a double-blind, placebo-controlled trial. He finds that the drug seems to have some effect on blood pressure, but it is insignificant ($p > 0.15$). His recommendation is to discontinue testing the drug because it does not work. If the drug does work, what mistake has the experimenter made?

(A) A type I error
(B) A type II error
(C) Overly stringent p-value criteria
(D) No mistake made
(E) Experimenter bias

Question 465

A 34-year-old woman presents with marked fatigue and blurry vision in the right eye. She also claims that she had a strange tingling sensation in her right leg 4 months ago, which went away after a month, for which she did not seek care. You notice that her speech is mildly dysarthric. On examination, there is mild decreased sensation in the right leg and papillitis on funduscopic examination of the right eye. Visual acuity is 20/20 in the left eye and 20/400 in the right. A brain biopsy stained for myelin reveals the appearance shown below.

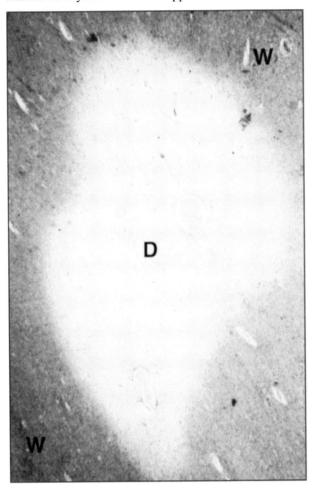

Which of the following is most likely to be true?

(A) The woman has had multiple strokes as a result of embolization of deep venous thrombi
(B) MRI of the brain is likely to be normal
(C) Cerebrospinal fluid examination would reveal increased IgG
(D) A fulminant, progressive course is the norm in this condition
(E) The woman is from an area near the equator

Question 466

A 62-year-old man presents with widespread bullae of various size all over his body, some of which have burst and are now superficial skin erosions that have crusted over. He says that the first "blisters" started in his mouth and were not painful until they ruptured. A few weeks later, the skin eruption started. He takes no medications and has had no unusual environmental exposures. The epidermis is detached easily from the skin. Which of the following is true of the most likely condition?

(A) It is usually seen in children.
(B) A biopsy stained for antibody likely would yield a lace-like immunofluorescence pattern.
(C) The condition is treated with wide-spectrum antibiotics.
(D) The condition is self-limiting and only of cosmetic concern.
(E) Corticosteroids are contraindicated because they often increase the number of lesions and make existing lesions larger.

Question 467

Which of the following is **not** likely to be a cause of chronic sinusitis?

(A) *Streptococcus pneumoniae*
(B) *Moraxella catarrhalis*
(C) Anaerobic bacteria
(D) *Staphylococcus aureus*
(E) Rhinovirus

Question 468

Which of the following bacteria is paired correctly with a reasonable empirical antibiotic choice?

(A) Streptococcal cellulitis—aztreonam
(B) Gonococcal urethritis—trimethoprim/sulfamethoxazole
(C) *Haemophilus* pneumonia—penicillin G
(D) *Borrelia burgdorferi*—doxycycline
(E) *Mycoplasma* pneumonia— piperacillin

Question 469

Which of the following is the most common primary tumor of the liver?

(A) Hepatoma
(B) Hepatocellular carcinoma
(C) Hemangioma
(D) Hepatoblastoma
(E) Cholangiosarcoma

Question 470

A 24-year-old woman with no history of medical problems presents for mild right upper quadrant pain. Her only medication is oral contraceptive pills. An ultrasound reveals a 1-cm, homogeneous, round solid mass lesion adjacent to the liver capsule. Given the hsitory of oral contraceptive use, what is the lesion most likely to be?

(A) Hepatocellular carcinoma
(B) Focal nodular hyperplasia
(C) Hemangioma
(D) Hepatic adenoma
(E) Hepatoblastoma

Question 471

A 41-year-old man is noted to have a hemoglobin of 10 gm/dL and hematocrit of 32% on a routine preoperative screen. What test should you order next?

(A) Sigmoidoscopy plus barium enema
(B) Total colonoscopy
(C) Complete blood count and peripheral smear
(D) Iron, ferritin, and total iron-binding capacity
(E) Folate and vitamin B_{12} levels

Question 472

Which of the following complications is most likely to be a result of uremia?

(A) Hypokalemia
(B) Pericarditis
(C) Increased tendency for clot formation
(D) Increased incidence of autoimmune disease
(E) Metabolic alkalosis

Question 473

A 28-year-old woman with no medical history presents with a nontender but mildly enlarged thyroid gland, elevated thyroid-stimulating hormone level, severe fatigue, bradycardia, menorrhagia, and marked cold intolerance. What is the most likely diagnosis?

(A) Hashimoto's thyroiditis
(B) Subacute thyroiditis
(C) Euthyroid sick syndrome
(D) Plummer's disease
(E) Surreptitious ingestion of thyroxine

Question 474

Which of the following would be **least** likely in the setting of severe liver failure?

(A) Jaundice
(B) Hyperglycemia
(C) Disseminated intravascular coagulation
(D) Encephalopathy
(E) Hypoalbuminemia

Question 475

Which of the following is true of hepatitis A?

(A) It may lead to liver failure and death.
(B) It usually is contracted through sexual contact.
(C) It causes cirrhosis in a significant minority of individuals.
(D) Chronic infection can be treated with interferon.
(E) The enzyme elevation seen with hepatitis A is distinct from other sources of hepatitis.

Question 476

When comparing a purely restrictive lung disease with a purely obstructive lung disease, which of the following is true?

(A) The forced expiratory volume in 1 second (FEV_1) is higher in restrictive disease.
(B) Restrictive disease is a more common cause of respiratory morbidity.
(C) Restrictive disease allows patients to have a higher exercise tolerance.
(D) The prognosis is better with an obstructive disease.
(E) None of the above

Question 477

A 3-day-old infant has dyspnea and tachypnea. On examination, you hear a loud, constant, machinelike murmur in the upper left sternal border and bilateral rales in the lower lung fields. After stabilization, which of the following is the appropriate first step to treat the most likely underlying disorder?

(A) Prostaglandin administration
(B) Indomethacin administration
(C) Propranolol administration
(D) Surgical correction
(E) Phototherapy

Question 478

A 32-year-old woman comes to the office complaining of palpitations. On examination, she has a fixed, split S2 and a mild flow murmur at the upper left sternal border. An electrocardiogram shows a right axis deviation. What is the most likely underlying cardiac disorder?

(A) Mitral valve prolapse
(B) Moderate-to-severe anemia
(C) Ventricular septal defect
(D) Atrial septal defect
(E) Pulmonic stenosis

Question 479

A 72-year-old man presents with the painful rash (shown in figure), which developed over a 2-3 day period.

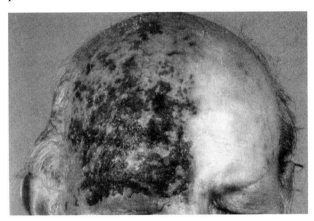

What is the most likely cause?

(A) A sexually transmitted disease
(B) A bacteria acquired from contact with another infected person
(C) A reactivated virus acquired during childhood
(D) A bacteria acquired from contact with an animal
(E) A bacteria acquired from an insect bite

Question 480

A 13-year-old obese boy is brought in by his mother for the sudden onset of right knee pain. The child limps, seeming to want to avoid weight bearing on the right leg. The knee is normal in appearance and has a full range of motion. The range of motion in the hip is limited and painful. The child is afebrile and has a normal leukocyte count. Based on this information, which of the following is the most likely cause of the child's symptoms?

(A) Slipped capital femoral epiphysis
(B) Legg-Calvé-Perthes disease
(C) Osgood-Schlatter disease
(D) Congenital hip dysplasia with subsequent osteoarthritis
(E) Septic arthritis of the hip

Question 481

A gravida 2, para 1, 32-year-old woman presents to the labor and delivery ward in early labor. She has had no prenatal care and mentions a history of hepatitis. A laboratory examination reveals hepatitis B surface antibody negative status and hepatitis B surface antigen positive status. Which of the following is true?

(A) The woman most likely was vaccinated against hepatitis B and does not have chronic hepatitis.
(B) The infant should receive hepatitis B immune globulin after birth.
(C) The infant should be vaccinated against hepatitis B starting at age 6 months.
(D) The woman had hepatitis B in the past, but it has resolved.
(E) The mother should receive hepatitis B immune globulin during labor.

Question 482

Which of the following is true concerning the TORCH syndromes?

(A) An affected child may appear normal at birth.
(B) Rubella is most dangerous when the mother becomes infected in the third trimester.
(C) Herpes is the most common of the TORCH infections.
(D) Cytomegalovirus often is obtained through maternal exposure to cats.
(E) Most TORCH infections cause mental retardation and macrosomia.

Question 483

What is the most likely diagnosis in a 24-year-old woman with a painless, discrete, sharply circumscribed, rubbery, mobile mass on examination of the right breast?

(A) Breast cancer
(B) Fibrocystic disease of the breast
(C) Breast abscess
(D) Fibroadenoma
(E) Fat necrosis of the breast

Question 484

A 36-year-old man comes to the emergency department complaining that people are "out to get him." He subsequently attacks a technician sent to draw his blood for routine laboratory studies. He is placed in four-point restraints and is severely agitated, appearing to react to visual or auditory hallucinations. Old chart review reveals a long history of substance abuse but no other medical or psychiatric history. On examination, the patient seems confused and has vertical and horizontal nystagmus. Which of the following is true regarding the substance that this patient has most likely abused?

(A) Urine acidification may hasten recovery.
(B) The patient needs to be on long-term antipsychotic therapy.
(C) The drug is not fatal in overdose.
(D) It is usually injected intravenously.
(E) Withdrawal may be fatal.

Question 485

Which of the following is true concerning mental retardation?

(A) The most common cause in males is fragile X syndrome.
(B) The number one known cause of preventable mental retardation is neglect.
(C) Most cases are mild and idiopathic.
(D) Klinefelter's syndrome often results in moderate-to-severe mental retardation.
(E) Most affected persons eventually require institutionalization.

Question 486

A 32-year-old man presents to the office complaining of recurrent thoughts of how dirty things are. He says he washes his hands 20 or 30 times a day, and his fear of bacteria is starting to interfere with his ability to do his job as an accountant. He is no longer able to handle money or use public doorknobs without first putting on surgical gloves. He says this problem started about 3 years ago but gradually has gotten worse. Which of the following is most likely to be true?

(A) The patient has obsessive-compulsive personality disorder.
(B) A sedative such as alprazolam is the treatment of choice.
(C) Behavioral therapy would be totally ineffective.
(D) A serotonin-specific reuptake inhibitor is often effective.
(E) The patient requires acute hospitalization and stabilization.

Question 487

A 52-year-old homeless alcoholic presents with high fever; productive cough with thick, reddish sputum; and dehydration. Sputum culture reveals a plump gram-negative rod with a thick capsule and mucoid appearance. Which is the most likely organism?

(A) *Escherichia*
(B) *Shigella*
(C) *Salmonella*
(D) *Klebsiella*
(E) *Pseudomonas*

Question 488

Which of the following conditions markedly increases the risk of developing hepatocellular carcinoma?

(A) Hemochromatosis
(B) Cystic fibrosis
(C) Chronic hepatitis A infection
(D) Industrial exposure to vinyl chloride
(E) Down syndrome

Question 489

Which malignancy has been associated with Epstein-Barr virus infection?

(A) Adenocarcinoma of the colon
(B) Oligodendroglioma
(C) Nasopharyngeal carcinoma
(D) Polycythemia vera
(E) Cervical cancer

Question 490

A 28-year-old woman presents with shortness of breath that has been gradually progressive. Chest radiograph reveals hyperinflation with diffuse bullous changes in the lungs. On lung spirometry, the patient's FEV_1/FEV (forced expiratory volume in 1 second/total forced expiratory volume) ratio is 0.28 (normal is > 0.70). The patient also has AST and ALT values that are twice the upper limit of normal, but a hepatitis panel is negative. She has smoked one-half pack of cigarettes per day for the past 3 years but denies alcohol use. What is the likely cause of this woman's respiratory problems?

(A) Alcoholism
(B) Smoking
(C) α_1-antitrypsin deficiency
(D) Wegener's granulomatosis
(E) Polyarteritis nodosa

Question 491

Which of the following is **not** considered a cyanotic heart disease?

(A) Tetralogy of Fallot
(B) Transposition of the great arteries
(C) Tricuspid atresia
(D) Patent ductus arteriosus
(E) Total anomalous pulmonary venous return

Question 492

What does the acronym *ABCDE* stand for in trauma management?

(A) Airway, breathing, circulation, deep tendon reflex, end-organ damage
(B) Airway, breathing, circulation, delivery, elevation
(C) Airway, breathing, core temperature, disability, early response
(D) Airway, bleeding, circulation, disability, exposure
(E) Airway, breathing, circulation, disability, exposure

Question 493

Which of the following is the most common overall cause of detectable subarachnoid hemorrhage?

(A) Bacterial infection
(B) Head trauma
(C) Viral infection
(D) Neoplasm
(E) Heparin

Question 494

What is the most common cause of postpartum hemorrhage?

(A) Placenta percreta
(B) Uterine atony
(C) Coagulation disorder
(D) Uterine inversion
(E) Vasa previa

Question 495

Which of the following is **not** considered likely to indicate rupture of the membranes (amniotic sac) in a pregnant patient?

(A) Pooling of amniotic fluid on speculum examination
(B) A woman telling you her water broke
(C) A positive Betke-Kleihauer test
(D) A ferning pattern when fluid collected during a sterile speculum examination is placed on a slide and allowed to dry
(E) A positive nitrazine test

Question 496

Select the four best vitamin or mineral supplements for a 16–year-old girl with cystic fibrosis.

(A) Vitamin A
(B) Vitamin B_1
(C) Vitamin B_2
(D) Vitamin B_6
(E) Vitamin B_{12}
(F) Vitamin C
(G) Vitamin D
(H) Vitamin E
(I) Vitamin K
(J) Iron
(K) Calcium
(L) Magnesium
(M) Folate
(N) Phosphate
(O) Niacin

Question 497

Select two supplements for a 67-year-old thin woman who smokes and takes a daily multivitamin.

(A) Vitamin A
(B) Vitamin B_1
(C) Vitamin B_2
(D) Vitamin B_6
(E) Vitamin B_{12}
(F) Vitamin C
(G) Vitamin D
(H) Vitamin E
(I) Vitamin K
(J) Iron
(K) Calcium
(L) Magnesium
(M) Folate
(N) Phosphate
(O) Niacin

Queston 498

Select one vitamin or mineral supplement for a sexually active 21-year-old woman who drinks three glasses of milk per day.

(A) Vitamin A
(B) Vitamin B_1
(C) Vitamin B_2
(D) Vitamin B_6
(E) Vitamin B_{12}
(F) Vitamin C
(G) Vitamin D
(H) Vitamin E
(I) Vitamin K
(J) Iron
(K) Calcium
(L) Magnesium
(M) Folate
(N) Phosphate
(O) Niacin

Question 499

Select one vitamin or mineral supplement for a 26-year-old man receiving a 6-month course of isoniazid after being exposed to tuberculosis and developing a positive PPD skin test.

(A) Vitamin A
(B) Vitamin B_1
(C) Vitamin B_2
(D) Vitamin B_6
(E) Vitamin B_{12}
(F) Vitamin C
(G) Vitamin D
(H) Vitamin E

(I) Vitamin K
(J) Iron
(K) Calcium
(L) Magnesium
(M) Folate
(N) Phosphate
(O) Niacin

Question 500

Select one vitamin or mineral supplement for a 48-year-old woman with known alcoholism who presents with confusion and ataxia.

(A) Vitamin A
(B) Vitamin B_1
(C) Vitamin B_2
(D) Vitamin B_6
(E) Vitamin B_{12}
(F) Vitamin C
(G) Vitamin D
(H) Vitamin E

(I) Vitamin K
(J) Iron
(K) Calcium
(L) Magnesium
(M) Folate
(N) Phosphate
(O) Niacin

BLOCK 10 ANSWER KEY

451. D	461. A	471. C	481. B	491. D
452. E	462. D	472. B	482. A	492. E
453. D	463. A	473. A	483. D	493. B
454. A	464. B	474. B	484. A	494. B
455. C	465. C	475. A	485. C	495. C
456. C	466. B	476. E	486. D	496. A, G, H, I
457. B	467. E	477. B	487. D	497. G, K
458. C	468. D	478. D	488. A	498. M
459. B	469. C	479. C	489. C	499. D
460. D	470. D	480. A	490. C	500. B

Refer to Answers and Explanations Section for Block 10

Pages 287–295

Figure credits

Question 465: Stevens A, et al: Nervous system. In Wheater's Basic Histopathology, 4th ed. New York, Churchill Livingstone, 2002, pp 268–283.

Question 479: du Vivier A: The dermatologic diagnosis. In du Vivier A (ed): Atlas of Clinical Dermatology, 3rd ed. New York, Churchill Livingstone, 2002, pp 1–21.

BLOCK 11

50 QUESTIONS

TIME ALLOWED: 60 MINUTES

Question 501

A 34-year-old woman with a long history of recurrent abdominal pain gets a plain abdominal radiograph, which reveals bilateral large calculi that fill and distend the renal pelvis and calices. Which of the following is most likely to be true?

(A) The woman has hypercalcemia
(B) The woman has hypocalcemia
(C) The woman has had recurrent *Proteus* urinary tract infections
(D) The woman has hyperuricemia and a history of arthritis
(E) The woman has factitious disorder

Question 502

A 62-year-old woman with a long history of smoking and leg "heaviness" presents with a painless lesion on the lateral aspect of her ankle and lower leg, which has developed over the past several months:

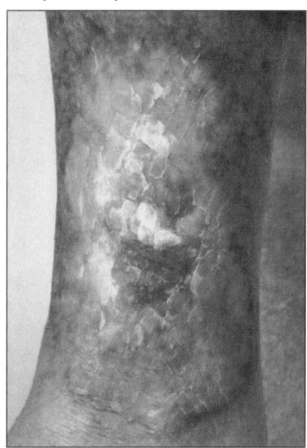

What is the most likely cause of this appearance?

(A) Arterial insufficiency
(B) Venous insufficiency
(C) Peripheral neuropathy
(D) Cardiac embolus traveling into the lower extremity
(E) Fungal infection

Question 503

A 59-year-old woman presents with concern over an area of skin on her left foot. She says a smaller lesion has been on her foot at this location for years, but recently has gotten bigger and started to itch and bleed.

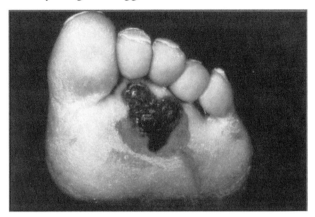

Which of the following is true regarding the most likely diagnosis?

(A) Prognosis is most closely related to the depth of invasion
(B) The fact that the lesion itches makes it more likely to be benign
(C) Surgical excision is contraindicated
(D) Intravenous antibiotic therapy is needed
(E) Local intralesional steroid injection is the treatment of choice

Question 504

Which of the following medications should be avoided in an asthmatic?

(A) Acetaminophen
(B) Penicillin
(C) Captopril
(D) Propranolol
(E) Ranitidine

Question 505

A 56-year-old man presents for an annual physical examination. His chest is wider in the anteroposterior direction than across, and he breathes with pursed lips. On a routine chest radiograph, the patient is noted to have hyperinflation of the lungs. Which of the following is most likely to be the cause of these findings?

(A) The patient had polio as a child.
(B) The patient is a smoker.
(C) The patient has cystic fibrosis.
(D) The patient has alpha-one antitrypsin deficiency.
(E) The patient uses illicit drugs.

Question 506

What congenital heart defect is associated with upper extremity hypertension in the presence of a normal or low blood pressure in the lower extremities?

(A) Patent ductus arteriosus
(B) Transposition of the great vessels
(C) Total anomalous pulmonary venous return
(D) Coarctation of the aorta
(E) Tetralogy of Fallot

Question 507

Which of the following would be expected to improve a symptomatic sinus bradycardia?

(A) Amiodarone
(B) Verapamil
(C) Procainamide
(D) Atropine
(E) Lidocaine

Question 508

A 31-year-old previously healthy woman with no medical history presents with anxiety, insomnia, heat intolerance, and new-onset atrial fibrillation. Which of the following is most likely to be true?

(A) The thyroid-stimulating hormone level is abnormally low
(B) The thyroid-stimulating hormone level is abnormally high
(C) The patient has unexplained weight gain
(D) The patient's symptoms are due to anxiety and panic attacks
(E) The patient's symptoms are due to a type IV hypersensitivity reaction

Question 509

A 42-year-old intravenous drug abuser has the following results from laboratory testing:

Hepatitis A IgM antibody	Negative
Hepatitis B surface IgG antibody	Positive
Hepatitis B surface antigen	Negative
Hepatitis B core IgG antibody	Positive
Hepatitis C antibody	Positive
AST	110 U/L (normal = 7–27)
ALT	112 U/L (normal = 1–21)

Which of the following is most likely to be true?

(A) The patient has chronic hepatitis B
(B) The patient has chronic hepatitis C
(C) The pattern of liver enzyme elevation indicates alcoholic hepatitis
(D) The patient's hepatitis B serology is due to vaccination
(E) The liver enzyme elevation is a laboratory error caused by dehydration

Question 510

Which of the following is true regarding inflammatory bowel disease?

(A) Crohn disease usually involves only the colon
(B) Ulcerative colitis is less likely to cause colon cancer than Crohn disease
(C) Transmural involvement is characteristic of ulcerative colitis
(D) The presence of skip lesions is more characteristic of Crohn disease
(E) Fistulas and abscess are more common with ulcerative colitis

Question 511

A 24-year-old Mediterranean woman is referred to your office because asymptomatic anemia is discovered on a routine complete blood count before elective plastic surgery. Laboratory values are as follows:

Hemoglobin	10 gm/dL
Mean corpuscular volume	78 µm/cell
White blood cell count	7200/µL
Platelets	324,000/µL
Hemoglobin A_2	7% (normal = 1.5–3.5)
Hemoglobin F	3.4% (normal = < 2)
Haptoglobin	140 mg/dL (normal = 40–336)
Coombs' test	Negative

What is the best way to treat this anemia?

(A) One-week course of oral iron therapy
(B) Three to six month course of oral iron therapy
(C) Correction of the underlying inflammatory disorder
(D) Administration of folate
(E) None of the above

Question 512

A 32-year-old woman with a history of gastrointestinal problems has a macrocytic anemia with several hypersegmented neutrophils on peripheral smear. Although otherwise healthy, she has fatigue secondary to the anemia. Physical examination reveals decreased position sense in the lower extremities, mild ataxia, and mild hyperreflexia. Which of the following tests is likely to reveal the cause of the patient's neurologic symptoms?

(A) Colonoscopy
(B) MRI of the brain
(C) Schilling test
(D) Cerebral angiogram
(E) Red blood cell folate level

Question 513

Which of the following is **not** likely to be seen in a nephritic syndrome, such as poststreptococcal glomerulonephritis?

(A) Oliguria
(B) Azotemia
(C) 6 gm of proteinuria per day
(D) Red blood cell casts seen in the urine
(E) Hypertension

Question 514

Which of the following is most likely to be found in the early stages of a nephrotic syndrome, such as minimal change disease?

(A) Lipiduria
(B) Hypertension
(C) Red blood cell casts
(D) Uremia
(E) Encephalopathy

Question 515

What is the preferred method of anesthesia in most obstetric patients who require it?

(A) General anesthesia
(B) Epidural anesthesia
(C) Spinal anesthesia
(D) Caudal anesthesia
(E) Paracervical block

Question 516

Which of the following is **not** a sign of placental separation?

(A) A fresh show of blood from the vagina
(B) Visualization of the uterus at the introitus
(C) Lengthening of the umbilical cord
(D) The fundus rising up
(E) The fundus becoming firm and globular

Question 517

Which of the following is indicated for a cervical chlamydial infection detected during pregnancy?

(A) Delay of treatment until after delivery
(B) Treatment with tetracycline
(C) Treatment with erythromycin
(D) Reconfirmation of the culture in the postpartum period because of a high false-positive rate during pregnancy
(E) Cotreatment for presumed gonorrhea infection

Question 518

A 21-year-old gravida 0, para 0, woman presents to your office because she thinks she has breast cancer. She notes bumps in both breasts that become tender around the time of menstruation. On examination, multiple cystic, tender lesions can be felt in both breasts without a dominant mass. What is the best course of action?

(A) Reassurance and scheduling of a follow-up appointment
(B) MRI of the breasts
(C) Fine-needle biopsy of both breasts
(D) Open breast biopsy of the largest lesion
(E) Mammography

Question 519

A thin 32-year-old woman with recently diagnosed schizophrenia and no other medical problems presents to the office complaining of amenorrhea, bilateral clear breast discharge, and decreased libido. She has been taking haloperidol for the last 3 months and seems coherent and appropriate. What is the most likely diagnosis?

(A) Delusional symptoms secondary to schizophrenia
(B) Malingering
(C) Hyperprolactinemia from haloperidol
(D) Breast cancer
(E) Polycystic ovary syndrome

Question 520

Which person would be **least** likely to develop a gram-negative pneumonia?

(A) A child with cystic fibrosis
(B) A homeless alcoholic
(C) A man with hypertension
(D) A hospitalized patient in the intensive care unit
(E) A woman with several episodes of vomiting while unconscious

Question 521

Which of the following patients does **not** have an indication for the *Streptococcus pneumoniae* vaccine?

(A) A 38-year-old male with HIV
(B) A 56-year-old woman with hypertension, diabetes, and renal insufficiency
(C) A 6-month-old child with sickle cell disease
(D) A healthy 69-year-old woman
(E) None of the above

Question 522

Which of the following conditions represents the most potent risk factor for testicular cancer?

(A) Family history of neoplasm
(B) Personal history of a hydrocele
(C) Personal history of corrected cryptorchidism
(D) Personal history of a varicocele
(E) Personal history of chemotherapy for an unrelated malignancy

Question 523

A 64-year-old male alcoholic presents with a chief complaint of 40-lb weight loss over the last 3 months and food "sticking" in his chest. He has smoked cigarettes for 50 years but has no other medical history. What is the most likely diagnosis?

(A) Barrett's esophagus
(B) Adenocarcinoma of the esophagus
(C) Squamous cell carcinoma of the esophagus
(D) Colon cancer
(E) Achalasia

Question 524

What is the most common location of primary brain tumors in children?

(A) Cerebral hemispheres
(B) Hypothalamus
(C) Rathke's pouch
(D) Posterior fossa
(E) Thalamus

Question 525

Which of the following is true concerning electromyography and nerve conduction studies?

(A) A demyelinating disorder causes increased conduction velocity and amplitude.
(B) A lower motor neuron lesion produces a lack of electric activity when the muscle is at rest.
(C) Repetitive stimulation of nerves often improves muscle contraction amplitude in myasthenia gravis.
(D) Primary muscle disorders usually result in a decreased contraction amplitude.
(E) A normal muscle has a large amount of random electric activity at rest.

Question 526

A 32-year-old woman presents with symmetric weakness in her legs 10 days after having an upper respiratory infection. The weakness came on in both feet and gradually ascended to involve the leg muscles below the knee over the next 24 hours. She denies any sensory changes. Physical examination reveals symmetric, bilateral muscle weakness below the knee with decreased reflexes and intact sensation. Which of the following is true concerning the most likely diagnosis?

(A) The patient needs immediate high-dose corticosteroids.
(B) Plasmapheresis may shorten the duration of symptoms.
(C) Cerebrospinal fluid is likely to show large numbers of lymphocytes and markedly increased pressure.
(D) CT scan or MRI of the brain is likely to show widespread demyelination.
(E) Nerve conduction velocity is likely to be normal.

Question 527

A 42-year-old man on no medications presents with an "itchy" skin rash on his back. He is otherwise in good health and appears to have good hygiene. He has multiple erythematous, oval, scaly patches on the back that appear parallel to the skin cleavage lines. There also are a few patches on the chest. He mentions that it started with one lesion 10 days ago on his left arm and that 1 week later, his whole back broke out. Which of the following is the treatment of choice for the most likely condition?

(A) Reassurance and supportive measures
(B) Excisional biopsy of the lesions
(C) Permethrin cream
(D) Intravenous corticosteroids as an inpatient for 10 days
(E) Oral fluconazole for 10 days

Question 528

A city being studied has a population of 100,000. Using culture as the gold standard test, 5000 people in the city are found to have chlamydial infection. A new DNA probe chlamydial test is positive on 4000 people in the city, of whom only 3000 tested positive by culture. What is the incidence of *Chlamydia* in this city?

(A) 4%
(B) 50/1000
(C) 50/10,000
(D) 5/1000
(E) Cannot be calculated from the information given

Question 529

A scientist decides to examine the risk of smoking in developing pancreatic cancer. He finds 100 cases of smokers who died and 200 cases of nonsmokers who died. By reviewing the hospital charts and autopsy records, the scientist determines the number of people in each group who died of pancreatic cancer. The cases are matched carefully so that there are no inequalities in terms of age, sex, or other demographics or habits. The scientist finds that four people in the smoking group died of pancreatic cancer versus two people in the nonsmoking group. Using the scientist's data, what is the relative risk of pancreatic cancer in smokers compared with nonsmokers?

(A) 1.5
(B) 2
(C) 3
(D) 4
(E) Cannot be calculated from the information given

Question 530

A teacher contacts you because she is worried about a student in her seventh-grade class. The child often comes into class after lunch seeming euphoric and unsteady on his feet, and seems to have a heightened sense of power and mildly slurred speech. She says the child is normal in the mornings and usually is back to normal within an hour after lunch. She does not note any symptoms of withdrawal (e.g., irritability, excessive fatigue) by the end of the day. Which of the following is the child likely to be abusing?

(A) LSD
(B) Cocaine
(C) Heroin
(D) Marijuana
(E) Inhalants

Question 531

A woman comes to the office because she is concerned about her 32-year-old husband, who occasionally wears her underwear under his normal male clothing. He does this only occasionally and in private, and she claims they have a normal sex life. He told her he does it because it makes him "feel sexy." It does not bother her husband, who is a successful stockbroker, but the woman is disturbed by it. Which of the following best describes the man's behavior?

(A) Homosexuality
(B) Fetishism
(C) Transsexual
(D) Transvestite
(E) Normal variant

Question 532

A 34-year-old woman comes to the office with a complaint of feeling anxious. What is the best initial question to ask the woman?

(A) "Does this condition run in your family?"
(B) "Could you tell me more about it?"
(C) "Do you have difficulty sleeping?"
(D) "What medications are you currently taking?"
(E) "Are you experiencing depression?"

Question 533

Which of the following substances is **not** a well-established teratogen?

(A) Isotretinoin
(B) Alcohol
(C) Cocaine
(D) LSD
(E) Trimethadione

Question 534

Which of the following is **false** concerning group B streptococcus in relation to pregnancy?

(A) It is a common cause of neonatal sepsis.
(B) It is a common cause of chorioamnionitis.
(C) It is a gram-positive cocci.
(D) Mothers with a positive culture for the organism should be treated during labor with amoxicillin.
(E) Its presence in the female genital tract indicates a maternal infection.

Question 535

Which of the following is true concerning pregnant HIV-positive mothers?

(A) It is okay for them to breast-feed.
(B) Transmission of the virus to the infant is unlikely.
(C) Antiretroviral medications should not be used in pregnant women.
(D) They should be screened for other sexually transmitted diseases even if asymptomatic.
(E) A positive ELISA HIV test in a neonate confirms maternal-fetal transmission of HIV.

Question 536

An otherwise healthy 50-year-old woman presents to the office complaining of irregular menstrual periods, hot flashes, and unpredictable mood swings. Which of the following is most likely to be true?

(A) She has uterine cancer.
(B) Her irregular menstrual periods are pathologic.
(C) Her follicle-stimulating hormone level is elevated.
(D) She has major depression.
(E) She has cervical cancer.

Question 537

A 14-year-old girl comes to the office complaining of amenorrhea. She says her first period was at the age of 11 and that they are normally regular. What should you do next to work up the amenorrhea?

(A) Order a urine human chorionic gonadotropin test.
(B) Administer progesterone.
(C) Order serum follicle-stimulating hormone and luteinizing hormone levels.
(D) Order a serum prolactin level.
(E) Order a serum thyroid-stimulating hormone.

Question 538

What is the preferred treatment for proliferative diabetic retinopathy?

(A) Laser burns applied to the entire periphery of the retina
(B) Focal laser burns to the involved area
(C) Intraocular methotrexate
(D) Reduction of insulin dose
(E) Vitrectomy

Question 539

Which of the following is the most likely cause of acquired legal blindness in an African-American adult?

(A) Glaucoma
(B) Type I diabetes
(C) Exudative ("wet") macular degeneration
(D) Trauma
(E) Retinal detachment

Question 540

Which of the following is **least** likely to cause death in the acute setting if treatment is delayed?

(A) Cardiac tamponade
(B) Pneumothorax
(C) Airway obstruction
(D) Epidural hematoma
(E) Aortic laceration

Question 541

Which of the following is true concerning abdominal trauma?

(A) With any gunshot wound to the abdomen, proceed directly to non-contrast abdominal CT.
(B) With any knife wound to the abdomen, proceed directly to non-contrast abdominal CT.
(C) With blunt abdominal trauma, if the patient is stable, abdominal angiography is preferred before surgery.
(D) If the patient with a normal physical examination is stable after blunt abdominal trauma, careful observation alone may be indicated.
(E) After blunt trauma, the combination of abdominal pain, hypotension, and left shoulder pain usually means a ruptured gallbladder.

Question 542

Which of the following is more consistent with a diagnosis of omphalocele than with gastroschisis in a newborn?

(A) Chromosomal aneuploidy
(B) There is no true hernia sac or membrane
(C) The umbilical ring is present
(D) There are no other anomalies
(E) The defect is to the right of midline

Question 543

A male newborn has respiratory distress after delivery, and when you listen to the chest, you hear what sounds like bowel sounds in the left thorax. Which of the following is the most likely condition?

(A) A Bochdalek-type diaphragmatic hernia
(B) Birth trauma
(C) A Morgagni-type diaphragmatic hernia
(D) A sliding-type hiatal hernia
(E) A paraesophageal hiatal hernia

Question 544

A previously healthy 11-month-old infant presents with bilious vomiting, maroon stools mixed with mucus, and a palpable sausage-shaped mass in the abdomen. What is the likely diagnosis?

(A) Intussusception
(B) Pyloric stenosis
(C) Intestinal atresia
(D) Meconium ileus
(E) Necrotizing enterocolitis

Question 545

Pain in the anatomic snuff-box after a fall on an outstretched hand likely represents fracture of which of the carpal bones?

(A) Hamate bone
(B) Triquetral bone
(C) Scaphoid bone
(D) Pisiform bone
(E) Lunate bone

Question 546

This substance has been shown to be teratogenic.

(A) Vitamin A
(B) Vitamin B_1
(C) Vitamin B_2
(D) Vitamin B_6
(E) Vitamin B_{12}
(F) Vitamin C
(G) Vitamin D
(H) Vitamin E
(I) Vitamin K
(J) Iron
(K) Calcium
(L) Magnesium
(M) Folate
(N) Phosphate
(O) Niacin

Question 547

A 57-year-old man presents with dementia, dermatitis, diarrhea, and stomatitis. Deficiency of which substance is most likely?

(A) Vitamin A
(B) Vitamin B_1
(C) Vitamin B_2
(D) Vitamin B_6
(E) Vitamin B_{12}
(F) Vitamin C
(G) Vitamin D
(H) Vitamin E
(I) Vitamin K
(J) Iron
(K) Calcium
(L) Magnesium
(M) Folate
(N) Phosphate
(O) Niacin

Question 548

A 42-year-old thin man with liver disease presents with new-onset diabetes and impotence. Derangement in which substance is most likely?

(A) Vitamin A
(B) Vitamin B_1
(C) Vitamin B_2
(D) Vitamin B_6
(E) Vitamin B_{12}
(F) Vitamin C
(G) Vitamin D
(H) Vitamin E
(I) Vitamin K
(J) Iron
(K) Calcium
(L) Magnesium
(M) Folate
(N) Phosphate
(O) Niacin

Question 549

A 47-year-old woman presents with difficulty seeing at night and scaly, dry skin. Deficiency of what substance is likely responsible?

(A) Vitamin A
(B) Vitamin B_1
(C) Vitamin B_2
(D) Vitamin B_6
(E) Vitamin B_{12}
(F) Vitamin C
(G) Vitamin D
(H) Vitamin E
(I) Vitamin K
(J) Iron
(K) Calcium
(L) Magnesium
(M) Folate
(N) Phosphate
(O) Niacin

Question 550

Acute elevation in pregnant women is often iatrogenic and may cause respiratory depression.

(A) Vitamin A
(B) Vitamin B_1
(C) Vitamin B_2
(D) Vitamin B_6
(E) Vitamin B_{12}
(F) Vitamin C
(G) Vitamin D
(H) Vitamin E

(I) Vitamin K
(J) Iron
(K) Calcium
(L) Magnesium
(M) Folate
(N) Phosphate
(O) Niacin

BLOCK 11 ANSWER KEY

501. C	511. E	521. E	531. E	541. D
502. B	512. C	522. C	532. B	542. A
503. A	513. C	523. C	533. D	543. A
504. D	514. A	524. D	534. E	544. A
505. B	515. B	525. D	535. D	545. C
506. D	516. B	526. B	536. C	546. A
507. D	517. C	527. A	537. A	547. O
508. A	518. A	528. E	538. A	548. J
509. B	519. C	529. E	539. A	549. A
510. D	520. C	530. E	540. B	550. L

Refer to Answers and Explanations Section for Block 11

Pages 297–305

Figure credits

Question 502: du Vivier A: Skin manifestations of disordered circulation. In du Vivier A (ed): Atlas of Clinical Dermatology, 3rd ed. New York, Churchill Livingstone, 2002, pp 563–577.

Question 503: du Vivier A: Collagen vascular disorders. In du Vivier A (ed): Atlas of Clinical Dermatology, 3rd ed. New York, Churchill Livingstone, 2002, pp. 201–228.

BLOCK 12

50 QUESTIONS

TIME ALLOWED:
60 MINUTES

Question 551

A 31-year-old woman who is 40 weeks' pregnant requires a cesarean section for failure to progress. She has made it clear to you that she is not to receive blood products under any circumstances because of religious concerns. You discuss the risks of hemorrhage and death, and she still refuses blood products but agrees to proceed with the surgery. During the cesarean section, the infant is delivered but acute, difficult to control hemorrhage develops. In your estimation, the woman requires a blood transfusion to survive. What is the appropriate next step?

(A) Call the woman's husband for permission to give blood products.
(B) Get permission from the courts to give blood products.
(C) Treat the patient as best as you can without giving blood products.
(D) Give the blood transfusion in the interest of saving the patient's life, and explain to the patient after the procedure why it was necessary.
(E) Give the blood transfusion but do not tell the patient.

Question 552

A 13-month-old girl is brought in by her father for a scheduled vaccination. The infant is healthy and has no significant medical history. She was formula fed until age 6 months, when solid foods were introduced gradually and well tolerated. The father is a dentist whom you know socially and is a concerned parent. The family lives in a prestigious old building that was built in the early 1900s. On examination, there are no abnormalities, and the child seems to be at a level of development appropriate for her age. Which of the following should be done at this time?

(A) Screening lead level
(B) Tuberculosis screening with a skin test
(C) Fluoride supplementation
(D) Screening for sickle cell disease
(E) Vitamin D supplementation

Question 553

A mother brings in her 5-year-old child for obesity. She is concerned that the child may have a disease causing the excessive weight. The child has not had any health problems and vaccinations are up-to-date. The child is not taking any medications. Family history is remarkable for hypertension, diabetes, and obesity. On examination, the child appears to be happy and at a developmental level appropriate for her age. Physical examination and vital signs are unremarkable. When compared with a standard national chart, the child's height is at the 45th percentile weight is at the 95th percentile. Laboratory tests reveal the following:

Hemoglobin	12 gm/dL (normal = 10.5–14)
Mean corpuscular volume	87 µm/cell
Sodium	137 mEq/L
Potassium	3.9 mEq/L
Chloride	102 mEq/L
CO_2 26 mEq/L	
BUN	8 mg/dL
Creatinine	0.8 mg/dL
Glucose	108 mg/dL (normal fasting = 70–110)

What is the most likely cause for the child's obesity?

(A) Cushing's syndrome
(B) Excessive growth hormone
(C) Diabetes mellitus
(D) Excessive caloric intake
(E) Hypothyroidism

Question 554

A 6-month-old infant is brought in by his mother because she thinks he might be "slow." The infant has no previous medical problems, and his vaccinations are up-to-date. His vital signs are within normal limits, and a physical examination is within normal limits. The infant, while prone, can lift his head up 90°, can roll front to back, can perform a voluntary grasp without voluntary release, can sit without support for several seconds, and frequently babbles unintelligibly. The infant does not understand one-step commands, is not able to say any words, and does not play pat-a-cake when prompted and shown how. What is the approximate developmental age of the infant?

(A) 1 month
(B) 2 months
(C) 4 months
(D) 6 months
(E) 12 months

Question 555

Which of the following is **false** regarding compartment syndrome?

(A) Patients often have pain with passive movement
(B) Compartment syndrome may occur after a technically successful revascularization procedure
(C) Paralysis is a late finding
(D) Absent pulses distal to the site of the affected muscle compartment is an early finding
(E) Treatment usually involves fasciotomy

Question 556

Which of the following is the most likely cause of an isolated oculomotor palsy with a normal and reactive pupil on the affected side in a 57-year-old man with hypertension and diabetes who has no other complaints or findings on physical examination?

(A) Microvascular complications of diabetes, hypertension, or both
(B) Stroke
(C) Brain tumor
(D) Cerebral aneurysm causing compression of the oculomotor nerve
(E) Exotropia

Question 557

What is the most likely cause of a visual field deficit in which the patient has lost vision in the lateral half of the visual field in both eyes?

(A) Lesion involving the temporal lobe
(B) Lesion involving the parietal lobe
(C) Pituitary tumor
(D) Bilateral optic neuritis
(E) Lesion involving the occipital lobe

Question 558

After severe trauma, a patient is found to have a large pleural effusion that turns out to be 1.5 L of blood with chest tube insertion. The bleeding is moderate but steady 4 hours later. The patient is receiving intravenous fluids and has received 2 units of blood. What is the next step in the management of this patient?

(A) Pleurodesis
(B) Repeat chest radiograph
(C) Thoracotomy
(D) Abdominal CT scan
(E) Transfuse 2 more units of blood

Question 559

Which of the following increases the risk of uterine atony?

(A) Mother between the ages of 20 and 30
(B) Prolonged use of oxytocin
(C) Oligohydramnios
(D) Term delivery
(E) Maternal obesity

Question 560

In which of the following scenarios should a pregnant woman receive Rh immune globulin (RhoGAM)?

(A) Mother Rh positive, father Rh negative, fetus Rh unknown
(B) Mother Rh negative, father Rh positive, fetus Rh unknown, Rh antibodies negative
(C) Mother Rh negative, father Rh positive, fetus Rh unknown, Rh antibodies positive
(D) Mother Rh negative, father Rh negative, fetus Rh unknown
(E) None of the above

Question 561

Which of the following is the correct order of the fetal positions during labor?

(A) Descent, internal rotation, flexion, external rotation, extension
(B) Internal rotation, descent, flexion, extension, external rotation
(C) Descent, flexion, internal rotation, extension, external rotation
(D) Flexion, extension, internal rotation, descent, external rotation
(E) Descent, flexion, internal rotation, external rotation, expulsion

Question 562

An abnormally thin 16-year-old female ballerina presents to the office complaining of six months of amenorrhea and feeling bloated. Which is the most likely diagnosis?

(A) Pregnancy
(B) Premenstrual syndrome
(C) Depression
(D) Anorexia nervosa
(E) Hypothyroidism

Question 563

Which of the following associations between a drug and one of its potential side effects is **incorrect**?

(A) Lithium—central diabetes insipidus
(B) Valproic acid—liver abnormalities
(C) Clozapine—bone marrow suppression
(D) Haloperidol—tardive dyskinesia
(E) Thioridazine—retinal pigment deposits

Question 564

A 26-year-old man is newly diagnosed with schizophrenia and given haloperidol. Two hours later, the patient has muscle spasms and a tightly clenched jaw. His head is turned to the right and seems fixed in position. Which intervention is appropriate?

(A) Stop the haloperidol.
(B) Decrease the haloperidol.
(C) Administer valproic acid.
(D) Administer benztropine.
(E) Switch the patient to clozapine.

Question 565

A small private hospital without a cardiac catheterization laboratory is tired of having patients go to the large public hospital down the street and designs an ad campaign that publishes their excellent myocardial infarction in-hospital mortality data in an attempt to get patients to come to their emergency department. The administrator for the large public hospital is alarmed to read the small hospital's mortality data in the newspaper because their mortality is lower than the large hospital's mortality for myocardial infarction. The administrator is worried because the small hospital usually transfers unstable patients to his larger hospital. Which of the following is most likely to explain the mortality statistic differences?

(A) Lead-time bias
(B) Recall bias
(C) Admission rate bias
(D) Nonrandom sampling
(E) Unacceptability bias

Question 566

Which of the following is true about prostate cancer?

(A) The incidence is less than the prevalence.
(B) The incidence and prevalence are equal.
(C) The incidence is greater than the prevalence.
(D) The incidence has been decreased by earlier detection.
(E) The prevalence decreases with age.

Question 567

A researcher does a retrospective study on smoking and pancreatic cancer. He compares 1000 people with pancreatic cancer to 1000 people without it. He finds that 100 people smoked in the cancer group and 10 smoked in the noncancer group. What is the odds ratio of pancreatic cancer in smokers based only on this information?

(A) Cannot be calculated from the information given
(B) 1.9
(C) 9
(D) 10
(E) 11

Question 568

Which of the following is **not** part of the normal aging process?

(A) Presbyopia
(B) Presbyacusis
(C) Decreased brain weight
(D) Slightly decreased ability to learn new material
(E) Increased basal metabolic rate

Question 569

A 40-year-old man is brought in by his wife for irregular mood swings and crying spells. He has no medical history. You notice irregular, spastic, involuntary movements in the patient's left hand and arm. A CT scan of the brain shows striking atrophy of the caudate nuclei bilaterally. Which of the following is most likely to be true?

(A) The patient has HIV.
(B) The patient has an inherited condition.
(C) The patient has Kayser-Fleischer rings in his eyes.
(D) The patient has an excessive amount of iron in his liver.
(E) The patient has suffered lacunar infarcts.

Question 570

A 7-year-old child is brought to the office by her mother. The mother claims the child seems to daydream excessively and sometimes completely ignores her. She mentions one episode in which the daughter started to answer a question the mother had posed, then stopped and would not respond to the mother, even after the mother shouted at her. The mother noticed that the child had unusual eyelid fluttering during the episode; 45 seconds later, the girl looked at the mother and finished the sentence she had started, not mentioning why she had ignored her mother. "Her eyes are open, so I know she can hear me," the mother exclaims. Their relationship is excellent, which makes the mother all the more concerned about this recent rebellious behavior. The girl seems healthy, active, and well adjusted, and physical examination is within normal limits. Which of the following is most likely to be true?

(A) This disorder almost never begins after the age of 20.
(B) The girl is normal.
(C) Seizure disorder is unlikely because of the lack of a postictal state.
(D) A routine chemistry profile is likely to be abnormal.
(E) This is an autosomal dominant condition.

Question 571

A 34-year-old man who is not on any medications and has not seen a physician in 10 years presents with what appears to be thrush. Which of the following is **least** likely to be true if the diagnosis is thrush?

(A) It represents a normal finding.
(B) It represents the presence of uncontrolled diabetes mellitus.
(C) It represents the presence of AIDS.
(D) It represents the presence of a blood dyscrasia.
(E) It represents the presence of an underlying immune disorder.

Question 572

A 6-year-old boy is brought in by his mother because of hair loss and a "skin tumor." On examination, there is a patchy area of hair loss on the side scalp with underlying skin that is erythematous and slightly scaly. Black dots can be seen on the affected skin, which appear to be the remnants of broken hairs. Under this area is the tumor, an erythematous, boggy mass.

Which of the following is true?

(A) The mass needs biopsy.
(B) Topical fluconazole usually is effective.
(C) If the scalp fluoresces under Wood's light, *Trichophyton* is the presumptive diagnosis.
(D) Systemic therapy is required.
(E) This condition is not contagious.

Question 573

A 25-year-old male patient with AIDS presents to the office because he was exposed to a neighbor's child with a chickenpox rash yesterday and wonders if he needs treatment. Which of the following is true?

(A) It is too late to give varicella-zoster immune globulin.
(B) The neighbor is not infectious once the initial chickenpox rash appears; you should query the patient about exposure a few days ago.
(C) The neighbor should be treated with acyclovir.
(D) The patient should receive the varicella vaccine.
(E) A Tzanck smear of the neighbor's skin is likely to show multinucleated giant cells.

Question 574

A 16-year-old boy who lives alone and is a full-time construction worker presents to the office with a painless lesion on the shaft of his penis. A single, erythematous, shallow ulceration with slightly raised margins and an indurated base is present. The patient admits to several episodes of recent unprotected sex with different partners. Which of the following is true?

(A) The treatment of choice is ceftriaxone.
(B) The causative organism grows well on chocolate agar.
(C) The patient's parents must be notified before treatment is given.
(D) The health department will likely need to be notified.
(E) The patient has a profound immunodeficiency.

Question 575

Which of the following is true concerning lung cancer?

(A) Small cell cancer often is curable surgically.
(B) Squamous cell carcinomas tend to start peripherally.
(C) Horner syndrome usually implies an apical tumor.
(D) Diaphragmatic paralysis can result from recurrent laryngeal nerve paralysis.
(E) Smoking is second only to asbestos as a risk factor for lung cancer.

Question 576

Which of the following is responsible for the most mortality in the United States?

(A) Alcohol
(B) Smoking
(C) Illicit drugs
(D) High cholesterol
(E) Viral infections

Question 577

Which of the following is the most common liver malignancy?

(A) Hepatocellular carcinoma
(B) Hemangioma
(C) Hepatoma
(D) Hepatoblastoma
(E) Metastasis

Question 578

A 42-year-old man develops chills, fever, and low back pain while receiving a blood transfusion for acute anemia secondary to trauma. What is the next step in the management of this patient?

(A) Take a culture of the transfused blood
(B) Start intravenous fluids and diuretics
(C) Stop the transfusion
(D) Administer corticosteroids
(E) Call the laboratory to make sure a proper cross-match was done

Question 579

Which of the following agents is best matched with a correct indication for its use?

(A) Fresh-frozen plasma for disseminated intravascular coagulation with bleeding
(B) Whole blood for symptomatic anemia secondary to autoimmune anemia
(C) Fresh-frozen plasma for hemophilia A
(D) Packed red blood cells for allergic, previously sensitized patients who need a transfusion
(E) Vitamin K for bleeding tendency secondary to severe liver disease

Question 580

A 72-year-old female nursing home patient with dementia presents with acute delirium. On examination, she is afebrile; urine and blood cultures are pending, and chest radiograph is negative. Laboratory tests reveal the following:

Hemoglobin	16 gm/dL
Mean corpuscular volume	90 μm/cell
Sodium	155 mEq/L
Potassium	3.8 mEq/dL
Chloride	121 mEq/L
CO_2	19 mEq/L
BUN	48 mg/dL
Creatinine	1.6 mg/dL
Urinalysis	Normal other than elevated specific gravity

An old emergency department record reveals a normal metabolic profile and renal function 3 months ago. What is the likely cause of the patient's renal insufficiency?

(A) Dehydration
(B) Acetaminophen abuse
(C) Glomerulonephritis
(D) Diabetic hyperosmolar, hyperglycemic state
(E) Nephrolithiasis

Question 581

What is the best way to differentiate between nephrogenic and central diabetes insipidus?

(A) Administer antidiuretic hormone and assess response
(B) Administer demeclocycline and asses response
(C) Administer a fluid challenge and asses response
(D) Assess the response to hypertonic saline
(E) Measure urine output with urine electrolytes

Question 582

Which of the following is **least** correct regarding gastroesophageal reflux?

(A) It is thought to be due to intermittent, inappropriate relaxation of the lower esophageal sphincter

(B) It may result in adenocarcinoma, which usually occurs in the mid-to-upper esophagus

(C) It may result in esophageal strictures

(D) It may result in a chronic cough

(E) It may result in asthma

Question 583

Which of the following is correct regarding peptic ulcer disease?

(A) A gastric ulcer can be classified as benign or malignant based on its location in most cases.

(B) Smoking is not related to causation or healing of peptic ulcer disease.

(C) Multiple duodenal ulcers in atypical locations, such as the distal duodenum, should increase the suspicion of a glucagonoma.

(D) Most peptic ulcers are located in the duodenum.

(E) Gastric ulcers are caused by gastric acid hypersecretion.

Question 584

Which of the following findings on physical examination is consistent with a lung consolidation from a lobar pneumonia?

(A) Increased breath sounds in the area of consolidation

(B) Increased tactile fremitus in the area of consolidation

(C) Decreased egophony in the area of consolidation

(D) Hyperresonant percussion note in the area of consolidation

(E) Decreased whispered pectoriloquy

Question 585

A 49-year-old man presents to the emergency department with a blood pressure reading of 240/156 mmHg in the right arm and 236/158 mmHg in the left arm. He has no medical history, and his only complaint is a headache. On physical examination, he has papilledema with no other findings. Which of the following treatment options is appropriate?

(A) Admit the man to the intensive care unit and lower the blood pressure to normal immediately with intravenous agents.

(B) Admit the man to the intensive care unit and lower the blood pressure to around 190/110 mmHg immediately with intravenous agents.

(C) Give the man a prescription for an oral antihypertensive, and arrange for office follow-up the next day.

(D) Give the man a prescription for an oral antihypertensive, and arrange for office follow-up in 1 week.

(E) Give the man a bolus of high-dose intravenous steroids, and check the urine for cocaine.

Question 586

What is the most common cause of death in people with untreated hypertension?

(A) Coronary disease

(B) Cerebrovascular accident

(C) Renal failure

(D) Encephalopathy

(E) Cancer

Question 587

A 62-year-old man with long-standing diabetes presents with acute-onset shortness of breath and "feeling sweaty." He is on multiple medications, including captopril, metformin, pioglitazone, and amlodipine, which he claims to have taken every day over the past several years. Physical examination and vital signs are within normal limits other than mild tachypnea and diaphoresis. Which condition is most important to rule out first in this scenario?

(A) Myocardial infarction

(B) Hyperkalemia

(C) Pericarditis

(D) Atrial fibrillation

(E) Third-degree heart block

Question 588

A 30-year-old woman presents with a chief complaint of dysphagia. Her difficulty is equal with solids and liquids and has become progressively worse. She denies any history of heartburn or weight loss. A barium swallow is done and reveals retained food in the esophagus with smooth distal tapering of the esophagus. Which of the following is true regarding the most likely diagnosis?

(A) The woman's condition is due to prolonged tobacco exposure.
(B) The woman has night sweats and high, spiking fevers.
(C) Esophagectomy is the treatment of choice.
(D) Endoscopy is contraindicated.
(E) Esophageal manometry is likely to be abnormal.

Question 589

A gravida 2, para 1, 25-year-old pregnant woman presents to the emergency department at 32 weeks' gestation with a blood pressure of 184/96 mmHg; 4+ proteinuria on urinalysis; and marked ankle, hand, and facial edema. The woman subsequently develops seizures in the emergency department. A magnesium sulfate infusion is started, and an ultrasound is performed. The fetus has no heartbeat and is not moving. The woman subsequently loses consciousness and is rushed to the intensive care unit. Which of the following most likely could have prevented this scenario?

(A) A low-salt diet
(B) The use of hydralazine to control blood pressure as soon as the woman came into the emergency department
(C) Regular prenatal care
(D) Regular use of prenatal vitamins
(E) Avoidance of alcohol use during pregnancy

Question 590

A 17-year-old woman comes to the office for primary amenorrhea. A pregnancy test is negative. She has normal adult female breast development but absent axillary and pubic hair with otherwise normal-appearing female external genitalia. The uterus is nonpalpable and absent on ultrasound examination, and the serum testosterone level is higher than the normal female range. Which of the following is likely to be true?

(A) The patient is a true hermaphrodite.
(B) The patient has 21-hydroxylase deficiency.
(C) The patient has an ovarian neoplasm.
(D) The patient has a male genotype.
(E) The patient is psychologically a male.

Question 591

A 24-year-old woman has secondary amenorrhea with a negative pregnancy test. If administration of progesterone fails to produce uterine bleeding, which of the following is a reasonable diagnostic possibility?

(A) Polycystic ovary syndrome
(B) Ectopic pregnancy
(C) Turner's syndrome
(D) Premature ovarian failure
(E) Hyperthyroidism

Question 592

What is generally the first step in the workup of an infertile couple in which history and physical examination of a normally menstruating woman reveal no abnormalities?

(A) Laparoscopy
(B) Progesterone challenge
(C) Semen analysis
(D) Hysterosalpingogram
(E) CT scan of the pelvis

Question 593

What is the most likely cause of dysfunctional uterine bleeding in 28-year-old woman with a normal physical examination and no other complaints?

(A) Polycystic ovary syndrome
(B) Hypothyroidism
(C) Oral contraceptive pills
(D) Physiologic dysmenorrhea
(E) Gynecologic cancer

Question 594

Most common cause of renal cell carcinoma

(A) Smoking tobacco
(B) Ethanol abuse
(C) Obesity
(D) Previous radiation therapy
(E) Previous chemotherapy
(F) Eating a high-fat, low-fiber diet
(G) Maternal diethylstilbesterol exposure
(H) Sunlight exposure
(I) *Schistosoma* infection

Question 595

Most common cause of pancreatic carcinoma

(A) Smoking tobacco
(B) Ethanol abuse
(C) Obesity
(D) Previous radiation therapy
(E) Previous chemotherapy
(F) Eating a high-fat, low-fiber diet
(G) Maternal diethylstilbesterol exposure
(H) Sunlight exposure
(I) *Schistosoma* infection

Question 596

Most common cause of bladder carcinoma

(A) Smoking tobacco
(B) Ethanol abuse
(C) Obesity
(D) Previous radiation therapy
(E) Previous chemotherapy
(F) Eating a high-fat, low-fiber diet
(G) Maternal diethylstilbesterol exposure
(H) Sunlight exposure
(I) *Schistosoma* infection

Question 597

Most common cause of endometrial carcinoma

(A) Smoking tobacco
(B) Ethanol abuse
(C) Obesity
(D) Previous radiation therapy
(E) Previous chemotherapy
(F) Eating a high-fat, low-fiber diet
(G) Maternal diethylstilbesterol exposure
(H) Sunlight exposure
(I) *Schistosoma* infection

Question 598

Most common cause of thyroid carcinoma

(A) Smoking tobacco
(B) Ethanol abuse
(C) Obesity
(D) Previous radiation therapy
(E) Previous chemotherapy
(F) Eating a high-fat, low-fiber diet
(G) Maternal diethylstilbesterol exposure
(H) Sunlight exposure
(I) *Schistosoma* infection

Question 599

Most common cause of cervical carcinoma

(A) Smoking tobacco
(B) Ethanol abuse
(C) Obesity
(D) Previous radiation therapy
(E) Previous chemotherapy
(F) Eating a high-fat, low-fiber diet
(G) Maternal diethylstilbesterol exposure
(H) Sunlight exposure
(I) *Schistosoma* infection

Question 600

A 52-year old man has occult blood detected in his stool during a routine screening rectal examination. A colonoscopy is performed and reveals an irregular focal polypoid lesion in the mid-ascending colon. A biopsy is performed. A representative slide from the biopsy is shown below.

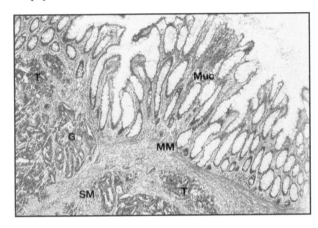

What is the preferred initial treatment for this condition?

(A) Antibiotics
(B) Surgery
(C) No treatment needed
(D) Chemotherapy
(E) Corticosteroids

BLOCK 12 ANSWER KEY

551. C	561. C	571. A	581. A	591. D
552. A	562. D	572. D	582. B	592. C
553. D	563. A	573. E	583. D	593. A
554. D	564. D	574. D	584. B	594. A
555. D	565. C	575. C	585. B	595. A
556. A	566. A	576. B	586. A	596. A
557. C	567. E	577. E	587. A	597. C
558. C	568. E	578. C	588. E	598. D
559. B	569. B	579. A	589. C	599. A
560. B	570. A	580. A	590. D	600. B

Refer to Answers and Explanations Section for Block 12

Pages 307–315

Figure credit

Question 600: Stevens A, et al: Neoplasia. In Stevens A, et al (eds): Wheater's Basic Histopathology, 4th ed. Churchill Livingstone, 2002, pp 68–85.

BLOCK 13

50 QUESTIONS

TIME ALLOWED:
60 MINUTES

Question 601

Which of the following patients **least** requires colonic examination with either barium enema and flexible sigmoidoscopy or colonoscopy?

(A) A 59-year-old man with occult blood in the stool and weight loss
(B) A 31-year-old woman with familial adenomatous polyposis who has not seen a physician in 10 years
(C) A 68-year-old woman who notes her stools are now pencil thin and black
(D) A 31-year-old man with Peutz-Jeghers syndrome who has not seen a physician in 10 years
(E) A 42-year-old man with severe ulcerative colitis for 17 years who had a colonoscopy 5 years ago

Question 602

A 72-year-old man presents with the complaints of urinary hesitancy, dysuria, and low back pain. On rectal examination, the prostate is enlarged and nodular. A pelvic radiograph reveals the presence of two dense, irregular, fairly homogeneous bone lesions involving the second and fourth lumbar vertebrae. Which of the following is likely to be true?

(A) The serum prostate-specific antigen level is increased.
(B) The back pain is due to osteoporosis.
(C) The patient has metastatic colon cancer.
(D) The patient has a primary bone cancer.
(E) Traditional chemotherapy agents are the only hope for treatment.

Question 603

Which of the following paraneoplastic syndromes is matched correctly with the type of cancer with which it is commonly associated?

(A) Syndrome of inappropriate antidiuretic hormone secretion—squamous cell carcinoma of the lung
(B) Eaton-Lambert syndrome—thymoma
(C) Hypercalcemia secondary to parathyroid hormone production—squamous cell carcinoma of the lung
(D) Cushing syndrome secondary to adrenocorticotropic hormone production—large cell carcinoma of the lung
(E) Polycythemia secondary to erythropoietin production—medullary thyroid carcinoma

Question 604

A 17-year-old black man started taking trimethoprim-sulfamethoxazole yesterday for sinusitis, and this morning he is in your office complaining of shortness of breath and fatigue. He has never taken sulfa antibiotics or trimethoprim before. You note some pallor of the sclera and borderline tachycardia, but the examination is otherwise unremarkable. Complete blood count reveals hemoglobin of 11 g/dL with normal white blood cells and platelet counts. On peripheral blood smear, reticulocytosis and bite cells are noted. What is the most likely cause of this patient's anemia?

(A) A genetic disorder
(B) Antibody-mediated red blood cell destruction secondary to sulfamethoxazole
(C) Antibody-mediated red blood cell destruction secondary to trimethoprim
(D) Disseminated intravascular coagulation
(E) Occult blood loss

Question 605

A 3-year-old girl is brought in by her mother for high fever. The child has no medical history and is on no medications, but the mother notes that the child has been somewhat lethargic in the past week. On examination, the child is lethargic, the pharynx is markedly erythematous, the heart is tachycardic, and the sclera are pale. Temperature is 103°F. Laboratory tests reveal the following:

Hemoglobin	6 gm/dL
Mean corpuscular volume	90 µm/cell
White blood cell count	920/µL
Platelet count	34,000/µL
Reticulocyte count	0.5% (normal = 0.5–2.5)

What is the most likely cause of the child's anemia?

(A) Chronic disease
(B) Child abuse causing internal hemorrhage
(C) Autoimmune disorder
(D) Iron deficiency
(E) Bone marrow infiltration with leukemia

Question 606

A 65-year-old man with a long history of urinary hesitancy presents with acute renal failure and anuria for 24 hours with no other symptoms or history. What is the most likely cause?

(A) Nephrolithiasis
(B) Benign prostatic hypertrophy
(C) Poststreptococcal glomerulonephritis
(D) Goodpasture's syndrome
(E) Wegener's granulomatosis

Question 607

Which of the following may be an effective treatment for nephrogenic diabetes insipidus?

(A) Hydrochlorothiazide
(B) Demeclocycline
(C) Lithium
(D) Antidiuretic hormone (vasopressin)
(E) Calcitonin

Question 608

What is the most likely cause of severe, symptomatic, intermittent hypertension with a marked elevation of urinary metanephrines?

(A) Pheochromocytoma
(B) Cushing syndrome
(C) Carcinoid syndrome
(D) Renal artery stenosis
(E) Hyperaldosteronism

Question 609

Which of the following is true regarding chronic pancreatitis?

(A) The most common cause is gallstones.
(B) Pancreatic calcifications usually indicate that progression to pancreatic cancer has occurred.
(C) B-vitamin supplements often are needed to prevent vitamin deficiencies.
(D) It may cause diabetes.
(E) Constipation is a common complaint.

Question 610

A 32-year-old woman presents with a chief complaint of diarrhea and bloating for the last 2 weeks. The woman claims she has had intermittent diarrhea and bloating since her teenage years, similar to her current complaints. On further questioning, the woman mentions taking a course of ciprofloxacin for a urinary tract infection 1 month ago. The woman is afebrile, and physical examination is remarkable only for mild, diffuse abdominal tenderness without rebound or guarding during palpation. She denies symptoms of reflux or peptic ulcer disease and claims to have a normal appetite. A sigmoidoscopy is unremarkable. What is the most likely diagnosis?

(A) Appendicitis
(B) Irritable bowel syndrome
(C) Crohn disease
(D) Ulcerative colitis
(E) Pseudomembranous colitis secondary to *Clostridium difficile* overgrowth

Question 611

A 72-year-old woman with a history of dementia develops hypoxemia while in the ICU being treated for severe sepsis from a urinary tract infection. A chest radiograph shows diffuse, asymmetric pulmonary edema with a normal cardiac silhouette. The patient has mottled skin, intercostal retractions, and scattered rales. Administration of 100% oxygen and diuretics does not improve oxygenation. What is the most likely cause of the hypoxemia?

(A) Seeding of the lungs with septic emboli
(B) Adult respiratory distress syndrome
(C) Community-acquired pneumonia
(D) Congestive heart failure
(E) Myocardial infarction

Question 612

A 32-year-old otherwise healthy woman comes into the office complaining of a skin rash on her legs 3 weeks after visiting her grandmother in the San Joaquin Valley area of California. She also mentions a dry, nonproductive cough and headache. Examination reveals bilateral red, tender nodules on the extensor surfaces of the shins. What would be the most likely infectious organism?

(A) *Histoplasma capsulatum*
(B) *Coccidioides immitis*
(C) *Blastomyces dermatitidis*
(D) *Paracoccidioides brasiliensis*
(E) *Cryptococcus neoformans*

Question 613

A 64-year-old man who has been smoking two packs of cigarettes per day since he was a teenager gets a routine preoperative chest radiograph that shows a 3 cm, round, ill-defined lesion in the left lower lobe as well as severe emphysematous changes. A chest radiograph done 1 year ago did not show the lesion. The patient denies any symptoms other than his usual chronic cough and shortness of breath and denies any sick contacts. What is the most likely diagnosis?

(A) Tuberculosis
(B) Community-acquired pneumonia
(C) Lung cancer
(D) Pulmonary hamartoma
(E) Coccidioidomycosis

Question 614

Which of the following is the best medication for immediate relief from an acute asthma exacerbation?

(A) Zafirlukast
(B) Prednisone
(C) Cromolyn
(D) Albuterol
(E) Ipratropium

Question 615

Which of the following is true concerning polyhydramnios?

(A) It is defined as an amniotic fluid volume greater than 750 mL
(B) It is associated with renal agenesis
(C) It often results in pulmonary hypoplasia
(D) It may cause maternal dyspnea
(E) The mainstay of therapy is amniotomy

Question 616

A 19-year-old gravida 1, para 1, woman becomes markedly dyspneic, tachypneic, tachycardic, and hypotensive after delivery of a healthy infant at 40 weeks' gestation. She complains of chest pain, and her skin becomes mottled. Two minutes later, the woman goes into shock and dies. An autopsy is most likely to reveal which of the following?

(A) Amniotic fluid pulmonary embolus
(B) Myocardial infarction
(C) Acute necrotizing bacterial pneumonia
(D) Acute fatty liver of pregnancy
(E) A hydatiform mole

Question 617

A 26-year-old pregnant woman comes to the office for a routine prenatal examination at 34 weeks and has no complaints. Her blood pressure is 166/92 mmHg. On previous visits, the woman was normotensive. She also has 4+ proteinuria on a routine urinalysis and marked ankle edema. Which of the following is true?

(A) The woman should return in 1 week for a remeasurement of her blood pressure.
(B) The woman should return in 1 month for a remeasurement of her blood pressure.
(C) The woman should be admitted to the hospital for rest, observation, and blood pressure control.
(D) The woman should be given enalapril and return in 1 week for a remeasurement of her blood pressure.
(E) The woman should have an immediate cesarean section for preeclampsia.

Question 618

Which of the following is true concerning uterine leiomyomas?

(A) They are the most common indication for hysterectomy.

(B) Malignant transformation occurs in only about 20% of cases.

(C) They tend to regress during pregnancy.

(D) They are not a cause of infertility.

(E) Oral contraceptive pills are a first-line treatment to reduce their size.

Question 619

A 41-year-old woman complains of dysmenorrhea and menorrhagia with a sensation of pelvic "fullness." On examination, the uterus is slightly enlarged, is normal in overall shape and position, and has a boggy consistency. Dilation and curettage reveals no evidence of cancer. A hysterectomy is performed. A sample slide from deep within the myometrium is shown below:

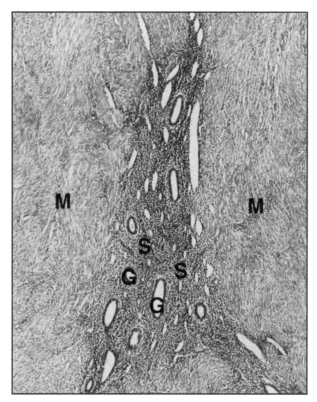

Which of the following is the most likely condition?

(A) Endometrial carcinoma

(B) Leiomyosarcoma

(C) Endometriosis

(D) Adenomyosis

(E) Menopause

Question 620

Which of the following may help a patient with a severe exacerbation of congestive heart failure requiring hospital admission to the intensive care unit secondary to borderline cardiogenic shock?

(A) Metoprolol
(B) Corticosteroids
(C) Milrinone
(D) Diltiazem
(E) Lidocaine

Question 621

Which of the following is **least** likely to cause secondary hypertension?

(A) Hypothyroidism
(B) Hyperadrenalism
(C) Psychogenic polydipsia
(D) Hyperthyroidism
(E) Cocaine abuse

Question 622

A sexually active 54-year-old man presents to the emergency department with pain and swelling in the right knee. The knee has limited movement secondary to pain, and the skin overlying the joint is erythematous. Arthrocentesis is performed, and the fluid is examined using polarized light microscopy. Needle-shaped crsytals with negative birefringence are identified. Which of the following is **incorrect** regarding the most likely condition?

(A) Antibiotics would not be helpful.
(B) Allopurinol is a first-line treatment to relieve the patient's current symptoms.
(C) Alcohol abuse and male sex are risk factors for this condition.
(D) Colchicine is a first-line treatment to relieve the patient's current symptoms.
(E) None of the above

Question 623

A 62-year old patient presents with early satiety and a 40-lb weight loss over the past 3 months. An upper GI barium series is performed. An image of the stomach from the procedure is shown below:

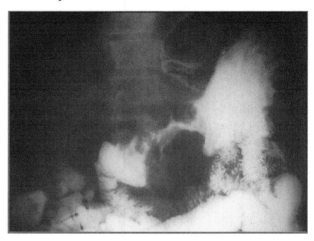

Which of the following would be **unexpected** given the epidemiology of the most likely condition?

(A) The patient is Japanese.
(B) The patient is male.
(C) A biopsy reveals adenocarcinoma.
(D) The patient is older than age 50.
(E) None of the above

Question 624

A 45-year-old woman is admitted for a modified radical mastectomy for a breast mass determined by biopsy to be cancer. After the surgery, pathology reveals that 2 of 8 lymph nodes in the axilla are positive for cancer. When you tell the patient, she is devastated. She is discharged the next day, and you see her 1 week later in your office for follow-up. The woman looks as though she has been crying recently and says she has no appetite whatsoever. She has not been sleeping well and feels isolated and depressed. She denies acute suicidal ideation, saying she is "too chicken" to commit suicide but wishes she could "end it all."

You ask about her wishes for further treatment of her malignancy, and she hands you a copy of a living will, which she drafted this morning. The living will essentially refuses all interventions and all care, including supportive care, if the patient should need it. What is the next appropriate step regarding the living will?

(A) Refer the patient for psychiatric evaluation of depression and postpone evaluation of her living will

(B) Put the living will in the chart and honor it

(C) Call the next of kin to ascertain what they think of the living will

(D) Prescribe an antidepressant, and tell the patient it is a multivitamin

(E) Admit the patient to the hospital, against her will if necessary, and begin appropriate treatment for the malignancy and her depression as you see fit

Question 625

You are seeing a 28-year-old schizophrenic man who currently is on olanzapine. He admits to not taking the medication lately because it clouds his thinking. He claims to be doing well now because he thinks he has identified his problem. His "problem" is a 22-year-old woman who lives across the street from the patient.

The patient claims that she has been orchestrating a nationwide conspiracy to torment him. He says he is going to "take care" of the woman and take care of his problems. When you ask the patient what he means by taking care of the woman, he makes a gesture of slitting his throat with an imaginary knife. When you try to talk him out of it, he laughs and says that you could not possibly understand the ramifications of his "mission" to "eliminate" the root of his problems. The patient has a history of violence when off his medications. What is the next appropriate step?

(A) Have the patient admitted to an inpatient psychiatry unit, against his will if necessary, and alert the authorities of the patient's plan.

(B) Have the patient admitted to an inpatient psychiatry unit, against his will if necessary, but do not alert the authorities because of physician-patient confidentiality.

(C) Try to convince the patient to take his medications and schedule a follow-up appointment in 48 hours.

(D) Give the patient a depot injection of haloperidol and schedule follow-up in 1 week.

(E) Call the woman across the street to alert her and schedule a follow-up appointment in 1 week, after convincing the patient to take his medicine.

Question 626

Which of the following skills is **least** likely to have been mastered by a 3-year-old child?

(A) Shoelace tying

(B) Running well

(C) Understanding one-step commands without the use of gestures

(D) Ability to build a tower of 6 blocks

(E) Good use of a cup and spoon

Question 627

A 3-year-old child presents to the emergency department with a high fever and respiratory distress. The child apparently was fine until about 12 hours ago when she began developing a fever, which progressed rapidly to high fever (103° F) and rapid, labored respirations. The child is not coughing, but you notice her appearance is toxic and she is drooling. What is the next step in management?

(A) Prepare to establish an airway.
(B) Examine the throat and perform throat culture.
(C) Order a CT scan of the neck.
(D) Order routine serum chemistries and blood cultures.
(E) Ask the child to describe her symptoms in her own words.

Question 628

A Mexican immigrant woman who came to the United States just 2 days ago brings in her 3-year-old child with a fever that began this morning. She says the child was fine yesterday. On examination, the child has a grayish, tough, fibrous inflammatory exudate on the pharynx, tonsils, and uvula and a fever of 102.5° F. What is likely to be the best initial treatment?

(A) Antitoxin
(B) Acyclovir
(C) Ribavarin
(D) Fluconazole
(E) Ciprofloxacin

Question 629

A lesion of which of the following peripheral nerves may produce wristdrop?

(A) Median
(B) Ulnar
(C) Radial
(D) Musculocutaneous
(E) Axillary

Question 630

All of the following are reasons to do an open fracture reduction instead of closed reduction **except**:

(A) Multiple areas of skeletal trauma, to allow mobilization at the earliest possible point in time
(B) Extremity function requiring perfect function, as in a professional athlete
(C) Fractures in children, to ensure proper development of immature bones
(D) Compromised blood supply
(E) Compound (open) fracture

Question 631

Which of the following is **least** consistent with cataracts as a cause of decreased vision?

(A) Gradual onset
(B) History of corticosteroid use
(C) Normal red reflex
(D) Bilateral involvement
(E) Normal appearance of the retina

Question 632

Which of the following is **inconsistent** with retinal detachment as a cause of loss of vision?

(A) Severe pain
(B) Sudden onset
(C) Seeing flashes of light
(D) Seeing floaters of black spots in the field of vision
(E) Unilateral involvement

Question 633

A gravida 1, para 1, 26-year-old obtunded woman has a positive qualitative urine pregnancy test, vaginal bleeding, abdominal pain with rebound tenderness, and a cursory uterine ultrasound that fails to reveal a fetus inside the uterus. The woman is hypovolemic by physical examination and has a blood pressure of 86/38 mmHg with a sinus tachycardia of 148 beats/min. Which of the following is the next step in her management?

(A) Laparotomy
(B) Confirmation of pregnancy with quantitative human chorionic gonadotropin test
(C) CT scan of the abdomen and pelvis
(D) Administration of intravenous fluids and repeat examination in one hour
(E) Culdocentesis

Question 634

Which of the following choices is **least** likely to increase the risk of ectopic pregnancy?

(A) History of pelvic inflammatory disease
(B) Use of an intrauterine device for contraception
(C) History of a previous ectopic pregnancy
(D) Nulliparity
(E) History of recent tubal sterilization

Question 635

Which of the following abortion definitions is correct?

(A) Threatened abortion—uterine bleeding at 16 weeks with cervical dilation but without passage of any products of conception
(B) Incomplete abortion—uterine bleeding at 25 weeks with passage of some of the products of conception through the cervix
(C) Inevitable abortion—uterine bleeding at 12 weeks without cervical dilation
(D) Missed abortion—fetal death at 10 weeks without maternal or physician detection and without expulsion of tissue for 3 weeks
(E) Complete abortion—intentional termination of pregnancy at 26 weeks because of a maternal request for termination

Question 636

Which of the following is a **contraindication** to labor induction?

(A) Prior cesarean section with a vertical uterine incision
(B) History of genital herpes
(C) Term pregnancy
(D) Nulliparity
(E) Preeclampsia

Question 637

Withdrawal from which of the following drugs may be fatal?

(A) Caffeine
(B) Cocaine
(C) Heroin
(D) Phencyclidine (PCP)
(E) Barbiturates

Question 638

A 22-year-old man presents to the emergency department complaining of a heart attack. He says he is going to die and has severe chest pains and shortness of breath. He appears quite anxious and is tachycardic and tachypneic. Medical history is insignificant. Electrocardiogram, cardiac enzymes, and complete metabolic profile are within normal limits. Arterial blood gas reveals a mild primary respiratory alkalosis without metabolic compensation. The patient starts to feel better a few minutes later. He says this is the third time these symptoms have occurred in the last 2 months, with negative tests each time. His heart rate and respiratory rate return to normal, and a physical examination is within normal limits. He denies psychiatric problems. Which of the following is most likely to be true?

(A) The patient is afraid to leave his house.
(B) The patient has a pulmonary embolus.
(C) The patient has generalized anxiety disorder.
(D) The patient has hyperthyroidism.
(E) β-blockers, nitrates, and aspirin are indicated.

Question 639

A 59-year-old man comes to the office because he has mistaken other women for his wife twice in the last 2 weeks even though she died 3 weeks ago. He starts to cry and tells you he thinks he's "cracking up." He knows his wife is dead and that he did not actually see her but admits to missing her terribly. Which of the following is most likely based on the information given?

(A) Psychotic depression
(B) Schizophrenic break
(C) Normal grief
(D) Pathologic grief
(E) Adjustment disorder

Question 640

Which of the following medications is most likely to cause priapism?

(A) Propranolol
(B) Prazosin
(C) Isotretinoin
(D) Trazodone
(E) Primidone

Question 641

Which of the following substances can be given safely to someone on tranylcypromine?

(A) Meperidine
(B) Amphetamines
(C) Nifedipine
(D) Wine
(E) Fluoxetine

Question 642

Which of the following is true concerning the negative predictive value of a test?

(A) It is the likelihood of a person having a negative test given his or her risk factors.
(B) The negative predictive value decreases with decreasing prevalence of disease in a population.
(C) An overly sensitive test increases the negative predictive value.
(D) It is determined by dividing the number of persons with a negative test by the whole population.
(E) The negative predictive value is not affected by the prevalence.

Question 643

How does changing the fasting glucose cutoff value from 140 mg/dL to 126 mg/dL affect the epidemiology of diabetes mellitus and the test itself?

(A) It decreases the positive predictive value of the test.
(B) It increases the number of false-negative results.
(C) It decreases the negative predictive value of the test.
(D) It increases the risk of diabetes.
(E) It makes the test more specific.

Question 644

A city being studied has a population of 100,000. Using culture as the gold standard test, 5000 people in the city are found to have chlamydial infection. A new DNA probe chlamydial test is positive on 4000 people in the city, of whom only 3000 tested positive by culture. What is the specificity of the new DNA probe test?

(A) 50%
(B) 60%
(C) 75%
(D) 80%
(E) > 95%

Question 645

A group of scientists decide to examine the risk of smoking in developing pancreatic cancer. They follow 30,000 people from the age of 20 until their death and separate the people into two groups—smokers and nonsmokers. There are 10,000 smokers and 20,000 nonsmokers. By reviewing the hospital charts and autopsy records after all the people have died, the scientists determine the number of people in each group who died of pancreatic cancer. The groups were matched carefully before the study started so that there are no inequalities in terms of age, sex, or other demographics or habits. The scientists finds that 300 people in the smoking group died of pancreatic cancer versus 200 people in the nonsmoking group. Using the scientist's data, what is the attributable risk of smoking in causing pancreatic cancer?

(A) 12.5/1000
(B) 20/1000
(C) 30/1000
(D) 40/1000
(E) Cannot be calculated from the information given

Question 646

After a stroke, a patient has trouble reading and doing math. Localize the deficit.

(A) Frontal lobes
(B) Dominant temporal lobe
(C) Dominant parietal lobe
(D) Nondominant parietal lobe
(E) Occipital lobes
(F) Midbrain
(G) Pons
(H) Medulla
(I) Cerebellum

Question 647

After a car accident, a patient is impulsive, uninhibited, and labile emotionally. Localize the deficit.

(A) Frontal lobes
(B) Dominant temporal lobe
(C) Dominant parietal lobe
(D) Nondominant parietal lobe
(E) Occipital lobes
(F) Midbrain
(G) Pons
(H) Medulla
(I) Cerebellum

Question 648

A chronic alcoholic is ataxic and mildly dysarthric. Localize the deficit.

(A) Frontal lobes
(B) Dominant temporal lobe
(C) Dominant parietal lobe
(D) Nondominant parietal lobe
(E) Occipital lobes
(F) Midbrain
(G) Pons
(H) Medulla
(I) Cerebellum

Question 649

A patient can talk, but his speech is incoherent and he has trouble understanding others. Localize the deficit.

(A) Frontal lobes
(B) Dominant temporal lobe
(C) Dominant parietal lobe
(D) Nondominant parietal lobe
(E) Occipital lobes
(F) Midbrain
(G) Pons
(H) Medulla
(I) Cerebellum

Question 650

A 52-year-old man presents to you for gradual onset of worsening shortness of breath over the past several months. He is a long-standing smoker but has no other significant past medical or social history. Examination of the man's fingers reveals the appearance shown below:

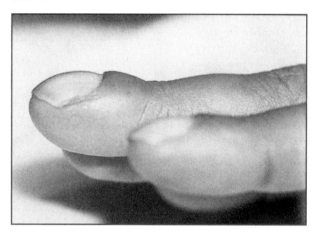

Which of the following is **incorrect** regarding the finding shown in the figure above?

(A) It most likely related to a complication of smoking in this patient
(B) It can be due to cardiovascular disease
(C) It can be due to gastrointestinal disease
(D) It can be due to pulmonary disease
(E) None of the above

BLOCK 13 ANSWER KEY

601. D	611. B	621. C	631. C	641. C
602. A	612. B	622. B	632. A	642. C
603. C	613. C	623. E	633. A	643. A
604. A	614. D	624. A	634. D	644. E
605. E	615. D	625. A	635. D	645. B
606. B	616. A	626. A	636. A	646. C
607. A	617. C	627. A	637. E	647. A
608. A	618. A	628. A	638. A	648. I
609. D	619. D	629. C	639. C	649. B
610. B	620. C	630. C	640. D	650. E

Refer to Answers and Explanations Section for Block 13

Pages 317–325

Figure credits

Question 619: Stevens A, et al: Female reproductive system. In Stevens A, et al (eds): Wheater's Basic Histopathology, 4th ed. New York, Churchill Livingstone, 2002, pp 198–215.

Question 623: Katz DS, Math KR, Groskin SA (eds): Radiology Secrets. Philadelphia, Hanley & Belfus, 1998, p 138.

Question 650: du Vivier A: The skin and systemic disease. In Atlas of Clinical Dermatology, 3rd ed. New York, Churchill Livingstone, 2002, pp 509–561.

50 QUESTIONS

**TIME ALLOWED:
60 MINUTES**

Question 651

A mother brings in her 1-year-old son for high fevers and "a seizure" at home. The infant has been acting completely normal and does not seem sick except for feeling warm and having the high fever, which the mother measured at 104° F at home last night. The infant has not had any change in feeding habits. At about the time the mother decided to bring in the infant, he had generalized shaking over his entire body that lasted 1 minute and was associated with incontinence. The infant was slightly lethargic after the event but was back to normal within 15 minutes.

The mother mentions a neighbor's child who also had a high fever that went away after a few days and who developed a rash but never seemed sick. On examination, the infant is alert and attentive. His temperature is 103.8° F, but the rest of the physical examination is normal. What is the best next step in the management of the infant?

(A) Perform lumbar puncture.
(B) Admit the child to the hospital for a fever of unknown origin workup.
(C) Administer acetaminophen.
(D) Administer phenytoin.
(E) Administer broad-spectrum antibiotics.

Question 652

A neonate has fever, lethargy, and seizures 1 week after being delivered at home. The infant was normal at birth and seemed healthy, according to his mother. The mother had a painful genital rash at the time of delivery that has resolved without treatment. The infant currently has a vesicular rash with all the lesions appearing roughly the same age, fever, conjunctivitis, mild jaundice, and irritability. An electroencephalogram shows diffuse abnormalities, and an MRI of the brain reveals multiple areas of inflammation scattered throughout the brain. Which of the following is most likely to be true?

(A) The child would benefit from acyclovir
(B) The child has a congenital metabolic disorder
(C) The child would benefit from broad-spectrum antibiotics
(D) The child's cerebrospinal fluid is likely to show an elevated white blood cell count with at least 75% neutrophils
(E) The mother has a history of gonococcal infection

Question 653

Which of the following disorders is most often associated with myocardial infarction in children younger than 10 years of age?

(A) Duchenne muscular dystrophy
(B) Familial hypertriglyceridemia
(C) Kawasaki disease
(D) Myotonic dystrophy
(E) Neurofibromatosis

Question 654

Which of the following is usually the underlying pathophysiologic mechanism resulting in the condition known as a *Charcot joint?*

(A) Infection
(B) Trauma
(C) Disuse atrophy secondary to pain or immobility
(D) Loss of proprioception and/or pain perception
(E) Improper fracture reduction

Question 655

Which of the following would be an **unusual** finding with a lumbar disk herniation at the L5–S1 level?

(A) Decreased ankle jerk
(B) Sciatica with straight-leg raise
(C) Weakness of plantar flexors in the foot
(D) Urinary retention
(E) Decreased strength in the gastrocnemius muscle

Question 656

Which of the following is true regarding chemical burns to the eye?

(A) Acid burns generally cause more damage than alkaline burns.
(B) Irrigation should be done only with sterile water.
(C) Neutralization with a solution of opposite pH gives the best long-term results.
(D) You should not obtain a full medical history before instituting treatment.
(E) Irrigation should be done only with sterile normal saline.

Question 657

Which of the following characteristics may be found with orbital cellulitis but is not generally seen with pre-orbital (preseptal) cellulitis?

(A) Proptosis
(B) Fever
(C) Swollen lids
(D) Chemosis
(E) History of trauma

Question 658

What is the initial imaging study of choice in the setting of acute head trauma?

(A) CT scan without intravenous contrast
(B) CT scan with intravenous contrast
(C) MRI
(D) Plain skull radiographs
(E) Positron emission tomography scan

Question 659

In which of the following patients is flail chest most likely to be seen?

(A) A patient with penetrating trauma to the left chest
(B) A patient with an acute pulmonary embolus
(C) A patient with blunt trauma to the superior abdomen
(D) A patient with several adjacent ribs broken in multiple places
(E) A patient with severe asthma

Question 660

Which of the following is **least** appropriate as an initial step in the workup and management of third-trimester bleeding in a 34-year-old gravida 3, para 2, woman?

(A) Urine drug screen
(B) Intravenous fluids
(C) Bimanual pelvic examination
(D) Complete blood count
(E) Establish maternal and fetal monitoring

Question 661

Which of the following is the **least** appropriate intervention in a gravida 1, para 0, 34-year-old woman with moderate pulmonary stenosis, preeclampsia, and a blood pressure of 174/94 mmHg who goes into labor after 33 weeks' gestation?

(A) Instigating tocolysis with ritodrine
(B) Placing the mother in the lateral decubitus position
(C) Administering oxygen through nasal cannula
(D) Giving hydralazine for blood pressure control
(E) Administering corticosteroids

Question 662

Which of the following is **not** an indication for a cesarean section delivery?

(A) Fetal scalp pH of 7.0 and persistent late decelerations seen on the fetal heart monitor
(B) Shoulder dystocia with failure to progress for 8 hours
(C) A vertex presentation with early decelerations
(D) Complete placenta previa
(E) Pregnancy of 44 weeks' gestation and failure of labor induction attempts

Question 663

Which of the following side effects is **not** generally seen with tricyclic antidepressants?

(A) Blurry vision when reading
(B) Lowering of the seizure threshold
(C) Sedation
(D) Orthostatic hypotension
(E) Bradycardia

Question 664

A 47-year-old woman comes to the office complaining of being tired all the time. She claims to have insomnia, poor appetite, random crying spells, and weight loss over the last 3 months. She has quit her job because she feels unable to concentrate and mentions that the world probably would be better off without her. Physical examination is within normal limits other than a restricted, depressed affect. Which of the following is true concerning the most likely diagnosis?

(A) It is more common in men than women
(B) The best treatment is psychotherapy
(C) The condition may be caused by cancer
(D) If changed, the appetite always is decreased, but appetite may be normal
(E) The presence of hallucinations would rule out this disorder

Question 665

Which patient is at the greatest risk for committing suicide?

(A) A 16-year-old girl who is mad at her parents and just broke up with her boyfriend
(B) A 32-year-old man who was just denied a promotion at work and is contemplating a divorce
(C) A 33-year-old married woman with two children who was just diagnosed with terminal cancer
(D) A 46-year-old woman with no psychiatric history whose husband just died
(E) A 72-year-old male widower suffering from depression, alcoholism and debilitating arthritis

Question 666

A city being studied has a population of 100,000. Using culture as the gold standard test, 5000 people in the city are found to have chlamydial infection. A new DNA probe chlamydial test is positive on 4000 people in the city, of whom only 3000 tested positive by culture. What is the positive predictive value of the new DNA probe test?

(A) 50%
(B) 60%
(C) 75%
(D) 80%
(E) > 95%

Question 667

An 83-year-old woman is killed in a car accident. Before her death, she suffered from progressively worsening memory loss and behavioral changes over several years for which she never sought medical treatment. At autopsy, her brain had prominent cortical atrophy with neuorfibrillary tangles and amyloid deposition.

Which of the following is **false** regarding the most likely neurologic disorder that affected this woman?

(A) It typically occurs in the elderly
(B) Neurofibrillary tangles and amyloid deposition are typically seen
(C) Recent memory is characteristically spared
(D) Gradual progression is the norm
(E) None of the above

Question 668

Which of the following is **not** a normal change in sexual functioning in the elderly?

(A) Lack of sexual desire
(B) Increased time before erection can be achieved after an orgasm in men
(C) Decreased vaginal lubrication in women
(D) Delayed orgasm
(E) Increased time to achieve an erection in men

Question 669

A 46-year-old man is brought to the emergency department because of a severe headache and subsequently loses consciousness after his eyes roll back into his head, developing clonic muscle contractions and urinating in his pants. Which of the following is correct?

(A) Malingering is likely
(B) The patient should be placed flat on his back
(C) The seizure is likely to stop on its own
(D) A finger should be inserted into the mouth to straighten the tongue
(E) Death occurs mainly as a result of primary brain damage from the seizure activity

Question 670

Which of the following is **least** likely to be associated with a peripheral neuropathy?

(A) Vitamin B_1 (thiamine)
(B) Lead
(C) Vitamin B_6 (pyridoxine)
(D) Folate
(E) Guillain-Barré syndrome

Question 671

Which of the following is true regarding clinical findings with cranial nerve lesions?

(A) With a hypoglossal nerve lesion, the tongue deviates to the side opposite the lesion.
(B) With a spinal accessory nerve lesion, a person has trouble turning the head to the same side as the lesion.
(C) Benign causes of an oculomotor nerve lesion usually do not affect the pupil.
(D) With a vestibulocochlear nerve lesion, hyperacusis usually occurs.
(E) A facial nerve lesion can be designated as an upper or lower motor neuron lesion based on whether or not the facial weakness is bilateral.

Question 672

A 19-year-old man comes to the office complaining of "zits." Over most of his face, he has comedones, papules, pustules, inflamed nodules, and inflammatory skin changes including some scarring. Which of the following is true?

(A) The patient should decrease the amount of sweet and salty food he eats.
(B) The patient should exercise to help reduce the number of lesions.
(C) The agent of choice in this setting is oral isotretinoin.
(D) This condition is thought to be caused partially by bacteria.
(E) Excessive masturbation often is associated with this condition.

Question 673

A 2-month-old infant is brought in by his mother because of "white stuff" in his mouth. Creamy white patches are seen on the tongue and buccal mucosa, and thrush is suspected. Which of the following is most likely to be true if thrush is the diagnosis?

(A) The mother has a sexually transmitted disease
(B) Antibiotic prophylaxis should be given to close contacts of the infant.
(C) You should be able to scrape the white patches off.
(D) Oral griseofulvin is a potential treatment option.
(E) The cause is usually *Trichophyton rubrum*.

Question 674

A patient with severe, widespread second-degree burns develops a fever and has what appears to be some bluish-colored pus with a fruity aroma present on the burned skin. What is the most likely organism?

(A) *Staphylococcus aureus*
(B) *Streptococcus* species
(C) *Pseudomonas* species
(D) *Staphylococcus epidermidis*
(E) *Corynebacterium* species

Question 675

A 49-year-old, otherwise healthy woman develops severe diarrhea and fever approximately 1 week after receiving oral amoxicillin for a sore throat. Assuming the two events are related, which of the following is likely to be true?

(A) She has developed poststreptococcal diarrhea
(B) She was misdiagnosed and has end-stage HIV infection (AIDS)
(C) She has an Epstein-Barr virus infection
(D) Sigmoidoscopy would show pseudomembranes
(E) Clindamycin is the treatment of choice

Question 676

A patient presents to the emergency department with severe nausea and vomiting that started roughly 4 hours after eating reheated leftover fried rice from her favorite Chinese restaurant. She felt completely normal before eating the rice. What is the most likely cause of her symptoms?

(A) Hepatitis A
(B) *Bacillus cereus*
(C) *Salmonella*
(D) Norwalk virus
(E) *Escherichia coli*

Question 677

Which exposure or history is **least** associated with an increased risk of bladder cancer?

(A) *Schistosoma haematobium* infection
(B) Smoking
(C) Aniline dye exposure
(D) Chronic alcoholism
(E) Chronic cyclophosphamide abuse

Question 678

What is the most likely cause of gastroenteritis in a young child?

(A) *Campylobacter*
(B) *Shigella*
(C) Virus
(D) *Salmonella*
(E) *Escherichia*

Question 679

A 63-year-old smoker presents with seizures, and CT scan reveals a 2-cm mass in the right parietal lobe. What is the most likely primary tumor?

(A) Meningioma
(B) Oligodendroglioma
(C) Choroid plexus papilloma
(D) Astrocytoma
(E) Acoustic neuroma

Question 680

Which of the following is true concerning reduction of disease incidence?

(A) Birth control pills can lower the risk of endometrial cancer.
(B) Maternal folate can lower the risk of having a child affected by Down syndrome.
(C) A thin body habitus protects against the development of osteoporosis.
(D) Early surgical correction of cryptorchidism with orchiopexy eliminates the increased testicular cancer risk seen in infants with cryptorchidism.
(E) Having several children decreases the risk of cervical cancer.

Question 681

Which of the following is thought to have the most significant influence on cervical cancer risk?

(A) High socioeconomic status
(B) Age greater than 70
(C) Alcohol abuse
(D) Nulliparity
(E) Sexual promiscuity

Question 682

A 67-year-old man presents with the sudden onset of blindness in the right eye. He has no pain. Visual acuity is 20/30 in the left eye and light perception only in the right eye. Funduscopic examination reveals the following appearance of the fundus:

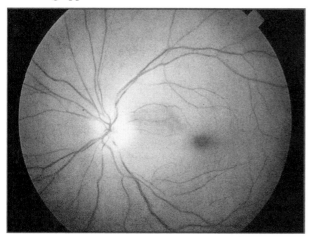

What is the most likely diagnosis?

(A) Central retinal artery occlusion
(B) Central retinal vein occlusion
(C) Retinal detachment
(D) Papilledema
(E) Acute glaucoma

Question 683

A mother brings in her neonate 3 days after birth because of red eyes that started 1 day ago. The infant was noted to have a normal ocular appearance during a routine neonatal nursery examination an hour after birth. The child has a copious purulent discharge bilaterally and significant conjunctival injection. What is the most likely diagnosis?

(A) Chemical conjunctivitis
(B) Chlamydial conjunctivitis
(C) Gonococcal conjunctivitis
(D) Viral conjunctivitis
(E) Allergic conjunctivitis

Question 684

What is the preferred surgical procedure to correct severe gastroesophageal reflux that fails multiple attempts at medical therapy?

(A) Vagotomy
(B) Vagotomy with proximal antrectomy
(C) Partial esophagectomy
(D) Myotomy
(E) Nissen fundoplication

Question 685

Which of the following is **least** correct regarding necrotizing enterocolitis in infants?

(A) It is most likely in premature infants.
(B) The risk is increased in low birth weight infants.
(C) The incidence is highest in infants aged 3 to 5 months.
(D) Pneumatosis intestinalis is one of its features that can be detected on x-ray
(E) It may cause shock and death.

Question 686

A 62-year-old heavy smoker with long-standing emphysema presents to the emergency department with increased shortness of breath and a change in his chronic cough. He relates several stories of how he has survived many bad exacerbations of his disease and seems to be in good spirits. His respiratory rate is 22 breaths/min and he is afebrile. Arterial blood gases reveal the following:

pH	7.33 (normal = 7.35–7.45)
PaO$_2$	54 (normal = 85–100)
PaCO$_2$	55 (normal = 35–45)
HCO$_3$	38 (normal = 24–28)

Which of the following is the next appropriate step?

(A) Immediate intubation with hyperventilation
(B) Immediate intubation with a regular respiratory rate
(C) Immediate intubation with high positive end-expiratory pressure
(D) Administration of oxygen via nasal cannula
(E) Starting broad-spectrum antibiotics

Question 687

A 47-year-old man has a myocardial infarction and is admitted to the ICU. He is currently asymptomatic after morphine and nitroglycerin are administered but has occasional, single premature ventricular complexes once or twice per minute on the rhythm strip. What is the best strategy to manage the premature ventricular complexes in this setting?

(A) Observation
(B) Lidocaine
(C) Amiodarone
(D) Procainamide
(E) Propafenone

Question 688

A 57-year-old obese man with no medical history presents with a long history daytime somnolence and morning headaches. His wife complains that he snores loudly and sometimes seems to stop breathing during the night. On examination, the patient is morbidly obese and has a crowded-appearing pharynx. His lungs are clear to auscultation. His cardiac evaluation reveals a parasternal heave, loud P_2 heart sound, and a right-sided S_4 heart sound. Which of the following conditions is the patient most likely to have?

(A) Narcolepsy
(B) Emphysema
(C) Cor pulmonale
(D) Chronic respiratory alkalosis
(E) Primary pulmonary hypertension

Question 689

Which of the following is **not** a first-line agent in the treatment of mild, stable congestive heart failure?

(A) Beta blockers
(B) Digoxin
(C) Angiotensin-converting enzyme inhibitors
(D) Dietary salt restriction and smoking cessation
(E) Cardiac rehabilitation with a supervised exercise program

Question 690

A 26-year-old gravida 2, para 1, woman at 40 weeks' gestation has been receiving an oxytocin infusion for the past hour because of failure to progress. She begins to develop painful, frequent, and poorly coordinated uterine contractions. Which of the following should be done next?

(A) Perform immediate cesarean section.
(B) Increase the oxytocin infusion rate.
(C) Stop the oxytocin infusion.
(D) Apply prostaglandin E_2 gel.
(E) Administer intravenous 5% dextrose in water.

Question 691

A 31-year-old, sexually active nulliparous woman in excellent health presents with a chief complaint of painful sexual intercourse. She mentions dysmenorrhea with perimenstrual spotting. On examination, the right adnexae is mildly tender to palpation, the uterus is retroverted, and there are nodularities felt in the area of the left uterosacral ligament. Which of the following is true regarding the most likely diagnosis?

(A) The woman is nulliparous because of a chromosomal disorder.
(B) The tumor is likely to have teeth or hair (or both) within it.
(C) Her symptoms are secondary to human papillomavirus.
(D) Laparoscopy is the gold standard for diagnosis.
(E) Most patients are less than 30 years old.

Question 692

Which of the following is **false** concerning *Gardnerella vaginalis*?

(A) Metronidazole is the treatment of choice
(B) Sexual partners need treatment
(C) Potassium hydroxide applied to a sample of the discharge tends to cause a fishy odor
(D) It is associated with clue cells
(E) The discharge tends to be grayish in color and malodorous

Question 693

Which of the following describes syphilis accurately?

(A) The initial lesion is usually a painful genital ulcer.
(B) A maculopapular rash on the palms and soles is nearly pathognomonic of primary syphilis.
(C) The causative agent is a gram-negative coccobacillus.
(D) Tertiary syphilis may result in dementia.
(E) The fluorescent treponemal antibody absorption test (FTA-ABS) is a commonly used screening test for syphilis.

Question 694

A city being studied has a population of 100,000. Using culture as the gold standard test, 5000 people in the city are found to have chlamydial infection. A new DNA probe chlamydial test is positive on 4000 people in the city, of whom only 3000 tested positive by culture. What is the negative predictive value of the new DNA probe test?

(A) 50%
(B) 60%
(C) 75%
(D) 80%
(E) > 95%

Question 695

A 57-year-old male diabetic who is hypertensive and smokes describes new-onset, poorly localized burning in the chest associated with exertion. What is the most likely cause of the patient's chest pain?

(A) Coronary artery disease or ischemia
(B) Pericarditis
(C) Panic attack
(D) Esophageal motility disorder
(E) Peptic ulcer disease
(F) Gastroesophageal reflux
(G) Pleuritis
(H) Musculoskeletal disorder

Question 696

A 28-year-old woman complains of intermittent, disabling sharp, substernal chest pressure or pain associated with cold beverages. What is the most likely cause of the patient's chest pain?

(A) Coronary artery disease or ischemia
(B) Pericarditis
(C) Panic attack
(D) Esophageal motility disorder
(E) Peptic ulcer disease
(F) Gastroesophageal reflux
(G) Pleuritis
(H) Musculoskeletal disorder

Question 697

A 38-year-old man with no medical problems other than a sore throat 1 week ago and a negative social history describes fairly rapid onset of shortness of breath with minimal exertion and constant, low-grade, sharp substernal chest pain for the past 24 hours. His father died of a heart attack in his late 60s. What is the most likely cause of the patient's chest pain?

(A) Coronary artery disease or ischemia
(B) Pericarditis
(C) Panic attack
(D) Esophageal motility disorder
(E) Peptic ulcer disease
(F) Gastroesophageal reflux
(G) Pleuritis
(H) Musculoskeletal disorder

Question 698

A 42-year-old male coffee drinker with no medical problems describes burning in the chest at night while trying to fall asleep. What is the most likely cause of the patient's chest pain?

(A) Coronary artery disease or ischemia
(B) Pericarditis
(C) Panic attack
(D) Esophageal motility disorder
(E) Peptic ulcer disease
(F) Gastroesophageal reflux
(G) Pleuritis
(H) Musculoskeletal disorder

Question 699

A 62-year-old female smoker with diabetes and strong family history of heart attacks relates shortness of breath when angry associated with a strange "twinge" in her chest. What is the most likely cause of the patient's chest pain?

(A) Coronary artery disease or ischemia
(B) Pericarditis
(C) Panic attack
(D) Esophageal motility disorder
(E) Peptic ulcer disease
(F) Gastroesophageal reflux
(G) Pleuritis
(H) Musculoskeletal disorder

Question 700

A 51-year-old unkempt homeless man presents with severe pruritus. Examination of the skin reveals burrow formation in the finger web spaces, volar surface of the wrist and thighs. A scraping of the contents of a burrow reveals the organism shown below:

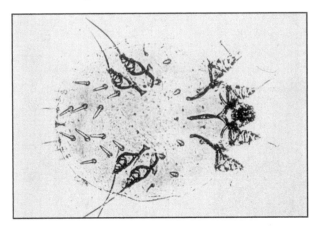

Which of the following is **false** concerning this condition?
(A) It is caused by *Sarcoptes scabei*
(B) Bed sheets and linens should be washed to help prevent recurrence
(C) Treatment of close contacts helps prevent recurrence
(D) Permethrin is an effective treatment
(E) Oral therapy is a required part of successful treatment

BLOCK 14 ANSWER KEY

651. C	661. A	671. C	681. E	691. D
652. A	662. C	672. D	682. A	692. B
653. C	663. E	673. C	683. C	693. D
654. D	664. C	674. C	684. E	694. E
655. D	665. E	675. D	685. C	695. A
656. D	666. C	676. B	686. D	696. D
657. A	667. C	677. D	687. A	697. B
658. A	668. A	678. C	688. C	698. F
659. D	669. C	679. D	689. B	699. A
660. C	670. D	680. A	690. C	700. E

Refer to Answers and Explanations Section for Block 14

Pages 327–335

Figure credits

Question 682: Vander JF, Gault JA (eds): Ophthalmology Secrets. Philadelphia, Hanley & Belfus, 1998.

Question 700: du Vivier A: Infestations of the skin. In du Vivier A (ed): Atlas of Clinical Dermatology, 3rd ed. New York, Churchill Livingstone, 2002, pp 331–341.

50 QUESTIONS

**TIME ALLOWED:
60 MINUTES**

Question 701

A 24-year-old woman comes to the emergency department with suicidal ideation. She claims she was about to jump off a building but decided to come in for help. Her affect is depressed, and she cries frequently and expresses feelings of hopelessness and worthlessness multiple times during the interview. You call the staff psychiatrist for further evaluation. While waiting to be examined by the staff psychiatrist, the patient decides to leave, after saying "it's hopeless anyway." What should you do next?

(A) Let the patient go
(B) Try to talk the patient out of leaving, but if she refuses to stay, you are required by law to let her go
(C) Try to talk the patient out of leaving, but if she refuses to stay, she should be admitted involuntarily
(D) Give the patient an antipsychotic
(E) Prescribe an antidepressant for the patient, and insist that she follow up in 24 hours with the mental health clinic after calling to obtain an appointment for her

Question 702

A father brings in his 2-year-old daughter for cough and fever. The child was well until 2 days ago, when she began to have a runny nose and sore throat and felt warm. This morning, the child developed a brassy cough and hoarseness, so the father brought her in for some antibiotics. On examination, you note mild inspiratory stridor, and the prominent "barking" cough. What is the most likely agent causing the child's symptoms?

(A) Respiratory syncytial virus
(B) Group A streptococcus
(C) *Staphylococcus aureus*
(D) *Bordetella pertussis*
(E) Parainfluenza virus

Question 703

A mother brings her 6-month-old infant to the office for fever and vomiting. The infant was healthy until 3 days ago, when she began having runny nose, irritability, and low-grade fever. The infant now has a temperature of 103.1° F and is tachypneic, tachycardic, hypotensive, and markedly lethargic. On examination, the infant has poor muscle tone and seems unaware of her environment, which the mother says is quite unlike the infant when she is healthy. The infant becomes quite irritable and cries when you shine a penlight to check for pupillary reflex, which seems intact. The pharynx is erythematous. What should you do next?

(A) Perform lumbar puncture and begin antibiotics if the results are suspicious for bacterial infection
(B) Prescribe penicillin and see the infant back in a few days
(C) Establish intravenous access, and begin intravenous fluids and empirical antibiotics
(D) Ask the mother if she may have had a sexually transmitted disease during delivery of the infant
(E) Give prophylactic phenytoin

Question 704

Which of the following is a correct association regarding fetal heart and maternal uterine contraction monitoring?

(A) Late decelerations usually indicate head compression.
(B) Early decelerations usually indicate uteroplacental insufficiency.
(C) Variable decelerations usually indicate cord compression.
(D) Short-term variability is a worrisome pattern on a fetal heart strip.
(E) More than three heart rate cycles per minute when looking at long-term variability on a fetal heart strip is normally an indication to do fetal scalp pH monitoring.

Question 705

Which of the following is **least** likely to result from a pregnancy complicated by diabetes?

(A) Prolonged fetal hyperglycemia postpartum
(B) Fetal macrosomia
(C) Fetal cardiovascular defects
(D) Fetal respiratory distress syndrome
(E) Maternal polyhydramnios

Question 706

Which of the following agents can be used to induce labor?

(A) Prostaglandin E_2
(B) Ritodrine
(C) Oxygen
(D) Intravenous fluids
(E) Indomethacin

Question 707

In an adult who has never had abdominal surgery or significant trauma before, what is the most likely cause of a small bowel obstruction?

(A) Adhesions
(B) Incarcerated hernia
(C) Colonic neoplasm
(D) Malrotation with midgut volvulus
(E) Peritonitis

Question 708

Which of the following is **not** generally used in the management of a small bowel obstruction?

(A) Intravenous fluids
(B) Nasogastric tube
(C) Laparotomy if peritoneal signs develop
(D) Decompression with an endoscope if patient is stable
(E) Asking the patient not to eat or drink anything

Question 709

Which of the following best reflects the prevalence of hemophilia?

(A) Males have a higher prevalence
(B) Females have a higher prevalence
(C) Roughly equal prevalence in both sexes

Question 710

Which of the following best reflects the prevalence of depression?

(A) Males have a higher prevalence
(B) Females have a higher prevalence
(C) Roughly equal prevalence in both sexes

Question 711

Which of the following best reflects the prevalence of Hirschsprung disease?

(A) Males have a higher prevalence
(B) Females have a higher prevalence
(C) Roughly equal prevalence in both sexes

Question 712

Which of the following best reflects the prevalence of schizophrenia?

(A) Males have a higher prevalence
(B) Females have a higher prevalence
(C) Roughly equal prevalence in both sexes

Question 713

Which of the following best reflects the prevalence of alcoholism?

(A) Males have a higher prevalence
(B) Females have a higher prevalence
(C) Roughly equal prevalence in both sexes

Question 714

Which of the following best reflects the prevalence of systemic lupus erythematosus?

(A) Males have a higher prevalence
(B) Females have a higher prevalence
(C) Roughly equal prevalence in both sexes

Question 715

Which of the following best reflects the prevalence of AIDS?

(A) Males have a higher prevalence
(B) Females have a higher prevalence
(C) Roughly equal prevalence in both sexes

Question 716

Which of the following best reflects the prevalence of phenylketonuria?

(A) Males have a higher prevalence
(B) Females have a higher prevalence
(C) Roughly equal prevalence in both sexes

Question 717

A 28-year-old woman develops diarrhea, abdominal bloating, fatigue over months and now has a pruritic skin rash on her elbows (see figure). Stool examination is negative for pathogens and blood, but the fecal fat content is significantly elevated.

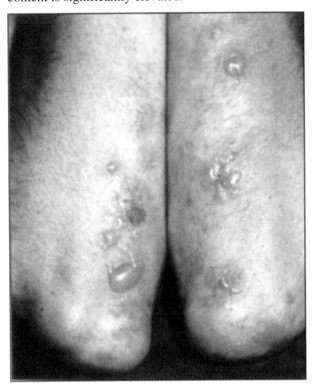

Which of the following is **least** correct regarding the condition responsible for this patient's gastrointestinal and skin complaints?

(A) Small bowel biopsy typically reveals blunting and flattening of mucosal villi, elongated crypts, and an inflammatory infiltrate of the lamina propria

(B) The skin rash is due to a herpes virus infection

(C) The condition increases the risk of small bowel lymphomas

(D) The cause is a dietary intolerance

(E) Human leukocyte antigen (HLA) testing suggests a genetic predisposition

Question 718

A man has thickened, distorted discolored, crumbling toenails with debris under the edges that developed over the past several weeks. The man says the changes are painless. Pulses are normal in both lower extremities, but maceration and scaling is present in the web spaces between the toes, which the patient says is pruritic. The remainder of the physical examination is within normal limits.

What is the most likely etiology for these findings?

(A) Atherosclerotic disease
(B) Venous insufficiency
(C) A fungal infection
(D) A bacterial infection
(E) A malignancy

Question 719

A city being studied has a population of 100,000. Using culture as the gold standard test, 5000 people in the city are found to have chlamydial infection. A new DNA probe chlamydial test is positive on 4000 people in the city, of whom only 3000 tested positive by culture. What is the prevalence of chlamydia in this city?

(A) 4%
(B) 50/1000
(C) 50/10,000
(D) 5/1000
(E) Cannot be calculated from the information given

Question 720

A retired professional boat captain presents with the lesion on his lip shown below. He is a self-proclaimed lover of the outdoors and otherwise healthy.

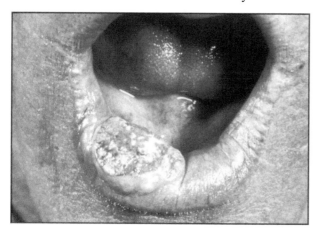

Which of the following is **least** correct regarding the most likely subtype of skin malignancy?

(A) Cumulative ultraviolet light exposure is a risk factor
(B) It is more commonly seen in light-skinned individuals
(C) Affected persons are at increased risk to develop *de novo* skin malignancies later in life
(D) It essentially never metastasizes
(E) Premalignant changes known as actinic keratosis not uncommonly precede this malignancy

Question 721

Which of the following is true regarding headaches?

(A) The most common cause is migraines.
(B) Cluster headaches are so called because they occur primarily at night.
(C) The presence of Kernig's sign should make you consider meningitis.
(D) Auras and family history are common with cluster headaches.
(E) Tension headaches occur mainly in patients with a psychiatric history.

Question 722

Which of the following is useful to distinguish between delirium and dementia?

(A) Presence of hallucinations
(B) Difficulty with orientation
(C) Sundowning (worsening of symptoms at night)
(D) HIV-positive status
(E) Normal arousal and attention level

Question 723

Which of the following is accurate regarding syncope?

(A) The most common cause is cardiac.
(B) The most common cause is infectious.
(C) The most common cause is embolic.
(D) Transient ischemic attacks are unlikely to cause syncope if involving the anterior circulation.
(E) History is generally not useful in determining the cause.

Question 724

A 25-year-old married diabetic woman comes to the office complaining of vaginal itching and a whitish discharge. She was treated 1 week ago for bronchitis with tetracycline. What is the most likely cause of this woman's current complaint?

(A) *Candida*
(B) *Trichomonas*
(C) Gonorrhea
(D) *Chlamydia*
(E) *Gardnerella*

Question 725

A 17-year-old woman complains of abdominal pain over the past week that she describes as dull and fairly constant. She says the pain is aggravated by sexual intercourse. A urine pregnancy test is negative. On examination, the patient has left adnexal tenderness, cervical discharge and pain when the cervix is moved. The patient's temperature is 101.2° F and she has leukocytosis. Which of the following is true regarding the most likely diagnosis?

(A) It is the most common cause of preventable infertility.
(B) It is rarely seen in women unless they use an intrauterine device for birth control.
(C) The bone marrow is infiltrated with immature-appearing cells.
(D) The most common cause is *Staphylococcus aureus*.
(E) Treatment often involves the use of methotrexate.

Question 726

A 25-year-old woman presents with a chief complaint of a rash on her elbows. She has dry, well-circum-scribed, silvery, scaling plaques on the extensor surfaces of both elbows, which are nonpruritic. Her mother had a similar rash when she was younger. Which of the following would **not** increase suspicion of the most likely diagnosis?

(A) Positive family history
(B) Pitting of the fingernails
(C) Black race
(D) Arthritis
(E) The patient's age

Question 727

Which of the following is **least** associated with hirsutism?

(A) Polycystic ovary syndrome
(B) Minoxidil
(C) Cushing syndrome
(D) Chronic liver disease
(E) Cyclosporine

Question 728

Which of the following is true regarding ovarian neo-plasms?

(A) Meigs' syndrome is metastasis of stomach cancer to both ovaries
(B) A Krukenberg tumor is an ovarian fibroma plus ascites and right hydrothorax
(C) Sertoli-Leydig cell tumors cause feminization and precocious puberty
(D) Death from epithelial malignancies is often due to complications of bowel obstruction
(E) Most ovarian malignancies are germ cell tumors

Question 729

A 32-year-old male nurse presents with a chief complaint of intermittent confusion and sweating. He was noted to have passed out on the job 2 days ago after similar symptoms, and a finger-stick at that time revealed a glucose level of 30 mg/dL. He is not diabetic and denies taking insulin. He is dramatic in his description of his symptoms but denies weight loss or other problems on review of systems. He begins to feel confused in front of you, and you draw some stat laboratory tests as a nurse gives the patient some fruit juice, which makes him feel better. The laboratory tests reveal the following:

Hemoglobin	16 gm/dL
White blood cell count	7800/μL
Glucose	36 mg/dL
C-peptide	Elevated
Sulfonylurea level	Undetectable
Insulin level	Elevated
Lactate level	Normal
Ketones, serum	Normal

What is the most likely diagnosis?

(A) Factitious disorder
(B) Surreptitious ingestion of chlorpropamide
(C) Insulinoma
(D) Glucagonoma
(E) Somatization disorder

Question 730

A 24-year-old woman with a negative review of systems is noted to have anemia on a complete blood count. The peripheral smear shows several spherocytes. The osmotic fragility test is negative, the mean corpuscular volume is within normal limits, the Coombs' test is positive, and the reticulocyte count is elevated. Which of the following is the most likely cause of the patient's anemia?

(A) Hereditary spherocytosis
(B) Hereditary elliptocytosis
(C) Autoimmune hemolysis
(D) Glucose-6-phosphate dehydrogenase deficiency
(E) Menstrual blood loss

Question 731

A 68-year-old, poorly controlled diabetic woman with coexisting hypertension and has chronic renal insufficiency. After severe pneumonia requiring ICU treatment for 2 weeks, the patient's creatinine increases from a baseline of 2.5 mg/dL to 3.5 mg/dL. A month after full recovery from the infection, the patient presents to the office complaining of weakness and fatigue. Examination shows no change from baseline except for mild scleral pallor. Laboratory tests reveal the following:

Hemoglobin	9 mg/dL
Mean corpuscular volume	88 µm/cell
White blood cell count	5000/µL
Reticulocyte count	0.7% (normal = 0.5–2.5)
Coombs' test	Negative
Ferritin	140 ng/mL (normal = 50–300)
Iron-binding capacity	300 µg/dL (normal = 250–410)
Peripheral smear	Within normal limits
Creatinine	3.7 mg/dL (normal = 0.6–1.5)

Which of the following is most likely to correct this patient's anemia?

(A) Iron
(B) Folate
(C) Correction of the underlying chronic inflammatory process
(D) Erythropoietin
(E) Corticosteroids

Question 732

A 32-year-old normally healthy woman has developed gradually worsening fatigue over the last 3 months. Her husband made her come in because he does not think she is her usual energetic self. She denies any other symptoms other than black, tarry stool. On examination, the sclera and mucous membranes are markedly pale, but a full physical examination is otherwise within normal limits. Stool occult blood testing is positive. A colonoscopy is performed and reveals bleeding from a vascular ectasia, which is cauterized. Post-colonoscopy laboratory values, which were stable over the next 40 hours, are shown below:

Hemoglobin	8.1 gm/dL
Mean corpuscular volume	68 µm/cell
White blood cells	7800/µL
Platelet count	520,000/µL
Iron	7 µg/dL (normal = 50–150)
Ferritin	8 ng/mL (normal = 50–300)
Total iron binding capacity	496 µg/dL (normal = 250–410)

What is the next best step in the management of this patient?

(A) Transfuse 2 units of packed red blood cells immediately.
(B) Transfuse 1 unit of packed red blood cells and begin iron therapy.
(C) Give high dose iron for one week
(D) Give oral iron therapy for 3 to 6 months.
(E) Give intravenous iron therapy for 1 week, then oral supplements indefinitely.

Question 733

A 48-year-old woman is treated for a right breast cancer with a modified radical mastectomy and a brief course of traditional chemotherapy for positive lymph nodes. Two years later, she presents with a chief complaint of fatigue, bone pain and weight loss for the past month. Physical examination is within normal limits other than borderline tachycardia. Laboratory tests reveal the following:

Hemoglobin	7.3 gm/dL
Mean corpuscular volume	93 μm/cell
White blood cell count	2900/μL
Platelets	90,000/μL
Reticulocyte count	0.7% (normal = 0.5–2.5)
Peripheral smear	3+ anisocytosis; 3+ poikilocytosis; 2+ nucleated red blood cells; 2+ giant, bizarre-appearing platelets; occasional myelocyte

What is the most likely diagnosis?

(A) Aplastic anemia
(B) Hodgkin lymphoma
(C) Acute lymphoblastic leukemia
(D) Metastatic breast cancer
(E) Folate deficiency

Question 734

A 34-year-old man comes to the emergency department with acute renal failure thought to be due to rhabdomyolysis induced by running a marathon 5 days ago in hot weather. Creatinine is 6.0 mg/dL, BUN is 71 mg/dL, pH is 6.9, and potassium is 8.2 mEq/L. The electrocardiogram shows tall, peaked T waves, widening of the QRS, and loss of P waves. On examination, he has crackles bilaterally up to the midlung fields and is moderately tachypneic with mild respiratory distress. He is given 2 ampules of bicarbonate, and the electrocardiogram remains unchanged. What is the best next step in the management of this patient?

(A) Provide oral potassium binder.
(B) Provide urgent hemodialysis.
(C) Admit for observation and supportive measures.
(D) Establish intravenous access and administer fluids.
(E) Intubate the patient and hyperventilate him.

Question 735

What is the most likely diagnosis in a 48-year-old, previously healthy man who develops a bloody nasal discharge and acute renal failure with a positive cytoplasmic-type antineutrophil cytoplasmic antibody titer?

(A) Poststreptococcal glomerulonephritis
(B) Goodpasture's syndrome
(C) Wegener's granulomatosis
(D) Nephrotic syndrome
(E) Metastatic renal cell carcinoma

Question 736

What is the best thing to do for a patient with renal insufficiency before doing a contrast-enhanced CT scan study of the brain?

(A) Order a skull radiograph.
(B) Administer an antihistamine.
(C) Administer intravenous fluids.
(D) Administer corticosteroids.
(E) Do a skin test to determine allergy to iodine.

Question 737

A 42-year-old woman presents for headaches with no other symptoms and is found to have a blood pressure of 186/108 mmHg. Her blood pressure was normal 6 months ago in the clinic. Physical examination reveals moderate ankle edema bilaterally but is otherwise normal. Laboratory tests reveal the following:

Hemoglobin	14 gm/dL
Mean corpuscular volume	86 μm/cell
Sodium	150 mEq/L
Potassium	2.9 mEq/L
Chloride	115 mEq/L
Renin	Low
Albumin	4.2 g/dL (normal = 3.5–5.0)
Total protein	8.0 g/dL (normal = 6.0–8.4)

What is most likely to be true?

(A) There is an adrenal mass
(B) There is an abdominal bruit present on physical examination.
(C) The patient has congestive heart failure.
(D) The patient has nephrotic syndrome.
(E) The patient is dehydrated.

Question 738

A 39-year-old woman presents with moon facies, fatigue, proximal muscle weakness, new-onset hypertension, and menstrual disturbances. What is the best test to order first?

(A) 24-hour urine for free cortisol
(B) MRI or CT scan of the brain
(C) Random total cortisol level
(D) Skin biopsy
(E) Antinuclear antibody titer

Question 739

Which of the following is **least** likely to be caused by long-term corticosteroid therapy?

(A) Thrombocytopenia
(B) Hirsutism
(C) Depression
(D) Osteoporosis
(E) Proximal muscle weakness

Question 740

A 32-year-old woman has severe, prolonged hypotension associated with postpartum hemorrhage during a cesarean section requiring transfusion of 8 units of blood. Three weeks later, she complains of severe fatigue and inability to breast-feed because of lack of milk flow when her infant attempts to nurse. Laboratory testing reveals undetectable serum thyroid-stimulating hormone level. What diagnosis should be considered?

(A) Sheehan syndrome
(B) Turner syndrome
(C) Noonan syndrome
(D) Postpartum depression
(E) Trousseau syndrome

Question 741

Which of the following findings would you **not** expect to find in Graves' disease?

(A) The thyroid has decreased radioactive iodine uptake on a nuclear scan (*cold* scan).
(B) Nontender goiter
(C) Pretibial myxedema
(D) Thyroid-stimulating antibodies
(E) Lid lag

Question 742

Which of the following is true regarding diarrhea?

(A) Diarrhea in children almost always is due to bacterial gastroenteritis.
(B) Diarrhea resulting from malabsorption often stops if the person stops eating.
(C) The hallmark of giardiasis is sigmoid colon involvement with characteristic inflammation.
(D) White blood cells in the stool usually indicate a secretory diarrhea resulting from bacterial toxins.
(E) Colon cancer does not cause diarrhea.

Question 743

In which of the following causes of a gastrointestinal bleed is the patient most likely to relate a history of pain?

(A) Esophageal varices
(B) Diverticulosis
(C) Vascular ectasia
(D) Internal hemorrhoids
(E) External hemorrhoids

Question 744

Which of the following conditions is most highly associated with achlorhydria?

(A) Gastroesophageal reflux disease
(B) Duodenal ulcer
(C) Zollinger-Ellison syndrome
(D) Pernicious anemia
(E) Achalasia

Question 745

Which of the following is true regarding duodenal peptic ulcers?

(A) Food characteristically makes symptoms worse initially.
(B) This condition most commonly is seen in individuals older than age 70.
(C) Recurrence rates can be reduced by treating *Helicobacter pylori* infection.
(D) The gastric acid secretion is almost always markedly elevated.
(E) They are less common than gastric ulcers.

Question 746

With which of the following conditions is a hiatal hernia most commonly associated?

(A) Gastric ulcer
(B) Duodenal ulcer
(C) Gastroesophageal reflux
(D) Hernia strangulation
(E) Zollinger-Ellison syndrome

Question 747

What is the most likely cause of an exacerbation of congestive heart failure in a previously stable patient?

(A) Medication or diet noncompliance
(B) Myocardial infarction
(C) Anemia
(D) Thyrotoxicosis
(E) Arrhythmia

Question 748

Which of the following symptoms or signs is more suggestive of left-sided heart failure than right-sided heart failure?

(A) Orthopnea
(B) Fatigue
(C) Jugular venous distention
(D) Peripheral edema
(E) Anorexia

Question 749

Which of the following signs or symptoms would be **least** expected with aortic stenosis?

(A) Angina
(B) Murmur radiating into the axilla
(C) Harsh systolic ejection murmur
(D) Left-sided S_3 heart sound
(E) Cardiomegaly

Question 750

A 35-year-old woman with a long-standing history of type I diabetes mellitus presents for a routine eye examination. She has no visual complaints. Dilated funduscopic examination reveals dot-blot hemorrhages, microaneurysms, and yellowish exudates. No macular edema or neovascularization are detected. What is the best treatment for this patient's ocular condition?

(A) Tight blood glucose control with a strict diet, exercise, and insulin regimen
(B) Panretinal photocoagulation
(C) Surgical retinal reattachment
(D) Steroid eye drops
(E) Lumbar puncture to lower cerebrospinal fluid pressure after obtaining a CT or MRI scan of the head to rule out an intracranial mass

BLOCK 15 ANSWER KEY

701. C	711. A	721. C	731. D	741. A
702. E	712. C	722. E	732. D	742. B
703. C	713. A	723. D	733. D	743. E
704. C	714. B	724. A	734. B	744. D
705. A	715. A	725. A	735. C	745. C
706. A	716. C	726. C	736. C	746. C
707. B	717. B	727. D	737. A	747. A
708. D	718. C	728. D	738. A	748. A
709. A	719. B	729. C	739. A	749. B
710. B	720. D	730. C	740. A	750. A

Refer to Answers and Explanations Section for Block 15

Pages 337–344

Figure credits

Question 717: Hoffbrand AV, Pettit JE: Megalolastic anaemias. In Hoffbrand AV, Pettit JE (eds): Color Atlas of Clinical Hematology, 3rd ed. St, Louis, Mosby, 2000, pp 57–70.

Question 720: du Vivier A: Non-melanoma skin cancer. In du Vivier A (ed): Atlas of Clinical Dermatology, 3rd ed. New York, Churchill Livingstone, 2002, pp. 163–200.

ANSWERS
AND
EXPLANATIONS

BLOCK 1

ANSWERS AND EXPLANATIONS

1. The answer is D. *(Medicine—Neurology)*

This patient most likely has narcolepsy, a sleep disorder that causes hypersomnia (i.e., increased sleeping or sleepiness). The disorder usually starts in adolescence or young adulthood. Patients often get sudden sleep attacks that are notable for their almost instantaneous onset of REM sleep (buzz phrase, *decreased REM latency*). These attacks may be dangerous because of the patient's inability to control or predict them, as in automobile accidents or the falling asleep at work described for this patient. Narcoleptic patients may experience **cataplexy**, which is momentary paralysis without loss of consciousness.

As in this patient, sleep paralysis, or inability to move on wakening or just before falling asleep, may occur. *Hypnopompic* (while waking up) and *hypnagogic* (while falling asleep) hallucinations are classically described. Treatment involves the use of stimulant-type drugs, such as modafinil, methylphenidate or dextroamphetamine, to allow daytime functioning. Continuous positive airway pressure breathing devices are used in the treatment of sleep apnea. This condition would be in the differential diagnosis and probably is more common. However, the body habitus (not obese) and description of sudden sleep attacks and "freezing attacks" of sleep paralysis make narcolepsy a better choice. Sleep apnea can occur at any age but is most common in the age 30 to 60 range. Diazepam and nortriptyline have sedative properties and would likely make things worse. Fluoxetine, an antidepressant drug in the serotonin-specific reuptake inhibitor (SSRI) class, may cause insomnia as an untoward effect, but it is not currently used to treat narcolepsy.

2. The answer is B. *(Medicine—Infectious Disease)*

This patient most likely has infectious mononucleosis due to the Epstein-Barr virus (EBV), which always should be in the differential diagnosis with upper respiratory infection symptoms, especially in a young adult. When these patients are given amoxicillin or ampicillin, $\geq 90\%$ develop a rash, usually maculopapular. *Streptococcus pyogenes* is probably more common than EBV infection but should have improved with antibiotics. EBV also may result in splenomegaly; lymphocytosis with toxic lymphocytes seen on peripheral smear; anemia, thrombocytopenia, or both; and hepatitis. Diagnosis is normally with a disposable heterophil-antibody agglutination test (monospot test), although serum heterophil or Epstein-Barr virus-specific antibody titers can be used if necessary. Treatment is supportive, and contact sports probably should be avoided because of the rare complication of splenic rupture when splenomegaly is present. Though an amoxicillin allergy is possible it is not the best answer for two reasons: it does not explain the patient's persistent symptoms and she did not have a problem when she took penicillin in the past.

3. The answer is A. *(Psychiatry—Child and Adolescent)*

Tourette's syndrome is a neurologic disorder that almost always begins before the age of 14, usually in 8- to 10-year-olds. Initial symptoms of facial motor tics (e.g., eye blinking, shoulder shrugging, head shaking, lip smacking) often are followed by more complex symptoms, including vocal tics (barking or grunting noises, throat clearing, short repeated phrases), and as many as one-third of patients develop coprolalia, or intermittent bursts of swearing. This condition tends to be lifelong, with exacerbations and remissions, and if symptoms are severe, antipsychotics (e.g., haloperidol) can be used. Behavioral therapy may be effective and should be tried because long-term therapy with antipsychotics may result in tardive dyskinesia. Fire setting and cruelty to animals should make you think of conduct disorder, the pediatric precursor to antisocial personality disorder. Though bed-wetting and separation anxiety disorder (choice D) are common in pediatric patients, they are often seen in younger children and not specifically related to the given presentation.

4. The answer is E. *(Psychiatry—General)*

This woman is in the midst of a manic episode, giving her a diagnosis of bipolar I disorder. An episode of mania is all that is required to make a diagnosis of bipolar disorder, although episodes of depression often precede or follow episodes of mania (making choice A incorrect). Bipolar disorder is a mood disorder, not a personality disorder, although lithium is a first-line agent in treatment (thus, choice C is incorrect). Symptoms and signs may include abnormally elevated mood, grandiosity, pressured speech, flight of ideas, distractibility, increased goal-directed activity (work or school, social, sexual), *shopping sprees* (a dead giveaway, though my wife doesn't seem to have mania), and marked impairment in social functioning. Roughly 50% of bipolar patients have a first-degree relative affected by a mood disorder, giving bipolar disorder one of the highest levels of genetic association of all psychiatric disorders (choice D is incorrect). In addition to several of the classic manic symptoms, the patient in the question also has impairment in functioning (trouble at work) because of her symptoms, making this mania rather than hypomania.

When symptoms of mania or depression become severe, psychotic symptoms often occur. These symptoms may require hospitalization and treatment with an antipsychotic, such as haloperidol or risperidone, in addition to a mood stabilizer, such as lithium (the gold standard) or valproic acid. Carbamazepine and other antiepileptics, such as gabapentin, are second-line agents. Bipolar II disorder involves hypomania (mild manic symptoms) coexisting with depressive episodes. Buspirone (choice B) is a nonsedating anxiolytic that is useful for generalized anxiety disorder but not effective in the treatment of mania.

5. The answer is E. *(Surgery—Trauma)*

The patient most likely has a pneumothorax that is turning into a tension pneumothorax. In the setting of blunt trauma to the chest, decreased breath sounds with a hyperresonant percussion note on the affected side equals pneumothorax. The development of neck vein distention and worsening shortness of breath most likely indicates the development of a tension pneumothorax. A hemothorax causes decreased breath sounds with a *dull* percussion note. Cardiac tamponade usually occurs after penetrating trauma to the left chest in the area of the heart and does not affect breath sounds normally, although it can result in neck vein distention (treated with pericardiocentesis, choice B). Intubation with positive-pressure ventilation (choice D) often is used with an open pneumothorax, in which a chest wall opening allows air into the thoracic cavity, and with significant pulmonary contusion and/or "flail" chest (multiple contiguous complex rib fractures that result in a section of the chest moving paradoxically during respiration).

Sending this patient for imaging studies in the radiology department (choices A and C) would be dangerous because deterioration already has begun (and radiologists rarely carry stethoscopes). Shock and death can occur without timely treatment in the setting of a tension pneumothorax. Needle thoracentesis, which involves placing a needle through the skin of the anterior or lateral chest wall, causes an audible rush of air and relieves the pneumothorax. A tube thoracostomy (chest tube) should then be placed.

6. The answer is A. *(Surgery—Trauma)*

The most likely diagnosis is cardiac tamponade, which in a trauma setting classically occurs with penetrating trauma to the left chest. Heart sounds often are distant, with normal breath sounds and percussion notes, unless a coexisting pneumothorax or hemothorax is present. Neck vein distention is classic, although it may be absent with marked hypotension. Imaging studies and further tests (choices B, C, and D) are not appropriate for this patient because he is deteriorating. If the patient is stable, echocardiography can be used to confirm the diagnosis before intervention. Treatment involves pericardiocentesis, or aspiration of the pericardial sac using a needle inserted just inferior to the xyphoid process and angled toward the heart. Needle thoracentesis (choice E) is used for pneumothorax or diagnostic pleural effusion, not tamponade.

7. The answer is C. *(Pediatrics—General)*

Greater than 50% of abused or neglected children are born prematurely or with low birth weight. Women are more likely to be the abuser than men (choice D is incorrect), and most abusers were abused themselves as children. The location and pattern of the bruises described would be highly unlikely in the setting of an accidental fall (choice A is incorrect). The interaction between mother and child, in which the child looks to the mother to answer questions, and the child's lack of eye contact would support, rather than go against, a diagnosis of child abuse (choice B is incorrect), though many children are shy in the clinical setting. Proof is not required to report child abuse (choice E is incorrect); rather, reporting is mandatory in the setting of *suspected* child abuse. You are not liable if your suspicion turns out to be false. Notice how in this question, the passage itself is not really needed to answer the question. By reading the question alone, you may have been able to save valuable time.

8. The answer is E. *(Medicine—Cardiology)*

The patient most likely has hypertrophic obstructive cardiomyopathy (HOCM), which often is an autosomal dominant condition (the family history and physical exam findings given in the question are classic). Molecular genetics has revealed multiple genetic abnormalities, including mutations in the genes coding for myosin (most common), troponins, and other cardiac muscle proteins. As a result of impaired left ventricular filling and outflow obstruction, patients often have symptoms with exertion. The usual murmur is a systolic murmur from outflow obstruction, which does not usually radiate. This murmur is increased by actions that decrease venous return (e.g., Valsalva maneuver), which increases the gradient across the obstruction. The S4 heart sound is due to ventricular hypertrophy and noncompliance. Sustained apical impulses are common, as are pulses with a brisk upstroke. The apical impulse and the pulse occasionally show a biphasic pattern, resulting from a *second effort* of the heart to eject blood past the hypertrophied myocardium. The hypertrophy of the left ventricle often is asymmetric, involving the septum to a greater degree than the free wall. Histopathologically, *myocardial fiber disarray* (i.e., disorganized architecture), severe myocyte hypertrophy, and interstitial fibrosis are seen.

Diagnosis may be suggested on an electrocardiogram, which shows left ventricular hypertrophy and deep Q waves in the lateral leads resulting from marked septal hypertrophy. Diagnosis is confirmed by *echocardiography* (choice A), the gold standard test, which shows the asymmetric hypertrophy. Chest radiographs often are normal because the hypertrophy inside the ventricular cavities may not cause cardiac enlargement until late in the course of the disease. Beta blockers (choice C) and centrally acting calcium channel blockers (choice D) are useful to slow down the heart and allow for adequate ventricular filling, which helps to overcome the narrowed outflow tract. These agents may also help control arrhythmias that can develop, in addition to the increasingly liberal use of pacemakers. Myomectomy/myoablation of the thickened septum may be useful in severe cases that are refractory to medical management. Positive inotropes (e.g., digoxin, dobutamine) and preload reducers (e.g., nitrates) should be *avoided* in these patients because they worsen the gradient across the obstruction and cause worsening of symptoms. Antibiotic endocarditis prophylaxis is appropriate for affected patients (choice B is incorrect), although the risk of endocarditis is considered only low to moderate.

9. The answer is B. *(Medicine—Neurology)*

Most intracerebral bleeds secondary to hypertension occur in the basal ganglia. Other common locations are the brain stem (pons most common, medulla rare), thalamus, and cerebellum. Treatment is largely supportive in this setting except for the rare instance of a large bleed that is surgically accessible (usually, a cerebellar bleed).

10. The answer is C. *(Medicine—Infectious Disease)*

In sexually active, promiscuous adults the most likely cause of septic arthritis is *Neisseria gonorrhoeae*. In other adult patients, the most common cause is *Staphylococcus aureus*. This patient should have blood cultures and urethral swabs in addition to joint fluid culture.

11. The answer is D. *(Medicine—Rheumatology)*

One of the hallmarks of osteoarthritis is that it typically lacks the marked inflammation (hot, swollen, erythematous joints) that often is seen in other causes of arthritis. Heberden's nodes are small palpable nodules at the distal interphalangeal joints, and Bouchard's nodes are located at the proximal interphalangeal joints. Bone spurs are typically seen on radiographs with osteoarthritis and are one of its diagnostic hallmarks. Evening or postuse worsening of symptoms is classic (versus morning stiffness with improvement in symptoms after moderate use in rheumatoid arthritis), and the incidence of osteoarthritis increases with age. Treatment is with acetaminophen or NSAIDs/aspirin.

12. The answer is C. *(Medicine—General)*

Allopurinol and probenicid are intended for maintenance of stable, symptom-free gout patients. When given during an acute attack, these agents often can worsen symptoms because a fall in uric acid levels acutely can precipitate more uric acid crystal deposition and inflammation. The other drug therapies (choices A, B and E) are useful during an acute attack of gout. Colchicine and indomethacin are typically used first with success, avoiding the need for corticosteroid injections in those wishing to avoid this invasive treatment. High levels of fluid intake (choice D) help to prevent uric acid kidney stone formation. Salicylates (e.g., aspirin) interfere with uric acid excretion and generally should be avoided in patients with gout. Other nonsteroidal anti-inflammatory agents do not have this property.

13. The answer is D. *(Obstetrics)*

This woman most likely has septic pelvic thrombophlebitis, an uncommon but classic obstetric/gynecologic topic. Her mild uterine tenderness went away; she has no vaginal discharge; and she already has received almost a week of broad-spectrum antibiotics, which should have cured an infection unless an abscess had developed. The negative CT scan rules out an abscess, leaving septic pelvic thrombophlebitis as the most likely diagnosis. Treatment is anticoagulation with heparin, which often eliminates the fever and can clinch the diagnosis retrospectively.

14. The answer is C. *(Medicine—Immunology)*

Immunoglobulin therapy should be avoided in individuals with IgA deficiency because anti-IgA antibodies may be present, causing an allergic reaction. IgA deficiency is the most common immunodeficiency, affecting roughly 1 in 500 people. It commonly leads to recurrent upper respiratory and gastrointestinal infections because IgA normally is secreted to prevent these infections. Although anaphylaxis can occur in anyone for various reasons, there is no reason to suspect any of the other conditions in this situation without a suggestive history.

15. The answer is A. *(Obstetrics)*

Whenever a child weighs more than 4000 gm (approximately 9.5 lb), maternal diabetes should be strongly suspected. Regular prenatal care would have detected the problem early and [hopefully] resulted in better blood glucose control, causing a smaller (i.e., normal) sized infant. There is no reason to suspect preeclampsia (which usually causes low-birth-weight infants and intrauterine growth retardation), Down syndrome, or a small pelvis (most women would have dystocia with an infant of this size). Diets should be avoided in the first 2 years of life to prevent growth abnormalities. At this age, children generally take in only the calories they need to sustain their own growth.

16. The answer is A. *(Pediatrics—Neonates)*

This patient with adrenogenital syndrome may die within the next few hours from adrenal insufficiency if corticosteroids are not administered. Hypertonic saline is inappropriate (choice C); however, intravenous rehydration with normal saline and possibly vasopressors may be required in this setting. The other choices are all reasonable once the child is stable, but the child is currently unstable. The most common form of adrenogenital deficiency is due to 21-hydroxylase deficiency (> 85% of cases), which causes virilization of female children with adrenal insufficiency, present in this case. The hyponatremia, hyperkalemia, hypotension, and tachycardia in the presence of ambiguous genitalia are diagnostic clues. A 24-hour urine study would detect an abnormally elevated level of 17-ketosteroids. Barr body determination would determine the true sex of the child, although the child is likely to be female in this setting. Questions like this can be frustrating because it seems as though there is more than one answer, and there is. But the best "next step," given the child's poor clinical condition, is to give corticosteroids.

17. The answer is C. *(Psychiatry—Child and Adolescent)*

This child has conduct disorder, the precursor to adult antisocial personality disorder, not oppositional defiant disorder. Treatment is generally ineffective, and antipsychotics are not indicated. Persons with antisocial personality disorder are at an increased risk of alcoholism (as are males with alcoholic fathers) and somatization disorders. These patients often are described as manipulative criminals without a conscience, although they can be quite charming when it is in their best interest. Oppositional defiant disorder describes children who rebel against authority but get along with their peers and do not engage in criminal behavior.

18. The answer is D. *(Surgery—General)*

This patient most likely has acute diverticulitis. His symptoms are mild, and he probably could be treated as an outpatient with empiric oral antibiotics (choice E is incorrect), such as ciprofloxacin and metronidazole to cover bowel flora, and a liquid diet that is advanced as tolerated to give the bowel time to quiet down. Colonoscopy (and barium enema) is generally avoided in the setting of suspected acute diverticulitis because of an increased risk of colonic perforation. Colon cancer screening, using a barium enema, flexible sigmoidoscopy, and/or colonoscopy is needed in this patient after the acute illness resolves. Colectomy is used in severe or repetitive cases of diverticulitis refractory to medical therapy and is not indicated in this patient. If intravenous fluids are given, which do not appear to be needed in this case, 5% dextrose in water should not be used (normal saline or $^1/_2$ normal saline would be preferred). Barium enema 2 weeks after symptom resolution can show diverticulosis and help rule out a more serious colon pathology. If diagnostic confirmation of diverticulitis is needed, a CT scan of the abdomen and pelvis with contrast should be ordered.

19. The answer is E. *(Pediatrics—General)*

This infant most likely has infant botulism obtained from ingesting honey. In the infant form of the disease, *Clostridium botulinum* organisms are ingested (usually via honey) and multiply in the gut, while producing toxins. This is slightly different from the adult form, which is due to ingestion of the preformed toxin. Treatment generally is supportive in the infant form, and hospitalization is required because of the possible development of respiratory failure from muscle paralysis.

Werdnig-Hoffmann disease (choice A) and other forms of spinal muscular atrophy tend to cause slowly progressive weakness over months, although symptoms may be present at birth. There is little in the question to suggest neglect, which is unlikely to cause such a dramatic change given normal previous visits. Abuse is a possibility, such as from bilateral subdural hematomas, but is not the best answer. Thyroid deficiency could present with similar physical findings, but the history should be one of gradual onset and slowly progressive symptoms. *Streptococcus* species do not generally produce toxins with primarily neurologic effects.

20. The answer is E. *(Pharmacology)*

Prednisone has multiple harmful effects when used in pharmacologic doses. Prednisone can cause osteoporosis; redistribution of fat with wasting of the extremities, increased abdominal obesity, and increased supraclavicular fat pad size; abdominal striae (as in this patient); hypertension; and worsening of diabetes (or cause diabetes in a susceptible patient). Other effects include an increased tendency toward infection; white cell count derangements; depression, mania, or psychosis; and fatigue and weakness (primarily in the proximal muscles). The risks always must be weighed against the benefits when initiating long-term steroid therapy.

This question highlights the usefulness of one technique of reading questions during examinations. In this question, all of the passage could be skipped except for the last sentence (the actual question), and the question could be answered correctly. Some advocate reading the actual question first, then going back to read the passage. This technique helps you focus on what the question is looking for (and may allow you to skim or skip the passage, as in this example).

21. The answer is C. *(Medicine—General)*

The patient has most likely had a congenital berry aneurysm rupture with resultant subarachnoid hemorrhage. Given the family history of kidney failure in two first-degree relatives, especially in a 36-year-old brother, polycystic kidney disease should be suspected as an underlying cause. In the scenario described, CT scan should be performed to look for subarachnoid blood, which would eliminate the need for a lumbar puncture. The history is not typical for acute bacterial meningitis (choice A). Anticoagulants (choice E) are contraindicated in the setting of a possible intracranial bleed, and carotid disease (especially bilateral) is highly unlikely in a patient this age (plus the symptoms are not typical of carotid occlusive disease). A cardiac source of the patient's symptoms is unlikely, so echocardiography (choice D) is unlikely to be diagnostically useful. Remember that subarachnoid hemorrhage can cause meningeal irritation and neck stiffness just like infectious meningitis.

22. The answer is E. *(Pediatrics—General)*

Although fertility is reduced in women with cystic fibrosis (roughly 50% are fertile) and pregnancy can be hazardous to maternal health, many women with cystic fibrosis have delivered healthy offspring. The infants would be expected to be healthy (unless the father is a carrier for cystic fibrosis), although all offspring would be carriers for cystic fibrosis. Of men with cystic fibrosis, 98% are infertile. Cystic fibrosis is an autosomal recessive condition (choices A and B are incorrect); both mother and father usually are carriers if a child gets the disease. After an affected child from two healthy adults, there is roughly a 25% chance (not 50%) that the next child would have cystic fibrosis. Diagnosis is made presumptively by elevated sodium or chloride in the sweat (not potassium). Genetic studies can be done to confirm the diagnosis and specific mutation type.

23. The answer is C. *(Pediatrics—General)*

The most common respiratory pathogens in cystic fibrosis are *Staphylococcus aureus* and *Pseudomonas aeruginosa*. Average life expectancy is around 30 years. Roughly 85% of patients with cystic fibrosis eventually develop exocrine pancreatic insufficiency. Cor pulmonale, diabetes, portal hypertension/cirrhosis, and bowel obstruction are other sequelae of cystic fibrosis. Meconium ileus in a newborn or rectal prolapse in an infant should make you suspect cystic fibrosis until proved otherwise.

24. The answer is B. *(Gynecology)*

This patient has bacterial vaginosis resulting from *Gardnerella vaginalis* overgrowth. The discharge is classically described as malodorous, thin, gray, and frothy with a positive *whiff test* (worsening odor after adding potassium hydroxide), with the presence of *"clue" cells* (epithelial cells covered by *Gardnerella* coccobacilli, giving them a granular appearance) and little inflammation (few white cells, little to no erythema). This is generally not a sexually transmitted disease (choice C is incorrect) and does not normally lead to pelvic inflammatory disease. The treatment of choice is metronidazole, not tetracycline.

25. The answer is D. *(Medicine—Rheumatology)*

This woman has dermatomyositis, a fairly uncommon connective tissue disease that classically causes proximal muscle weakness and tenderness; elevated creatine kinase levels resulting from muscle destruction; and a rash classically around the eyelids (i.e., heliotrope rash), hands, and elbows (Gottron's sign). Patients are at an increased risk of malignancy, although less than 10% of patients develop one. This patient also has anemia, which is likely anemia of chronic disease. Muscle biopsy is an important part of making the diagnosis because it is almost uniformly abnormal, with degeneration of muscle fibers, inflammation, centralization of nuclei and interstitial fibrosis. Electromyography is usually abnormal as well and classically shows spontaneous fibrillations with sharp waves; bizarre, high-frequency discharges; and small-amplitude, short-duration polyphasic motor unit potentials. A silent myocardial infarction and depression are unlikely as the cause of this woman's symptoms (and wouldn't explain the anemia or eyelid changes), although coexisting depression may worsen fatigue and should be asked about in more detail.

26. The answer is C. *(Medicine—Rheumatology)*

A positive rapid plasma reagin (RPR) or Venereal Disease Research Laboratory (VDRL) test, the nonspecific serum tests for syphilis, not gonorrhea, sometimes can be present in lupus. A positive blood test for gonorrhea would make you more inclined to consider septic arthritis in the differential diagnosis, although this would be an atypical presentation. Procainamide, hydralazine, and isoniazid (used in tuberculosis prophylaxis) are the three classic causes of drug-induced lupus. Alopecia and weight loss also are relatively common with lupus.

27. The answer is A. *(Medicine—General)*

This patient has hemochromatosis, which usually is an autosomal recessive disorder of iron metabolism causing excessive iron absorption and iron overload. This disorder can affect multiple organ systems, including the skin (greyish hue), pancreas (this disorder has been called *bronze diabetes*, and roughly 80% of affected persons develop insulin-requiring diabetes without treatment), liver (hepatitis, cirrhosis and hepatocellular carcinoma), joints (arthritis), heart (congestive failure, arrhythmias), and genitals (testicular atrophy, impotence and loss of libido). Men usually are affected at an earlier age than women, owing to the protective effect of monthly menstrual blood loss in women. Ocular involvement is not common in this disorder. Roughly half of these patients die from the complications of cirrhosis or hepatocellular carcinoma. The mainstay of treatment is phlebotomy to reduce iron stores in the body. Bone marrow transplant would not cure or improve this disorder. Complications that develop (e.g., cirrhosis, diabetes, heart failure) are treated in the same way as in the general population.

28. The answer is A. *(Ophthalmology)*

This patient has developed a right central retinal artery occlusion causing blindness secondary to temporal arteritis with probable coexisting polymyalgia rheumatica. Immediate corticosteroid therapy is indicated with suspicion of temporal arteritis to preserve vision (in this case, to preserve vision in the left eye because the right eye may not regain sight), even before the diagnosis is confirmed with a temporal artery biopsy, the gold standard for diagnosis. Again, more than one answer, but the single best answer for "what to do next" is an important distinction, since this is an ophthalmologic emergency. An ANA titer is not helpful (low sensitivity and nonspecific), and muscle biopsy (as well as electromyography) is normal in polymyalgia rheumatica. The patient's low-grade fever is most likely secondary to the active arteritis, and cultures are not indicated with the given description. Things in the vignette that should raise suspicion of temporal arteritis include age over 50, jaw claudication, scalp tenderness, and a markedly elevated sedimentation rate.

29. The answer is D. *(Medicine—General)*

This patient most likely had a transient ischemic attack secondary to a small cholesterol plaque embolus. He should have a carotid ultrasound (duplex) study to look for carotid artery stenosis; however, the decision whether or not to do a carotid endarterectomy should be withheld pending the results of the study. Carotid endarterectomy is an elective procedure generally reserved for stable patients; additionally, the patient may not have a surgical lesion.

The patient would benefit from being put on aspirin (after a CT scan is done to rule out an intracranial hemorrhage in this setting), a beta blocker (to reduce the incidence of a second heart attack and improve survival), and an angiotensin-converting enzyme inhibitor (to slow progression of nephropathy and neuropathy), if they can be tolerated. This patient needs a fasting lipid profile to determine the need for cholesterol-lowering therapy and should quit smoking. With his multiple atherosclerosis risk factors and clinical evidence of atherosclerosis, this patient needs aggressive medical management (and possible surgical intervention if testing reveals any surgically correctable lesions in the coronary or carotid arteries) to prevent further morbidity and death.

30. The answer is E. *(Ophthalmology)*

This patient has herpes simplex keratitis, which can lead to blindness, and needs an expert involved in her care. Erythromycin drops would not help, and corticosteroids should not be given in this setting because they may make the infection worse. For Step 2 purposes, you generally should avoid giving steroid eye drops to any patient. Referral to an optometrist for glasses is inappropriate because the vision may return to normal once the infection is treated. If any treatment is given before referring the patient to an ophthalmologist, it should be antiviral eye drops, such as idoxuridine or trifluridine. A patch over the eye would not be helpful, although it is useful in UV light-induced keratitis. The photophobia the patient is experiencing may indicate the development of iritis, a complication that can be treated with a cycloplegic agent such as atropine, to reduce discomfort.

31. The answer is A. *(Medicine—General)*

Most patients with cystic fibrosis have malabsorption that can lead to deficiencies of the fat-soluble vitamins (A, D, E, and K) secondary to exocrine pancreatic insufficiency. In the absence of pancreatic enzyme replacement, these vitamins are not absorbed effectively. Although a daily multivitamin may help some, it probably would not be enough in the absence of pancreatic enzyme therapy—usually high-dose supplementation is required. The patient's symptoms and signs are due to vitamin A deficiency (i.e., poor night vision, dry eyes, dry skin), vitamin D deficiency (osteopenia), and vitamin E deficiency (dry skin). The patient is most likely vitamin K deficient as a result of malabsorption and recent broad-spectrum antibiotics and probably has an increased bleeding tendency rather than a hypercoagulable state. There is little in the question that should make you consider psoriasis or the need for further antibiotics (the crackles probably are due to chronic lung scarring).

32. The answer is D. *(Medicine—Gastroenterology)*

This patient has Wilson disease, an autosomal recessive disorder characterized by excessive copper accumulation in the body. Penicillamine is a copper chelator used to treat the disorder. The diagnosis should be suspected because of the findings of liver disease, neurologic and psychiatric abnormalities, and a low level of ceruloplasmin. This patient undoubtedly has a Kayser-Fleischer ring around her corneas, which is virtually pathognomonic of Wilson disease. Iron therapy is not used, although zinc therapy may be helpful in patients who cannot tolerate penicillamine. It is unlikely that this patient has chronic viral hepatitis (she would not benefit from antiviral therapy), although with a positive surface antibody, she may have been vaccinated in the past (further serology would be needed to determine). In Wilson disease, the serum copper level may be high, low, or normal and is not a reliable test. A low ceruloplasmin level (main condition for which this test is useful, so if it is mentioned, think Wilson disease) is fairly sensitive, however, and a liver biopsy (the confirmatory diagnostic test) should reveal increased levels of hepatic copper stores.

33. The answer is A. (Dermatology)

A port-wine stain (nevus flammeus) is a permanent vascular malformation that results in a purple patch. When this abnormality occurs in the distribution of the trigeminal nerve, there is an association with the Sturge-Weber syndrome (encephalotrigeminal angiomatosis), one of the neurocutaneous syndromes (like tuberous sclerosis, von Hippel-Lindau syndrome, neurofibromatosis and ataxia-telangiectasia). Sturge-Weber syndrome consists of a port-wine stain in the trigeminal nerve distribution, ipsilateral meningeal angiomas (causes intracranial calcifications and commonly results in seizures), and angiomas of the choroid of the eye (may cause glaucoma). There is no cure. Tuberous sclerosis causes facial angiofibromas (adenoma sebaceum), which can resemble acne.

34. The answer is E. (Surgery—Vascular)

When considering deep venous thrombosis risk factors, it is helpful to remember *Virchow's triad* of venous stasis, endothelial damage, and hypercoagulable state. Causes of venous stasis include severe heart failure and immobilization. Causes of endothelial damage include trauma and hypercoagulable state can result from malignancy and congenital deficiencies that cause an increased tendency to form clots. Hypertension by itself is not thought to increase the likelihood of deep venous thrombosis.

35. The answer is B. (Medicine—General)

The patient shows symptoms and signs of hypocalcemia, which in adults often is from inadvertent surgical removal of the parathyroid glands during thyroid surgery. Trousseau's sign (carpopedal spasm with inflation of a blood pressure cuff) is present, and Chvostek's sign (facial muscle tetany from tapping on the facial nerve) probably could be elicited in this patient. Electrocardiogram normally shows QT interval prolongation in hypocalcemia versus QT interval shortening in hypercalcemia. By causing a respiratory alkalosis, hyperventilation shifts calcium to the intracellular space and may worsen or cause hypocalcemia symptoms and signs. There is little reason to suspect Graves' disease from the history, and corticosteroids are not indicated for hypocalcemia.

36. The answer is A. (Preventive Medicine)

This is one of those frustrating questions that can appear on Step 2, in which you think you know what the patient has, but the answer has nothing to do with the patient's condition. This question tests your ability to read quickly, avoid overaggressive interventions, and avoid missing an opportunity for preventive health maintenance. The patient has carpal tunnel syndrome. Choice A is correct because the patient needs colon cancer screening and the other choices are inappropriate. Carpal tunnel syndrome should always be treated conservatively first with wrist splints, nonsteroidal anti-inflammatory drugs, and rest. You would not refer a patient for bilateral wrist surgery without confirming the diagnosis with a nerve conduction study or electromyography and first treating conservatively.

An MRI of the brain is not indicated, although acromegaly (usually due to a pituitary adenoma) occasionally can cause carpal tunnel syndrome. Vasoactive intestinal peptide levels can be elevated in a rare pancreatic islet cell tumor known as a VIPoma, which primarily causes refractory diarrhea, not carpal tunnel syndrome. No symptoms or signs of gout are mentioned, thus allopurinol is not indicated.

37. The answer is A. (Surgery—General)

The patient has a classic history for appendicitis. Rovsing's sign is elicited by pressing on the left lower quadrant. A positive sign is present if the patient feels referred pain at McBurney's point in the right lower quadrant. Trousseau's sign is carpopedal spasm from a blood pressure cuff or tourniquet in hypocalcemia (different from Trousseau syndrome, which describes migratory thrombophlebitis secondary to visceral malignancy). Kernig's sign is positive in meningitis if a patient resists knee extension when the thigh is flexed. Murphy's sign is seen in cholecystitis and is inspiratory arrest that occurs if a hand palpates under the right rib cage. Grey Turner's sign is bluish discoloration of the flank from retroperitoneal hemorrhage (e.g., severe pancreatitis).

38. The answer is A. *(Urology)*

This patient most likely has a testicular torsion, a surgical emergency. In this condition, the sooner surgery is performed, the more likely it is that the testicle can be salvaged. Delay in surgery could result in testicular infarction. Prehn's sign is mentioned in the question, which entails elevating the testicle to see if pain is relieved. Pain often is relieved (positive sign) if the patient has epididymitis, the primary differential diagnosis in a case such as this, whereas the pain does not improve after this maneuver in testicular torsion. Scrotal ultrasound, when readily available, is used to confirm the diagnosis prior to surgical intervention and can also make the diagnosis of epididymitis and orchitis, the two primary differential considerations (both more common than torsion)

Epididymitis has a more gradual in onset and often is associated with urinary tract or urethritis symptoms. It also tends to be more common in men older than age 30, whereas torsion is more common in men younger than age 20. Laparotomy is not indicated; rather, local scrotal exploration with orchiopexy of *both* testicles to reduce the chance of a further episode of torsion is indicated if torsion is confirmed by ultrasound (or ultrasound is not available). Although mumps can cause orchitis, there is no suggestive history, and this condition is rare in the United States because of mandatory vaccination.

39–41. *(Obstetrics)*

The answers are the following: 39. I   40. J   41. E.

Many of the normal physiology changes in pregnancy become pronounced in the second trimester. The following are common laboratory test changes: erythrocyte sedimentation rate is markedly elevated (worthless test in pregnancy); thyroxine and thyroid-binding globulin increase (but free thyroxine is normal); hemoglobin increases, but plasma volume increases more so that the net result is a decreased hematocrit and hemoglobin. BUN and creatinine decrease, whereas the glomerular filtration rate increases (the high end of normal range for BUN and creatinine indicates renal disease in pregnancy). The alkaline phosphatase level increases markedly because of placental production. Mild proteinuria and glycosuria are normal in pregnancy. Electrolytes (e.g., sodium) and liver transaminases remain normal.

Cardiovascular changes include a slight decrease in blood pressure as well as a heart rate increase of 10 to 20 beats/min and stroke volume increase, which leads to a cardiac output increase of up to 50%. Pulmonary changes include increased minute ventilation due increased tidal volume with the same or only slightly increased respiratory rate, which leads to decreased CO_2. These changes together are result in physiologic hyperventilation and respiratory alkalosis, and are normal. The residual volume also decreases, in part due to a growing intraabdominal mass (i.e., fetus).

42–43. *(Psychiatry—General)*

The answers are the following: 42. G   43. I.

The factors associated with a good prognosis in schizophrenia include good premorbid functioning (most important), late onset, obvious precipitating factors, married, family history of mood disorders, positive symptoms, and a good support system. The factors associated with a poor prognosis in schizophrenia include poor premorbid functioning (most important); early onset; no precipitating factors; single, divorced, or widowed; family history of schizophrenia; negative symptoms; and poor support system.

44. The answer is A. *(Gynecology)*

This patient has multiple uterine leiomyomas, also known as fibroids or a fibroid uterus. These benign smooth muscle tumors are the most common neoplasms in women, with up to 20% of women harboring one or more fibroids by the age of 40, the large majority of which are asymptomatic. The malignant potential is less than 1% and some believe it is nonexistent. The size and location of these tumors generally determine whether or not they are symptomatic. Fibroids are classified by where in the myometrium they are located: submucosal (just beneath the endometrium, may protrude through the endometrium and into the endometrial canal in some cases), intramural (centered in the myometrium, as in the question figure), and subserosal, which describes tumors that arise near or from the outer surface of the uterine myometrium (may be exophytic and pedunculated). Submucosal fibroids are most likely to cause menstrual disturbances, because they can cause thinning and ulceration of the overlying endometrium due to pressure necrosis, whereas subserosal fibroids would be the least likely to cause such disturbances. A lower uterine or cervical fibroid can complicate pregnancy by obstructing the birth canal. The sheer size of fibroids can also cause symptoms–gynecologists all have their personal "whopper" stories (basketball-size tumors are not rare).

Fibroids are the most common indication for hysterectomy (the most common major surgery in women) and many are hormonally responsive, thus they may rapidly enlarge during pregnancy or estrogen therapy. Conversely, fibroids typically involute after menopause and often calcify (a characteristic appearance can be seen on plain abdominal or pelvic x-rays). Diagnosis is typically made with ultrasound. Treatment for these tumors is only needed in the setting of significant symptoms (e.g., anemia, chronic pelvic pain, bowel obstruction) or if they are so large they prevent an adequate pelvic exam (may mask ovarian tumors), since they are almost invariably benign. For unknown reasons, African-American women have an increased incidence and growth rate compared to white women.

45. The answer is E. *(Surgery—Vascular)*

The patient developed acute aortic dissection, which led to his presenting symptoms, widenened mediastinum on chest x-ray, and death (choice C is incorrect). In aortic dissection, which is strongly associated with hypertension (at least two-thirds of cases), blood (labeled "H" in the figure) breaks through the intima (labeled "In") and typically splits the media (labeled "M"; "A" labels the adventitia). Further downstream in the aorta, the dissection usually breaks back through the media and intima, establishing two vascular channels that blood can flow through (the "true"/original and "false"/new lumen). Marfan and Ehlers-Danlos syndrome are unusual (though classic) causes of aortic dissection (choice A is incorrect), in which case the dissection tends to affect younger adults and is often unassociated with hypertension. Though a DeBakey classification exists, the Stanford classification of aortic dissection is easier and more practical to use. Stanford type "A" dissections involve the ascending aorta or arch (begin proximal to the origin of the left subclavian artery) and have a very high mortality rate (> 50%); thus they are generally treated with immediate surgical repair. Standford type "B" aortic dissections begin distal to the left subclavian artery origin in the descending thoracic aorta and have a much lower mortality rate (roughly 10%); thus they are generally treated medically. In a recent series, roughly two-thirds of cases were type A and one-third were type B (choice D is incorrect). Roughly two-thirds of cases occur in men (choice B is incorrect).

Death can be due to aortic rupture, ischemia from retrograde or antegrade extension of the dissection to involve critical branches of the aorta (e.g., coronary, carotid, renal, and/or mesenteric arteries), or extension into the aortic root with resultant hemorrhage into the pericardial sac and cardiac tamponade.

46–50. *(Medicine—Oncology)*

The answers are the following: 46. B   47. F   48. E   49. B   50. C.

The discovery that environmental agents can lead to cancer is an important one, as it allows preventative measures to be employed. For example, abstinence (as well as condom use and monogamy) can reduce the incidence of cervical cancer and the hepatitis B virus vaccine and avoidance of alcohol and intravenous drug use can reduce the incidence of hepatocellular carcinoma. The following table includes the major currently known infectious etiologies of human malignancy (other viruses have been implicated in animals but are not included):

Agent	Associated Malignancies
Epstein-Barr virus	Nasopharyngeal carcinoma, African Burkitt lymphoma, lymphoproliferative disorder
Hepatitis B and C viruses	Hepatocellular carcinoma
Human herpesvirus 8	Kaposi's sarcoma
Human papillomavirus	Anal, cervical, and penile cancer

ANSWERS AND EXPLANATIONS

51. The answer is A. *(Surgery—Vascular)*

This patient has Leriche syndrome—buttock atrophy and claudication with impotence that are seen with aortoiliac occlusive disease due to atherosclerosis. Nonpalpable pedal and popliteal pulses and cool, shiny, hairless skin are other clues to the presence of significant atherosclerosis. Psychogenic causes are unlikely when erections cannot be achieved in any setting and there are no clues to suggest anxiety. Alcoholism is a possibility, but there are no clues that would make you choose this answer over atherosclerotic disease (which does have supportive clues). The patient has no symptoms of heart failure. Depression is a possibility, but there are no clues to its presence. Medications, especially those used to treat hypertension and depression, are notorious causes of sexual dysfunction and should be asked about in any patient with complaints of sexual dysfunction.

52. The answer is B. *(Surgery—Trauma)*

This child most likely has suffered a splenic injury/rupture, given her history of blunt abdominal trauma, left upper quadrant tenderness, referred pain to the left shoulder (Kehr's sign), and hemodynamic instability. Transfusion is indicated, but type O *negative* (positive may cause a reaction in the absence of known blood type information) blood should be used in this scenario, and this is only a temporizing measure until the patient can be transported to the operating room. Waiting for laboratory test results is not appropriate because the patient may die. Also, with acute hemorrhage, the hemoglobin and hematocrit may be normal until re-equilibration has occurred (may take 4–12 hours). The patient has not had a cardiac or respiratory arrest, so CPR is not indicated. The patient is having an obvious change in mental status, and any result from a mini-mental status examination would not change management at this time.

53. The answer is B. *(Medicine—General)*

This patient likely has a deep venous thrombosis (DVT), most likely in the thigh and possibly the calf. Women taking birth control pills have an increased tendency toward thrombosis, especially if they are older than 35 and smoke. Women who are older than age 35 should not be offered birth control pills if they smoke because of the markedly increased incidence of thrombosis, myocardial infarction, and death. Additionally, since a DVT has developed while the patient is on oral contraceptives, these will need to be stopped. Although venography is the gold standard for the diagnosis of DVT, it is invasive and should be reserved for cases in which the diagnosis is not clear. The DVT probably begins above the level of the calf because the thigh is swollen (and may be exclusively in the thigh), so a calf vein study would not be an adequate exam.

The diagnostic test of choice is a venous ultrasound or duplex scan because it is noninvasive and easier to perform. Although cellulitis would be in the differential diagnosis of an edematous, erythematous, painful leg, the history is much more suggestive of a DVT (long plane ride promoting venous stasis, birth control pills in a female smoker > 35 years old). Homan's sign, which was performed in the question and was negative, is a notoriously unreliable sign of DVT and is present in only about one third of cases. Treatment of DVT involves anticoagulation with some form of heparin, then crossover to warfarin for at least 3–6 months.

54. The answer is C. *(Neurosurgery)*

This patient is displaying the **Cushing reflex**, which occurs with markedly increased intracranial pressure, secondary to head trauma and probable delayed cerebral edema, hemorrhage, or both. The reflex consists of a triad including elevated blood pressure, bradycardia, and irregular respirations and indicates life-threatening levels of intracranial hypertension. There is no reason to suspect infection because the patient had a closed head injury and is afebrile. Hypoxia always is a possibility with acute delirium, but you would expect the patient to be breathing hard and fast consistently to improve oxygenation, and hypoxia would not explain the marked increase in blood pressure. Acute cocaine withdrawal, although it may cause delirium, does not present in this fashion. Intensive care unit delirium is a well-known phenomenon but is not enough to explain the blood pressure and irregular respirations. This patient needs prompt intubation and neurosurgical evaluation. Forced hyperventilation can lessen intracranial pressure temporarily; mannitol or furosemide can be used as well. A craniotomy may be required in severe cases.

55. The answer is B. *(Medicine—General)*

A smoker older than age 50 with painless jaundice, unexplained weight loss, depression, and a positive **Courvoisier's sign** (a palpable distended gallbladder) is considered to have pancreatic cancer until proved otherwise. In this scenario, the cancer invades and blocks the bile duct, causing the gallbladder to distend and the direct bilirubin to rise because it is blocked from being excreted. Lung cancer is theoretically possible with an occult small cell cancer and early metastases, but less likely, as this presentation would be very atypical for lung cancer (e.g., absence of pulmonary symptoms, bile duct blockage as the first indication of metastatic disease).

Hemochromatosis has a gradual, slow progression, and there were no clues to the presence of cirrhosis in the question (the spleen was not enlarged and no sequelae of portal hypertension were mentioned, liver exam was within normal limits). Primary sclerosing cholangitis tends to occur in younger people with inflammatory bowel disease (about half of cases are associated with IBD, typically ulcerative colitis) and tends to cause pruritus. Primary malignant bone tumors are unusual in adults and would tend to produce local bone symptoms. Do not let the alkaline phosphatase elevation fool you (can be elevated in bone disease or bile duct disease) because the elevated 5'-nucleotidase confirms that the origin of the alkaline phosphatase is bile duct pathology.

56. The answer is A. *(Surgery—General)*

The patient has a history of biliary colic and **Charcot's triad** of cholangitis—right upper quadrant pain, fever with chills, and jaundice. The dilated bile duct and gallstones on ultrasound are consistent with the diagnosis. Ultrasound is not accurate at visualizing stones within the common duct, so this finding should not steer you away from the diagnosis of choledocholithiasis (stone in the common bile duct).

Initial management of cholangitis should include intravenous fluids and antibiotics until the patient is stable. This woman shows possible signs of early septic shock (warm flushed skin, low-normal blood pressure in a woman that is normally hypertensive, and tachycardia), and blood cultures ideally should be drawn before antibiotics are started. CT scan and repeat blood cell counts are unnecessary tests at this point, and administering bile salts to dissolve stones is not done in the setting of acute cholangitis. Patients should be stabilized (i.e., infection controlled and blood pressure normalized) in this setting before surgical intervention is pursued. Once stable, surgery and/or endoscopic retrograde cholangiopancreatography with stone removal are reasonable therapeutic options.

57. The answer is A. *(Pediatrics—Neonates)*

This child has Down syndrome, with characteristic physical findings at birth, including **Brushfield's spots** in the eye. The karyotype normally involves trisomy 21, although other variants (e.g., translocations) may occur. Down syndrome becomes more common with an increasing age of the mother. Although the overall risk of having a child with Down syndrome is approximately 1/700, a woman at the age of 46 has a risk of roughly 1/20. Affected individuals have a markedly increased risk of leukemia, congenital heart defects (e.g., ventricular septal defects), and Alzheimer disease (if they survive to adulthood). There is no strong association with renal disease, and the average IQ of individuals with Down syndrome is around 50 (moderate mental retardation).

58. The answer is D. *(Pediatrics—Adolescent)*

Transient gynecomastia, which may involve tenderness, is normal during puberty. Reassurance is all that is needed. If you are going into plastic surgery, you may argue that **E** is correct, but for board purposes, do not encourage cosmetic surgery, especially in a condition likely to resolve on its own. Endocrine disorders are rare as causes of gynecomastia, and there are no other symptoms to steer you toward these *zebra* diagnoses. For those not familiar with the term *zebra*, it relates to the following medical wisdom: "When you hear the sound of hooves, think of horses, not zebras." Horses, or common diagnoses, are much more common than zebras, or rare diagnoses.

59. The answer is B. *(Medicine—General)*

This is a simple problem of mechanics. When an area of skin has pressure on it for too long, the skin begins to break down. Prophylactic antibiotics, artificial skin, hyperalimentation, and daily multivitamins are not effective measures. Early detection and application of artificial skin to erythematous areas may help slow progression of a decubitus ulcer, but the pressure must be taken off the skin. Special airflow mattresses are also available and help to prevent decubitus ulcers by automatically varying the pressure points.

60. The answer is B. (Pediatrics—General)

This infant has fetal alcohol syndrome with most of its classic manifestations, not any chromosomal abnormalities. He probably will never catch up to his peers in terms of mental development and probably is mentally retarded. Fetal alcohol syndrome is the most common cause of preventable mental retardation. No alcohol is good alcohol during pregnancy.

61-66. (Medicine—Infectious Disease)

The answers are the following: 61. A   62. A   63. A   64. D   65. A   66. F.

Chlamydia trachomatis has multiple serotypes. Serotypes A–C cause trachoma, a leading cause of blindness in developing countries. Serotypes D–K cause urethritis, pelvic inflammatory disease, and neonatal conjunctivitis in infants born to infected mothers. Serotypes L1 and L2 cause lymphogranuloma venereum, a sexually transmitted disease seen mostly in tropical areas that classically causes suppuration of inguinal lymph nodes. *Chlamydia* is the most common cause of pelvic inflammatory disease (PID), though many infections are polymicrobial and co-infection with *Neisseria* and *Chlamydia* are common. Of the three common types of neonatal conjunctivitis (chemical conjunctivitis from prophylactic drops, *Neisseria* and *Chlamydia*), *Chlamydia* characteristically has the latest time of onset, while chemical conjunctivitis almost always develops within the first 24-36 hours after birth (and there is a history of prophylactic eye drop use). Condylomata lata are hypertrophic, flattened papules seen in secondary syphilis, compared with condylomata acuminata, which are cauliflower-like appearing warts seen with human papillomavirus infection. Only *Trichomonas* is treated with metronidazole of the choices listed.

67. The answer is E. (Medicine—Hematology)

Given the child's age, race, family history, and symptoms, sickle cell anemia with dactylitis (*hand-foot* syndrome) as the first manifestation of the disease is the most likely diagnosis. Dactylitis in these cases is thought to be caused directly by sickle cell anemia, not a result of infection. The patient needs to be admitted to the hospital and given intravenous fluids and other supportive care. Although you always should think about child abuse, there is little to support its diagnosis in this case.

68. The answer is B. (Neurosurgery)

The other choices are the four classic signs of basilar skull fracture. Periorbital ecchymosis sometimes is called the *raccoon eyes* sign, and postauricular ecchymosis is sometimes called *Battle's sign*. Scalp ecchymosis may represent an underlying skull fracture of the calvaria, although often it simply represents a bruise or hematoma.

69. The answer is E. (Medicine—Rheumatology)

This patient has osteoarthritis with multiple Heberden's nodes. Because all nonsteroidal anti-inflammatory drugs can precipitate gastrointestinal bleeding, NSAIDs should be avoided in a patient with a history of a severe gastrointestinal bleed. Indomethacin is particular is quite potent and associated with a high incidence of GI complications. Joint aspiration and connective tissue disorder workup probably are not required in this clear-cut case of osteoarthritis. There is no reason to suspect that the patient is HLA-B27 positive. Osteoarthritis is the most common cause of arthritis (> 75% of cases), and its incidence and prevalence increase with age. Cyclooxygenase II selective inhibitors, such as celecoxib and rofecoxib, are a good choice of medication to try in a patient with a history of gastrointestinal bleeding because they seem to cause less GI bleeding and ulceration than older NSAIDs at recommended therapeutic doses, though the difference is not as great as initially believed. The addition of misoprostol to an NSAID regimen can also reduce the GI complication risk.

70. The answer is D. (Medicine—Rheumatology)

This woman most likely has rheumatoid arthritis, and these patients may develop pleuritis or pericarditis. The rheumatoid factor is positive in about 90% of adult patients at some point in time and is more likely positive than not in this woman (pediatric patients are less likely to have a positive rheumatoid factor). Given the multiple joint involvement, time course, and symmetric nature of the process, infection is unlikely. With typical bacterial joint infections (usually *Staphylococcus aureus* or *Neisseria gonorrhoeae* in sexually active younger patients), the neutrophil count is usually at least 75% of the total white blood cell count and gram stain is often positive. *M. tuberculosis* is unlikely in the absence of significant risk factors, has a predilection for the spine, and is most commonly monoarticular. Interestingly, only 50% of patients with tuberculous arthritis have demonstrable pulmonary involvement. Choice **E** describes gout, which this patient also is unlikely to have given her age, sex, and lack of metatarsophalangeal joint involvement in the big toe (i.e., podagra).

71. The answer is A. *(Radiology)*

Approximately 85% of kidney stones are radiopaque compared with only about 15% of gallstones. Free air under the diaphragm indicates the presence of pneumoperitoneum (not pneumothorax) and usually means there has been a perforation in an intraabdominal portion of the gastrointestinal tract. It is also normal to have pneumoperitoneum in the week or so after abdominal surgery. A pneumothorax usually causes collapse of a lung and air above the diaphragm. Loss (not increased conspicuity) of the psoas shadow on the right side may be a sign of appendicitis. Colon cancer, especially when early, usually cannot be seen on a plain radiograph, although the effects of colon cancer may be seen (e.g., bowel obstruction). Air-fluid levels in the small bowel may be normal, but when multiple and associated with abnormal bowel distention, they usually signify a bowel obstruction or an adynamic ileus, not diarrhea.

72. The answer is B. *(Medicine—Hematology)*

This patient has a macrocytic anemia most likely secondary to folate deficiency and alcoholism. Although vitamin B_{12} deficiency is possible, it often produces neurologic deficits, is not usually caused by a nutritional deficiency (the liver typically stores more than 1 year's worth), and is much less common than folate deficiency. The patient's pattern of liver enzyme abnormality, with AST being elevated by a 2:1 ratio over ALT, is consistent with alcohol-induced hepatitis, although a patient such as this is at risk for viral hepatitis, and screening would not be inappropriate. Someone who smells of alcohol and has had back pain for 15 years should not be given narcotics in the emergency room and is unlikely to have metastatic cancer.

73. The answer is A. *(Medicine—Hematology)*

This patient has iron-deficiency anemia, giving her a low iron level, low ferritin, and increased iron-binding capacity. Chronic inflammation (or anemia of chronic disease) tends to cause a decreased iron-binding capacity with a normal or increased ferritin level (an acute-phase reactant), although the iron level often is low. Hemolytic anemias are unlikely without a suggestive history and with a normal haptoglobin (may decrease with intravascular hemolysis), normal lactate dehydrogenase (general marker of cellular destruction), and normal peripheral smear (no schistocytes or bite cells). There is no particular reason to suspect thalassemia with no family history, recent onset of symptoms as an adult, normal peripheral smear, and normal iron levels, although it does cause a microcytic anemia. Anemia is a frustratingly large but high-yield topic and a common clinical problem.

74. The answer is C. *(Ethics)*

A living will should be respected even in the face of family members or others who disagree with it. A competent adult patient can make his or her own decisions and the question doesn't give you enough information to question the patient's competence when the will was drafted. The woman is understandably upset because she does not want to lose her husband. She needs calm reassurance, comforting, and understanding, but the patient's wishes must be respected. It is not necessary to contact an attorney or schedule a family meeting because the living will clearly states the patient's wishes. Being short or refusing to deal with the woman is the easy way out but is not appropriate in this setting. Avoid being rude, short, nasty or condescending to patients or their family members—especially when taking the USMLE!

75. The answer is C. *(Laboratory Medicine)*

There was probably hemolysis of the blood sample resulting in an elevated potassium level, a common laboratory problem. The patient does not appear to have renal or adrenal problems because BUN, creatinine, electrolytes, acid-base status, and electrocardiogram are normal. There is no reason to suspect multiple myeloma. Whenever an elevated potassium level does not make sense clinically, consider hemolysis. For example, it is highly unlikely that a potassium level this high would not cause symptoms or EKG findings. Also, in the absence of symptoms or EKG findings, urgent treatment is not needed. Remember the old clinical adage: "Treat the patient, not the lab value or x-ray result."

76. The answer is A. *(Ear, Nose, and Throat Surgery)*

Although the other choices can cause hearing loss, presbycusis, the normal sensorineural hearing loss that occurs with age, is the most common. Although there is a wide range of severity, the highest frequencies generally are affected first, and lower frequencies become involved gradually. Meningitis is probably the most common cause of acquired sensorineural hearing loss in children. Otosclerosis is fairly common but usually causes conductive hearing loss rather than sensorineural hearing loss. In this condition, the otic bones become stiffened and fused. Drug-induced causes of hearing loss are important to be aware of, but relatively uncommon. It can be frustrating when question ask for the most common etiology or condition, but this is often how a differential diagnosis is formed—i.e., from the most common and/or most likely to the least common and/or least likely. It is part of the transition from the books to the wards to learn that 95% of patients with hypertension have plain old boring essential hypertension and that you may never get to see an actual case of pheochromocytoma in your career.

77. The answer is E. *(Surgery—General)*

The importance of this question is to remember that all elevated amylase levels are not from the pancreas. Amylase also commonly increases as a result of damage to the gastrointestinal tract, salivary glands, or a ruptured tubal pregnancy and can be elevated in renal insufficiency. With a history of peptic ulcer disease and free air under the diaphragm, peptic ulcer causing duodenal or gastric perforation should be at the top of the list of differential diagnoses. Although you cannot rule out a pancreatic or hepatic abscess, these are uncommon, and there are no particular risk factors that are mentioned to make these likely. Pancreatitis should not cause free air under the diaphragm, a sign that usually comes from a perforation in the gastrointestinal tract. Alcohol-induced hepatitis also is likely, given the pattern of liver enzyme elevation, with a slightly elevated AST that is more than twice the value of the ALT. Perforated peptic ulcers can actually cause pancreatitis as well, though this is a rare cause of pancreatitis.

78. The answer is D. *(Laboratory Medicine)*

The point of this question is to make you remember that alkaline phosphatase can come from bone, placenta, or liver. Given a normal 5'-nucleotidase and normal liver enzymes and bilirubin, liver disease is unlikely. Although the question does not steer you toward any particular diagnosis, bone disease is more likely than liver or gallbladder disease as the cause of the elevated alkaline phosphatase in this patient. Pancreatic cancer is very unlikely in a 27-year-old woman.

79. The answer is A. *(Laboratory Medicine)*

In the setting of hypomagnesemia, hypokalemia is extremely difficult to correct (even high-dose potassium would not work). Hypomagnesemia is fairly common in alcoholics, owing to renal magnesium loss from an effect of alcohol on the kidney. There is no particular reason to suspect renal artery stenosis, which classically causes hypertension and a renal artery bruit, and can result in renal insufficiency and *increased* potassium levels when severe. Abdominal CT scan and corticosteroids are not indicated. If the magnesium is low, giving magnesium and potassium supplements together would correct the potassium.

80. The answer is D. *(Medicine—General)*

This patient most likely has a pulmonary embolus (PE), given the signs of deep venous thrombosis (swollen, tender calf) and respiratory alkalosis with hypoxia in the absence of wheezing or other signs of asthma exacerbation. CT scan of the chest has become an increasingly utilized test to diagnose pulmonary embolism, but must be performed with IV contrast to detect emboli. Additionally, high-resolution CT is a technique used to diagnose the cause of interstitial lung disease, not PE. Expiratory chest radiographs are sometimes used when a small pneumothorax is suspected, which would not cause the degree of hypoxia seen in this patient. Pulmonary function testing would not be helpful in this setting, although ordering a peak flow determination would rule out an asthma exacerbation, which is unlikely given the patient's comments and lack of response to metered dose inhaler therapy. Ventilation-perfusion scintigraphy is a sensitive technique to diagnose PE, though its specificity is relatively poor and less than CT with contrast. Thoracotomy with embolectomy is a rarely used, heroic attempt to save the life of a patient with a massive PE. Without a definitive diagnosis of PE and an unstable patient, this would be an inappropriate intervention. Additionally, percutaneous catheter-based techniques with mechanical and chemical thrombolysis are now preferred over open thoractomy in such situations.

81. The answer is B. *(General Knowledge and Principles)*

Any patient with asthma and nasal polyps should avoid aspirin because these patients tend to be sensitive to aspirin, and it often can precipitate a severe asthma exacerbation. There is no reason to suspect antisocial personality disorder and no particular reason to stop zafirlukast. Experimentation with tobacco, alcohol, and drugs is common and normal during adolescence, and the patient does not have a substance abuse disorder. The most common cause of death in adolescence is accidents, second is homicide, and third is suicide, though in African American males, homicide is the leading cause of adolescent death.

82. The answer is A. *(Pediatrics—General)*

Children should not be given aspirin for a fever because of the association with Reye's syndrome, which can occur up to the age of 18 or so. Reye's syndrome classically causes severe liver inflammation, encephalopathy, and intractable vomiting. Increased levels of ammonia are fairly common as well. Subacute meningitis and a brain tumor usually have a history of gradual worsening, not the sudden changes mentioned in the question. The lumbar puncture was normal. Meningococcemia is a possibility, and blood cultures should be obtained, but there is no mention of fever or hypothermia, and the level of liver derangement would be unusual unless coexisting shock were present. Skin petechiae are also common and classic with meningococcemia. Hypoglycemia is present but is a result of liver damage, not the primary event (i.e., hypoglycemia does not cause liver damage, but the reverse may be true).

83. The answer is D. *(Pharmacology)*

Acetaminophen does not have significant antiplatelet effects, whereas aspirin does. Acetaminophen is a much less potent peripheral anti-inflammatory agent compared with aspirin, although both have analgesic effects and are helpful in osteoarthritis. Both may cause vomiting in overdose.

84. The answer is C. *(Pharmacology)*

Oral contraceptive pills (OCPs) have many effects besides preventing pregnancy of which you need to be aware. They decrease the incidence of ovarian and endometrial cancers, dysmenorrhea, menorrhagia, functional ovarian cysts, and benign breast disease. OCPs are a frequent cause of secondary hypertension in women, are contraindicated in the presence of active liver disease, and may cause liver tumors (benign adenomas). OCPs commonly cause weight gain, edema, and bloating and increase the risk of thromboembolic disease, especially in women older than 35 who smoke (these women should not be offered OCPs). OCPs may worsen and/or cause migraines, seizures, dyslipidemia, and gallbladder disease.

85. The answer is C. *(Gynecology)*

Oral contraceptive pills (OCPs) are a common cause of secondary hypertension in women. If a woman on OCPs develops hypertension, she should stop the OCPs and have her blood pressure rechecked. It is not appropriate to start medication or lifestyle changes until a trial off of OCPs is attempted.

86. The answer is C. *(Pharmacology)*

Barbiturates, antiepileptics, and rifampin are the classic liver enzyme inducers, whereas cimetidine and ketoconazole are the classic liver enzyme inhibitors; this is important to remember because of drug-drug interactions. Penicillin, lansoprazole, and fluoxetine have little effect on liver enzymes.

87. The answer is C. *(General Knowledge and Principles)*

The only thing you have learned is that the patient responded to placebo. Patients with confirmed disease often respond to placebo, and this does not mean their pain is psychological. This experiment should not have been done in the first place and should not be continued. Sugar pills are not an accepted therapy for arthritis and should not be continued whether the patient is told the truth or not.

88. The answer is E. *(Emergency Medicine)*

All the other choices are appropriate because hypoglycemia or narcotic overdose may cause this scenario. Oxygen should be given and intravenous access should be obtained. There is no cause for sodium bicarbonate to be administered at this point. Sodium bicarbonate may be useful as a cardioprotective agent in hyperkalemia or tricyclic antidepressant overdose but is not administered blindly in a scenario such as this without further data, evidence, and/or failure of other therapies.

89. The answer is C. *(Medicine—General)*

The patient has hypercalcemia that most likely has caused nephrolithiasis to develop. The next thing to do is administer normal saline. Once the patient is well hydrated, further treatment may include loop diuretics (such as furosemide) or possibly pamidronate (second-line agent in this setting). Thiazide diuretics are contraindicated in the setting of hypercalcemia because they cause calcium retention. Patients should be encouraged to drink plenty of fluids. An abdominal radiograph should be done in an attempt to detect nephrolithiasis and to rule out other obvious causes for abdominal pain. If negative, an intravenous pyelogram or non-contrast CT or the abdomen and pelvis could be done if the suspicion of renal stones remained.

90. The answer is A. *(Dermatology)*

This patient has Kaposi's sarcoma, an AIDS-related condition that has recently (making it high-yield) been linked to human herpesvirus-8 infection. The classic history is a rash that won't go away despite multiple treatmentsin an AIDS patient. Before the AIDS epidemic, this malignancy was typically seen in elderly males of European origin or in Africans. The incidence of Kaposi' sarcoma in AIDS patients has declined significantly in the past few decades, probably due (at least in part) to the advent of highly active antiretroviral therapy (HAART) with three-drug regimens that allow the immune system to recover/ retain a higher level of functioning than when the AIDS epidemic began. In fact, AIDS-related Kaposi sarcoma may regress with the use of HAART and can be an indication for starting such therapy in patients who were previously undiagnosed or refused therapy. Herpes zoster (described in choice **B**) is a painful condition that, when it becomes disseminated (as it can in AIDS and other immunosuppressed states), causes toxicity and acute illness with systemic symptoms. Classic herpes zoster should be confined to one (or possibly two) dermatome (does not cross midline to a significant degree). In the absence of treatment, progression and systemic dissemination of Kaposi's occurs with visceral involvement. Pulmonary involvement in particular has a significant negative impact on prognosis. Local therapy may be appropriate for smaller isolated skin lesions but would not be a good option in the case patient, who has widely disseminated skin lesions. Caseous necrosis is not a histologic feature of Kaposi's sarcoma; rather it is usually seen with tuberculosis and deep fungal infections.

91. The answer is D. *(Dermatology)*

This patient has psoriasis, which usually starts in young adulthood and is more common in whites. It is thought to be a genetically related autoimmune type of disorder by most, and a family history can be obtained in about 30% of patients. Treatment is difficult and complex, but excisional biopsy and antifungals are not effective. Topical agents, such as corticosteroids, tar, and anthralin, with or without UV light therapy (e.g., UVB phototherapy or psoralens and UVA therapy) are used with varying success. This condition is not associated with visceral malignancy but is associated with other autoimmune phenomena and arthritis. A *Christmas tree* distribution sometimes is used to describe the classic appearance of pityriasis rosea on the back, not psoriasis. Psoriasis classically appears on the extensor surfaces of the elbows and knees and the scalp. The micrograph demonstrates a parakeratotic layer (labeled "P" on the figure), areas of nuclear debris from inflammatory cells or "microabscesses" (labeled "M"), dilated capillaries ("C"), edematous and expanded dermal papillae ("DP"), acanthosis (i.e. increased thickness in the stratum spinosum) with greatly elongated, narrow rete pegs ("R"), and a chronic inflammatory infiltrate in the upper dermis ("D").

92. The answer is B. *(Medicine—Oncology)*

Leukemia is the most common malignancy in children and adolescents, followed by lymphomas and central nervous system tumors.

93. The answer is D. *(Medicine—Nutrition)*

Vitamin C is involved in cross-linking collagen, and when deficient, the collagen problems can cause blood vessel fragility and petechial-type bleeding, classically in the gums, but also on the skin itself. Vitamin K deficiency causes deeper bleeding and bruising, not the petechial-type bleeding often associated with platelet disorders.

94. The answer is B. *(Medicine—Hematology)*

Although aspirin affects platelet function, it does not generally cause thrombocytopenia (i.e. causes a qualitative not quantitative platelet problem). The other listed agents are classic causes of drug-induced thrombocytopenia. Although usually benign, some cases of thrombocytopenia from heparin paradoxically can cause thrombosis; it usually is advised to monitor platelet counts of patients on heparin for several days and stop the infusion if thrombocytopenia develops.

95. The answer is D. *(Medicine—Hematology)*

Von Willebrand's factor, absent in the autosomal dominant disorder named after it, is needed for adequate platelet function and acts as a serum storage protein for factor VIII. In its absence, factor VIII levels are decreased, and patients classically have prolonged bleeding and partial thromboplastin times. Heparin is monitored with the partial thromboplastin time. The effect of newer low-molecular-weight heparins, such as enoxaparin, cannot be measured with this test. If needed, an antifactor Xa assay can be used to measure the effect of low-molecular-weight heparins. Warfarin prolongs the prothrombin time (but not bleeding time), and hemophilia A and B prolong the partial thromboplastin time, distinguished by a low factor VIII or IX, respectively.

96. The answer is E. *(Medicine—Hematology)*

This woman most likely has thrombotic thrombocytopenic purpura, a rare, potentially fatal disorder. The hallmarks are thrombocytopenia, fever, neurologic disturbances, and evidence of intravascular hemolysis (schistocytes, helmet cells, elevated reticulocyte count, elevated lactate dehydrogenase). Damage may occur to any organ from platelet plugs. Platelet transfusions can make the situation worse and should be avoided, and in any case, are typically reserved for platelet counts less than 20,000/μl, when the risk of intracranial hemorrhage becomes high. Plasmapheresis and plasma exchange often result in a remission, supporting the theory of an unknown platelet-aggregating factor in the blood as the cause.

97. The answer is B. *(Medicine—Cardiology)*

This patient most likely has viral pericarditis, usually caused by coxsackievirus or echovirus. This is the most likely diagnosis in a young person with a history of a recent upper respiratory infection, low-grade fever, pleuritic-type chest pain, and a pericardial friction rub (the scratchy sound). Electrocardiogram classically shows diffusely elevated ST segments in the precordial and limb leads, not Q waves. Myocardial infarction is extremely unlikely in this patient, given the age, lack of mentioned risk factors, and lack of *significant* family history (myocardial infarction in first-degree male relative < 55 years old or female relative < 65 years old). A stress test is not indicated at this time. Although endocarditis cannot be excluded entirely, there is little in the history to suggest a risk for endocarditis (e.g., dental surgery, intravenous drug abuse), and it is less likely given the friction rub. There is no reason to suspect a previously damaged heart valve, although abnormal valves are more likely to be affected by subacute endocarditis.

98. The answer is A. *(Obstetrics)*

Chorionic villus sampling can be performed at 9 to 12 weeks' gestation, whereas amniocentesis usually is not performed until 16 weeks. Chorionic villus sampling cannot detect neural tube defects and is associated with a higher miscarriage rate than amniocentesis, however. It is advocated primarily for women who are genetic carriers of a disease recognized after a previously affected child or strong family history. It allows women the option of a first-trimester abortion, but this is not done at the same time as the test. It is a separate procedure that must be decided on by the mother after she has received the test results, which normally take several days because cell culture is often performed.

99. The answer is D. *(Obstetrics)*

Maternal serum alpha-fetoprotein determinations ideally are done at 16 to 18 weeks' gestation. Low alpha-fetoprotein may mean Down syndrome, trisomy 18, fetal demise, or inaccurate dates (fetus is younger than estimated). High alpha-fetoprotein may mean neural tube defects (e.g., anencephaly, spina bifida), ventral wall defects (e.g., omphalocele, gastroschisis), multiple gestation, fetal demise, or inaccurate dates (fetus is older than estimated).

100. The answer is C. *(Pediatrics—Infectious Disease)*

Head lice, caused by *Pediculus capitis*, are common in normal school-age children and do not indicate poor hygiene or child abuse. They are self-limiting and do not cause growth or development problems. Permethrin cream is preferred over lindane because of possible neurotoxicity concerns with lindane if systemic absorption occurs. Decontamination of sources of reinfection is required for successful treatment.

BLOCK 3

ANSWERS AND EXPLANATIONS

101. The answer is C. *(Ethics)*

Only the patient, if he or she is competent, should decide whether or not information is withheld or disclosed. The family does not have a right to make that decision. When dealing with family members, however, you must remember their fears and concerns as well. Although you should ask the patient whether or not she wants to know the diagnosis, taking 5 minutes to discuss the family's fears with them may be all that is required to resolve this issue. Telling the patient anyway is partly correct, but not as good an answer as choice **C**. An attorney is not required in this situation (yet).

102. The answer is C. *(Pharmacology)*

Isoniazid, procainamide, and hydralazine are classic causes of drug-induced lupus, and methyldopa is a classic cause of autoimmune hemolytic anemia. Omeprazole has not been associated with autoimmune side effects.

103. The answer is B. *(Pediatrics—Neonates)*

The Apgar score is a general measure of well-being normally performed at 1 and 5 minutes after birth. Five categories are assessed, with a maximum of 2 points assigned for each category—possible scores range from 0 to 10, with 10 being the highest. The categories are respirations, heart rate, *color* (not grasp reflex), muscle tone, and reflex irritability. Studies have suggested that a low Apgar score at birth equates with a lower chance of good health at 1 year of age and later. The assessment of an infant begins before delivery is completed. You do not simply wait until 1 minute after birth to begin the assessment—an infant may need to be suctioned and intubated within 45 seconds of being born.

104. The answer is E. *(Pediatrics—Neonates)*

The child has caput succedaneum, a benign condition caused by the molding of the head to pass through the birth canal that resolves on its own and requires no further workup. This condition must be differentiated from a cephalhematoma, which is a periosteal hemorrhage sharply confined to one skull bone (commonly the parietal bone) that does not cross the midline. Although a cephalhematoma also is usually benign, it may indicate an underlying skull fracture, and a skull radiograph or CT scan of the head may be appropriate in this setting to rule out a skull fracture.

105. The answer is C. *(Preventive Medicine)*

This young woman has myopia, or near-sightedness, and glasses would improve her vision. This is one of those frustrating questions that makes sure you do not forget about health maintenance. All sexually active women, even if younger than age 18, should have an annual Pap smear. Reading glasses are for presbyopia, not myopia, and would not improve the patient's vision.

106. The answer is A. *(Emergency Medicine)*

This patient has developed neuroleptic malignant syndrome, a potentially fatal side effect of antipsychotic medication. Autonomic instability with high fevers, fluctuating hypertension, tachycardia, and tachypnea normally is present along with muscular rigidity and a markedly elevated creatine kinase secondary to muscle necrosis. The mainstay of therapy is to first stop the antipsychotic, then provide supportive care, including intravenous hydration, antipyretics, and cooling blankets. This syndrome is thought to be related to malignant hyperthermia, and some have used dantrolene with success, although many patients do well with supportive care alone. Sodium bicarbonate may be needed to prevent renal shutdown from myoglobinuria. Mortality is said to be 10%, and this syndrome may occur at any time during antipsychotic treatment, although classically it occurs when a patient has been recently started on antipsychotics.

107. The answer is C. *(Emergency Medicine)*

Infection of burns normally is secondary to *Staphylococcus aureus* or *Pseudomonas aeruginosa*. Third-degree burns involve all layers of epidermis and dermis (including nerve endings) and are classically *painless*. These burns generally require skin grafting. Second-degree burns involve the epidermis and part of the dermis, usually include blisters and open, weeping surfaces, and are very painful. Topical antibiotics are given prophylactically for second-degree and third-degree burns, but intravenous antibiotics are reserved for true infection. A tetanus booster should be given to all burn patients if it has been more than 5 years since their last booster.

108. The answer is A. *(Obstetrics)*

Renal agenesis causes oligohydramnios because the fetus swallows amniotic fluid but cannot excrete it. The end result of the oligohydramnios is hypoplastic lungs, neonatal respiratory distress, and characteristic (Potter's) facies known as Potter syndrome. In this condition, death usually results from severe respiratory insufficiency, which develops immediately after birth due to pulmonary hypoplasia (before uremia occurs). The other choices are all more likely to be associated with polyhydramnios.

109. The answer is B. *(Urology)*

This is an example of hyperacute rejection resulting from preformed antibodies, and the kidney needs to be removed because current methods of immunosuppression are not effective in this condition. This situation is different from acute rejection, mediated by T cells, and chronic rejection, mediated by T cells and antibodies, which often are responsive to immunosuppressant medication. Intravenous hydration is a good idea in this setting but does not stop the process. This episode would not prevent the patient from receiving another transplant in the future. Although macrophages are involved in most inflammatory processes, they are not thought to be primarily responsible for any of the forms of transplant rejection.

110. The answer is A. *(Surgery—Trauma)*

This patient needs a retrograde urethrogram to rule out a urethral injury before any attempt at bladder catheterization. Trauma patients with any of the following signs generally need a retrograde urethrogram before attempting bladder catheterization: high-riding or boggy prostate, blood at the urethral meatus, scrotal ecchymosis, or severe pelvic fracture. CT scan of the abdomen is a reasonable option but should be performed with contrast enhancement to help visualize vital structures. There is no clear indication for broad-spectrum antibiotics in this scenario with the information given.

111. The answer is D. *(Urology)*

This patient has acute urinary retention most likely secondary to prostatic enlargement. The first step in managing this patient is to drain the bladder to prevent potential permanent kidney damage. Because the transurethral (Foley) catheter could not be placed, a suprapubic (transabdominal) catheter is required. Although prostatectomy may be an option at a later time (transurethral resection of the prostate is usually preferred), current management should be focused on relieving the obstruction. An alpha-fetoprotein level would not be helpful; heparin would not be helpful. Renal artery stenosis would not cause the findings described in this patient (i.e., would not cause hydronephrosis or a distended bladder), although it is a potential cause of renal insufficiency/failure.

112. The answer is C. *(Medicine—Cardiology)*

This patient most likely developed a cardiac thrombus secondary to atrial fibrillation and now is having embolization of pieces of the thrombus. Deep venous thrombosis, if it embolized, would cause a pulmonary embolus, not systemic (arterial) emboli. The exception would be in the rare instance of some type of septal defect with right-to-left shunting that allowed for paradoxical systemic emboli to occur (highly unlikely). The patient lacks any signs of severe peripheral vascular disease, and this does not tend to present so suddenly in different parts of the body. Buerger's disease is a vasculitis usually seen in 20 to 40-year-old men who smoke. Temporal arteritis can cause strokes but usually does not affect the extremities, and the woman has no symptoms of polymyalgia rheumatica. This woman, given her history of rheumatic heart disease and probable atrial enlargement from mitral stenosis that caused the atrial fibrillation, probably should have been on warfarin rather than aspirin to prevent this very scenario from occurring.

113. The answer is A. *(Surgery—Vascular)*

This patient has claudication, the peripheral vascular disease equivalent of angina. Best initial management is conservative, including cessation of smoking, initiation of an exercise program, and control of other atherosclerosis risk factors (cholesterol, hypertension, and diabetes). Revascularization may be required eventually but carries a significant morbidity and mortality because of the presence of widespread atherosclerosis and should be reserved for severe, disabling symptoms or failure of conservative management. Urgent referral is inappropriate, although consulting a vascular surgeon would be appropriate. Heparin is not needed in this instance. This patient needs to be on aspirin to prevent a second heart attack and to reduce the risk of stroke. The patient also needs to be on carvedilol to decrease the risk of a second heart attack and control his hypertension. Because the patient is currently normotensive, increasing the dose of carvedilol is not needed at this time. Additionally, such a dose increase may theoretically worsen his claudication because beta$_2$-receptors stimulate vasodilation of the vessels that supply muscle beds and increase blood flow to muscles.

114. The answer is A. *(Surgery—Vascular)*

When carotid stenosis is greater than 70%, carotid arterectomy provides the best long-term prophylaxis against a stroke, especially in patients with symptoms (such as the transient ischemic attack the patient in the question experienced). Aspirin should be used if the stenosis is less than 50%, and the optimal therapy for 50–70% range stenosis is still being determined using randomized trials. Current data indicate that such patients should be managed medically in the absence of symptoms, with surgery contemplated on a case-by-case basis in those with symptoms referable to such a lesion. Warfarin can reduce stroke risk, but the risks generally outweigh the benefits when used in this setting. Bilateral carotid endarterectomy would not be advised because the right carotid artery does not have enough of a stenosis to derive much benefit from carotid endarterectomy. Simvastatin can also reduce stroke risk, but is not as effective as carotid endarterectomy for such a significant stenosis.

115. The answer is E. *(Medicine—General)*

This patient most likely has sinusitis, a common cause of headaches, with maxillary sinus tenderness and purulent nasal discharge. Cluster headaches display a pattern over months to years that involves several headaches over a period of days (clusters), then none for a period of time. Migraine headaches classically have an aura, are often unilateral, and may produce nausea and vomiting. There is no reason to suspect an immunodeficiency or any relation to the history of dysmenorrhea. The patient most likely would benefit from antibiotics.

116. The answer is E. *(Pediatrics—General)*

This child has recurrent otitis media, a common pediatric problem. The main complication is potential hearing loss with the possibility of developmental delay because of the hearing loss. There is no particular reason to suspect an immunodeficiency (which should cause infections in other areas) or child abuse. Leukemia and lymphoma are not thought to occur with increased frequency in children with recurrent otitis media, though they can certainly cause immunodeficiency (which, again, should cause other or more severe infections).

117. The answer is C. *(Medicine—Infectious Disease)*

Pseudomonas aeruginosa is one of the most commonly cultured organisms in otitis externa, along with *Staphylococcus aureus*. Culture usually is not performed in straightforward cases, however. The external ear canal is red, swollen, and erythematous, and manipulation of the auricle usually causes pain. There may be otorrhea, or discharge from the ear, as well. Treatment involves topical antibiotics with or without topical corticosteroids. Acetic acid may be used in place of corticosteroids to alter the pH of the canal, which seems to be helpful.

118. The answer is E. *(Pharmacology)*

Heparin can cause mild thrombocytopenia in 5% of patients after several days of therapy, but in a small percentage, the thrombocytopenia is severe and associated with paradoxic thrombosis. Cases of stroke and myocardial infarction have been reported. Heparin, in contrast to warfarin, does not cross the placenta and does not harm the fetus. The major risk with heparin is bleeding; however, this is not a true side effect but rather an exaggerated therapeutic effect.

119. The answer is E. *(Preventive Medicine)*

Treatment for mumps orchitis is seldom necessary in the United States because of widespread immunization. Mumps orchitis usually is unilateral and rarely results in the feared complication of sterility. Treatment is supportive with scrotal elevation, ice packs, and aspirin or other nonsteroidal anti-inflammatory medications. In this case, prevention is the best treatment.

120. The answer is C. *(Laboratory Medicine)*

This patient most likely has developed type II diabetes and is in the midst of a nonketotic, hyperglycemic, hyperosmolar state. Diabetic ketoacidosis occurs in type I diabetes and should cause a decreased CO_2 level (acidosis). When the glucose becomes markedly elevated, a reciprocal drop in sodium level occurs (the sodium decreases approximately 1.7 mEq for each 100 mg/dL increase of the glucose level > 200). This is not a true drop in the level of sodium in the body, and the level returns to normal with correction of the glucose level. Treatment includes large amounts of intravenous hydration with normal saline and, at the same time, insulin. The patient most likely has total body *depletion* of potassium, which is common in this setting. Prophylactic hypertonic saline should not be given for hyponatremia, as it may cause brainstem damage and coma (central pontine myelinolysis). A trial of vasopressin is used with diabetes insipidus to determine whether it is central or nephrogenic, and is not appropriate in this case.

121. The answer is E. *(Medicine—Infectious Disease)*

Otitis media most commonly is due to *Streptococcus pneumoniae*, *Haemophilus influenzae* or *Moraxella catarrhalis*. Empirical treatment should be directed toward these pathogens. Cefaclor, an oral second-generation cephalosporin, is a good choice. Vancomycin and gentamicin usually are given intravenously, making them inappropriate; vancomycin has poor gram-negative coverage, and gentamicin has poor gram-positive coverage. Fluconazole is an antifungal, and nitrofurantoin generally is used only for urinary tract infections.

122. The answer is E. *(Pediatrics—General)*

As a general rule of thumb, 75% of neck masses are benign in children, whereas 75% are malignant in adults older than age 40. Branchial cleft cysts are usually lateral in location and often present when they become infected. Thyroglossal duct cysts are in the midline and classically elevate with tongue protrusion due to their residual connection with the foramen cecum of the tongue. Lymphadenitis is a common cause of a neck mass in children and has many possible causes.

123. The answer is D. *(Pediatrics—General)*

Trauma, especially nose picking, is the most common cause of a nosebleed in children. Thrombocytopenia also can result in nose bleeding, such as from leukemia or idiopathic thrombocytopenic purpura. In adolescents, angiofibroma is a benign nasopharyngeal tumor that represents a classic (though rare) cause of nosebleeds.

124. The answer is B. *(Medicine—Immunology)*

In allergic rhinitis, there also usually is a history of seasonal flare-ups; boggy and bluish turbinates; onset before the age of 20; family history; and other allergic conditions, such as asthma or eczema.

125. The answer is A. *(Medicine—Neurology)*

Benign positional vertigo is a common disorder that can be recognized by the lack of hearing loss or tinnitus (which tend to occur in the other mentioned conditions) and the elicitation of symptoms by placing the patient in a certain position. The other listed conditions tend to cause symptoms regardless of the patient's position. Avoidance of the provocative position is the usual treatment for this disorder.

126. The answer is B. *(Pediatrics—General)*

Hearing loss is the most common sequela of meningitis in children, and formal testing should be performed after meningitis because children, in contrast with adults, often do not report their symptoms. The subsequent hearing loss may lead to developmental problems. Although more subtle cognitive deficits and mental retardation may occur because of meningitis, these can be detected by routine history and physical examination, with formal developmental testing reserved for difficult cases. Vision screening is important but can be done by the primary care provider using a standard vision chart. Repeat blood cultures are not required, and HIV testing would be done only in selective cases that seem suspicious (e.g., unusual organism growing in the cerebrospinal fluid culture, additional infections).

127. The answer is B. *(Pharmacology)*

Thioridazine, an older second-line antipsychotic, can cause retinal deposits that may cause vision problems but does not tend to affect hearing. Aminoglycosides in combination with loop diuretics increase the risk for hearing loss compared with either agent alone. Quinine toxicity can result in headaches, tinnitus, and hearing loss (called *cinchonism*). Aspirin toxicity commonly causes tinnitus and hearing loss, which often is reversible upon cessation of the drug.

128. The answer is B. *(Medicine—Cardiology)*

Although considered a first-line agent in the management of acute myocardial infarction, nitrates have not been shown to improve survival in the setting of or after a myocardial infarction. Beta blockers, aspirin, and angiotensin-converting enzyme inhibitors have been shown to improve survival in large, placebo-controlled studies. Smoking cessation improves survival in any setting.

129. The answer is B. *(Medicine—Cardiology)*

Although used for congestive heart failure, digoxin has not been shown to improve survival in congestive heart failure patients. Beta blockers, angiotensin-converting enzyme inhibitors, and spironolactone have been shown to improve survival in large-scale, controlled trials. Beta blockers generally should be avoided in unstable heart failure because they may worsen the ejection fraction when used acutely. Smoking cessation improves survival in any setting.

130. The answer is B. *(Ear, Nose, and Throat Surgery)*

Although all may result in facial nerve paralysis, Bell's palsy is the most common. Bell's palsy is thought to be due to reactivation of latent herpes virus infection. It classically presents as sudden-onset unilateral paralysis after an upper respiratory infection. Many cases resolve spontaneously within a few months, although permanent paralysis may result. If bilateral facial nerve paralysis occurs, Lyme disease and multiple sclerosis become more likely diagnoses. Brain stem infarction, similar to other potential causes of an upper motor neuron lesion affecting the facial nerve, generally would cause sparing of the forehead on the affected side unless it was right at the level of the nucleus. Lower motor neuron lesions cause the entire half of the face to be involved.

131. The answer is B. *(Medicine—Neurology)*

A proximal facial nerve lesion may result in paralysis of the stapedius muscle, causing hyperacusis, or an increased sensitivity to sound (things sound louder than they are). When the stapedius muscle contracts, the intensity of sound that stimulates the cochlear system is reduced. When this muscle is paralyzed, sound dampening does not occur. The vestibular branch of the eighth cranial nerve is involved in balance, not hearing or sound, and the other choices have nothing to do with hearing function.

132. The answer is A. *(Preventive Medicine)*

Folate supplements given to women have been shown to reduce the incidence of neural tube defects. Many neural tube defects begin in the first 30 days of pregnancy, before most women have had their first prenatal visit (and before many women know they are pregnant). Smoking cessation and maternal hypertension control are not thought to help prevent neural tube defects, although they are recommended for other reasons and would have a greater impact on the health of our society (particularly smoking cessation).

133. The answer is D. *(Medicine—Infectious Disease)*

This patient has a classic description of giardiasis, caused by the parasite *Giardia lamblia*. The organism infects the proximal small bowel, causing steatorrhea and often resulting in the appearance of unique-appearing cysts or trophozoite forms in the stool. The treatment of choice is metronidazole or furazolidone; the penicillin class is ineffective.

134. The answer is C. *(Medicine—Neurology)*

Cerebral perfusion pressure is equal to the blood pressure minus the intracranial pressure. If intracranial hypertension is present, the body raises blood pressure to maintain cerebral perfusion. Lowering the blood pressure in this setting is dangerous and should not be done unless the blood pressure is so high that it is causing clinically apparent damage to other organs (e.g., myocardial infarction, renal failure). Reverse Trendelenburg (head up) position and intubation often are first-line therapies, and diuretics often are used to lessen cerebral edema (mannitol is generally more effective than furosemide).

135. The answer is A. *(Surgery—Trauma)*

Shear injury is a common result of closed head injuries that may not show up on CT scan but may cause temporary or permanent neurologic deficits. Heparin is not indicated for head trauma and should never be started in this setting until an intracranial hemorrhage has been ruled out with a CT scan. Lumbar puncture should not be done in the setting of head trauma until a CT scan has been performed, and even then, is almost never indicated. A *blown* (fixed, dilated) pupil in the setting of a head injury normally indicates increased intracranial pressure and pending/early uncal herniation, which can lead to death. Most skull fractures are managed with observation and do not require surgical intervention unless there is impingement on brain parenchyma, an open fracture, a cerebrospinal fluid leak, or contamination (cleaning and débridement required). The calvaria is the roof of the skull, as opposed to the base of the skull.

136. The answer is A. *(Medicine—General)*

The patient most likely has podagra, or acute gout of the great toe. Given his lack of risk factors for septic arthritis, antibiotics are not necessary at this point. Allopurinol should **not** be given to someone in the midst of an attack of gout because this may worsen symptoms. Anti-inflammatory agents, such as indomethacin or colchicine, should be used in the acute setting. Allopurinol is a maintenance medication started after the acute attack has subsided.

The next thing to do would be arthrocentesis to confirm the diagnosis. The patient can have this done as an outpatient and does not require hospitalization. A good rule of thumb is that a hot, painful, swollen joint generally should be *tapped* (i.e. arthrocentesis should be performed) unless the diagnosis is clear. With gout, you would look for the joint fluid to contain needle-shaped crystals with negative birefringence by polarized microscopy. Thiazide diuretics, with their potential to increase uric acid levels, can precipitate an attack of gout in a susceptible individual. Elevated uric acid levels are not always found in those with gout, although they are usually present.

137. The answer is D. *(Psychiatry—General)*

This patient has a history consistent with posttraumatic stress disorder, which affects a large number of Vietnam veterans. In the history, look for a severely traumatic event (e.g., war, rape, natural disaster) with re-experiencing of the event (e.g., nightmares, flashbacks, illusions) and an attempt to avoid things that trigger a memory of the event. These patients often have chronic anxiety, hyperalertness, and a feeling of detachment from others. Treatment with sedatives, such as diphenhydramine and lorazepam, although a possible adjunct to other treatment modalities, is inappropriate in isolation and not the cornerstone of management. Many of these patients are prone to developing alcoholism and drug addiction to diminish their emotional pain.

Haloperidol is not indicated in this disorder unless frank psychosis develops (not present in this case), and electroconvulsive therapy is a second-line treatment for depression, usually used after a trial of medication is unsuccessful. Fluoxetine and other serotonin-specific reuptake inhibitors, however, have been shown to be beneficial in this condition. The best answer is **D** because group therapy with others who are experiencing similar problems is an effective therapy and may provide a support group, which many of these patients lack. Adjunctive medications, such as serotonin-specific reuptake inhibitors, are also commonly prescribed.

138. The answer is C. *(General Knowledge and Principles)*

A thoracentesis probably would relieve the patient's symptoms as well as provide important diagnostic information. The other options are premature, other than respiratory isolation, a reasonable precaution in many cases. Empirical tuberculosis therapy is not given—a diagnosis should be secured first. The causes of a pleural effusion are many, ranging from cancer and infection to autoimmune disorders and congestive heart failure. Evaluation of the pleural fluid can help narrow the differential diagnosis and guide further therapy. It also may reveal the underlying process, which can be obscured by the fluid on radiograph. Right and left decubitus views of the chest also would be helpful to evaluate the underlying lung parenchyma and to determine if the effusion is free-flowing or loculated. A CT scan of the chest may be of benefit after thoracentesis as well, but a PET scan is not indicated for work-up of a pleural effusion.

139. The answer is A. *(Orthopedic Surgery)*

The epidemiology of slipped capital femoral epiphysis is important to increase your suspicion of the condition. It tends to affect overweight boys between the ages of 9 and 13 and frequently causes a limp with pain in the ipsilateral knee, thigh, or groin (referred pain). Plain x-ray films are the initial diagnostic study of choice and are generally all that is needed to confirm the diagnosis. Early surgical pinning generally is employed to prevent further slippage of the femoral epiphysis with resultant abnormalities of the hip joint. Legg-Calvé-Perthes disease, or idiopathic avascular necrosis of the femoral head, can cause similar symptoms but tends to affect children between the ages of 4 and 9 and is not associated with obesity.

140. The answer is D. *(Orthopedic Surgery)*

This is primarily a result of coexisting morbidities (e.g., in the setting of trauma, visceral injury, or head injury; in the setting of hip fracture in the elderly, heart disease, and lung disease) or excessive bleeding and indicates a significant trauma force. In the elderly, insufficiency fractures of the pelvis (i.e., pubic rami) are common and often not associated with significant (or any) trauma.

141. The answer is C. *(Ophthalmology)*

Presbyopia, or hardening of the lens that decreases the ability to accommodate in near vision, is an almost universal complaint after the age of 50 and is considered a normal part of aging. Retinal detachment is a phenomenon that results in sudden symptoms, and it as well as macular degeneration would be expected to affect near and far vision (symptoms while driving a car). Cataracts and diabetes are possibilities but typically affect both near and far vision and are not as common as presbycusis. Patients with diabetes and cataracts may develop myopia because of lens distortion, making near vision easier than far. A common complaint of patients with cataracts is that driving becomes difficult at night because of the glare of oncoming headlights caused by the degenerative changes in the lens.

142. The answer is B. *(Pediatrics—Ophthalmology)*

An esotropia means that the affected eye deviates inward, whereas an exotropia means that the affected eye deviates outward. Either of these conditions is known as *strabismus* or *lazy eye*, and it is almost always abnormal after the age of 3 months, requiring referral to an ophthalmologist to prevent blindness (amblyopia). Because the visual neural connections are still actively developing until the age of 7 or 8, the brain learns to suppress the image from the affected eye because it cannot fuse the two incongruent images it receives from the eyes. This suppression leads to failure of the development of neural connections and permanent loss of vision in the affected eye that cannot be corrected with glasses (neural problem, not a refractive problem) later in life.

This condition is one of the reasons why vision screening is so important because early detection and treatment—which may involve eye patches, special glasses, or surgery—allow the affected eye to retain maximal vision. An oculomotor palsy normally causes the affected eye to look *down and out*. In the first 3 months of life, intermittent strabismus often is physiologic and requires only close monitoring and follow-up. Persistent abnormal eye deviation is abnormal at any age and requires prompt ophthamologic referral

143. The answer is A. *(Gynecology)*

This is a classic (are you getting tired of the word "classic" yet?) description and microscopic appearance of Paget's disease resulting from ductal breast carcinoma that extends into the skin, though only about half to two-thirds of women have a palpable breast mass at the time of presentation. Paget's cells (labeled "P" in the figure) are malignant epithelial cells with hyperchromatic nuclei and pale cytoplasm. Fibroadenoma and fibrocystic disease of the breast are unlikely to cause a new-onset breast mass in a postmenopausal woman and would not cause the described skin changes in the nipple. A chest wall sarcoma is a theoretic possibility, but this would be extremely rare and much less likely than Paget's disease. Cellulitis would not be expected to cause an underlying breast mass, unless it was a fluctuant (unlikely to be described as "solid") abscess.

144. The answer is C. *(Medicine—Neurology)*

The CT scan is compatible with a large, old stroke in the distribution of the right *anterior* cerebral artery (remember on a CT scan that the patient's right is on the left side of the image), which should cause left-sided symptoms due to decussation of the corticospinal tract fibers in the medulla. Age and hypertension are the biggest risk factors for stroke. Aspirin commonly is used for prevention and can result in a modest reduction in cerebrovascular accident incidence, but is not universally recommended to those over 50 due to the incidence of side effects and risks of bleeding in those at low risk of stroke. The woman is likely to have left leg weakness given the location of the stroke (remember the homunculus of the motor cortex? The foot and leg "hang" over the midline near the groove between the cerebral hemispheres).

145-150. *(Pharmacology)*

The answers are the following: 145. C 146. H 147. G 148. E 149. A 150. F.

Cyclophosphamide can cause hemorrhagic cystitis acutely and bladder carcinoma with chronic use. Vincristine primarily causes peripheral neuropathy, whereas vinblastine primarily causes myelosuppression. Isotretinoin is a vitamin A analogue used to treat severe acne that is teratogenic. Tetracycline should not be given to pregnant women or children younger than 8 years old unless absolutely necessary because of potential staining of the teeth in the child. Amiodarone has many side effects, including pulmonary fibrosis, corneal deposits, hypothyroidism or hyperthyroidism, liver dysfunction, and photosensitivity. Thioridazine is an antipsychotic that can be cardiotoxic in overdose and can cause retinal deposits. Cyclosporine is an immunosuppressive agent that is primarily nephrotoxic. Verapamil is a centrally-acting calcium channel blocker primarily used in patients with tachycardia and/or hypertension and dihydroxycholecalciferol is the active form of vitamin D in the human body.

ANSWERS AND EXPLANATIONS

151. The answer is A. *(Surgery—General)*

Smoking cessation is the best thing to keep patients healthy. *Post*operative incentive spirometry, early ambulation, and minimal use of narcotics also help but are less effective than smoking cessation at least 1 week (preferably ≥ 1 month) before surgery. Withholding all narcotics is harsh in many cases because patients may be in severe pain after surgery and is not as effective a measure as smoking cessation. Mechanical ventilation has complications of its own and is not used unless needed. Perioperative antibiotics rarely are indicated to prevent pulmonary complications.

152. The answer is C. *(General Knowledge and Principles)*

Do not let your base of medicine knowledge obscure your knowledge of everyday life. When a person yells and screams for a few hours, it is common to "lose" the voice or get hoarse. The time course makes the diagnosis clear, and reassurance is all that is needed. The man probably will have his normal voice back in a few days (unless his team makes the playoffs).

153. The answer is C. *(Surgery)*

In an unstable trauma patient, the ABCs (airway, breathing, circulation) should be followed first, in that order. All of these interventions are appropriate, but given the unstable nature of the patient, there is a certain order that should be followed. First, establish an airway and ensure adequate breathing (ventilation); then address circulation and neurologic disability (the "D" in "ABCD"). A history and physical examination are important, but immediate resuscitation and stabilization are needed to prevent death. In an ideal situation, more than one factor can be addressed at the same time, as more than one health care professional is available to assist the patient.

154. The answer is B. *(Surgery)*

Each of the choices is a possibility, but the description is classic for appendicitis, which is the most common of the listed conditions in this age group. Cholecystitis tends to cause right upper quadrant pain. Meckel's diverticulum often presents at a younger age but is a possibility as well. Small bowel obstruction pain classically remains poorly localized until late in its course.

155. The answer is B. *(Medicine—General)*

Hypercalcemia may cause pancreatitis, but pancreatitis is not thought to be caused by hypocalcemia. Hypocalcemia results from pancreatitis, however, and severe hypocalcemia is one of Ranson's criteria for determining prognosis. The other choices are known causes of pancreatitis. In the United States, alcohol and gallstones are the most common etiologies for pancreatitis, together causing roughly 85% of cases seen.

156. The answer is D. *(Surgery—General)*

Spontaneous bacterial peritonitis, a condition that occurs in patients with chronic ascites, is treated with antibiotics and supportive measures, not with laparotomy. The other causes are much more likely to need to be treated with laparotomy. The mechanism of small bowel obstruction often does not determine whether or not laparotomy is needed; the patient's condition (e.g., progression to peritonitis or bowel ischemia, failure to resolve with conservative management) is the determining factor. Diverticulitis often responds to antibiotics and temporary diet changes (e.g., initial trial of nothing by mouth or liquid diet) to allow the bowel to "rest," but perforation and abscess formation are not uncommon and may require laparotomy.

157. The answer is B. *(Obstetrics)*

There are many potential complications with multiple gestations. The higher the number of fetuses, the higher the risk of most of these complications. Maternal complications include an increased likelihood of anemia, hypertension, premature labor, postpartum uterine atony, postpartum hemorrhage, and preeclampsia. Fetal complications include an increased risk of polyhydramnios, malpresentation, placenta previa, abruptio placentae, velamentous cord insertion and vasa previa, premature rupture of the membranes, prematurity, umbilical cord prolapse, intrauterine growth retardation, congenital anomalies, and perinatal morbidity and mortality. The higher the number of fetuses, the lower the birth weight of each child is likely to be (the opposite of macrosomia).

158. The answer is D. *(General Knowledge and Principles)*

If the liver is in failure, vitamin K would be ineffective because the liver would be unable to synthesize clotting factors no matter how much vitamin K is present. Fresh frozen plasma is required in this setting to treat the clotting factor deficiencies that are likely to develop. The liver also stores glucose and is a major center for gluconeogenesis; glucose may be needed in liver failure. Intravenous fluids often are required for these patients, who have fluid shifts and electrolyte abnormalities. Addressing the underlying cause is generally a good thing in any condition.

159. The answer is B. *(Obstetrics)*

This woman has asymptomatic bacteriuria, which is treated during pregnancy because of the high rate of progression to pyelonephritis. This higher rate of progression compared with nonpregnant persons is thought to be due to several factors, including the gravid uterus compressing the ureters and progesterone's relaxing effect on the ureters. Ciprofloxacin and other quinolones should be avoided in pregnancy unless absolutely necessary because they may cause cartilage abnormalities in the fetus. This woman should have a culture done, but empirical treatment can be started before the results of the culture come back. Gram-negative rods are likely to be present, such as *Escherichia coli*, but other pathogens also would be treated. Watchful waiting normally is a good thing but could result in progression to a serious infection in this case.

160. The answer is C. *(Obstetrics)*

Hyperemesis gravidarum occurs in the first trimester, is more common in overweight younger women with their first child, is more common in whites than blacks, and is more common and severe in patients with an immature personality and multiple underlying social stressors. The criteria for hyperemesis are not strict and basically include intractable nausea and vomiting with an inability to keep food down that occurs in the first trimester. Some add weight loss of 5% or more and electrolyte disturbances to the diagnostic criteria. There is no reason to suspect a choriocarcinoma with the information given, although it could be a cause (rare, making it a less correct answer).

161. The answer is E. *(Psychiatry—Addiction Psychiatry)*

This question describes classic withdrawal from caffeine. Barbiturates and benzodiazepines tend to cause insomnia in withdrawal, not fatigue. LSD does not tend to cause any withdrawal symptoms. Marijuana tends to cause insomnia in withdrawal, although whether or not a true withdrawal syndrome exists is controversial. Any drug may cause irritability in withdrawal if the user craves the substance psychologically. Severe headaches, although nonspecific, are typical in caffeine withdrawal. The combination of all three symptoms and the high prevalence of coffee drinking make caffeine withdrawal the best choice.

162. The answer is E. *(Psychiatry—Addiction Psychiatry)*

The girl is likely to be abusing marijuana, the most commonly abused illicit drug. Symptoms of intoxication include conjunctival injection, time-space distortion, and the infamous "munchies" (desire to eat). Chronic use may produce what has been dubbed the amotivational syndrome, or a lack of motivation. Overdose is not fatal, although it may produce severe dysphoria. Physical withdrawal is not known to occur, but psychological cravings may be severe. Because it tends to cause users to eat, marijuana is sometimes used to help people gain weight and reduce nausea, not lose weight. This argument is used by some AIDS and cancer patients who are plagued by nausea as a reason to legalize personal use of marijuana.

163. The answer is B. *(Preventive Medicine)*

The top three causes of adolescent death in decreasing order are accidents, homicide, and suicide. These three causes account for approximately 75% of all adolescent deaths. In African-American adolescents, however, homicide is more common than accidents as a cause of death.

164. The answer is D. *(Pediatrics—General)*

This mother is impatient. Regular bedwetting is considered physiologic until at least age 3 and is not considered a disorder until age 5. Although a urinary tract abnormality is possible, the scenario described (with normal physical examination and normal urinalysis) makes it barely more likely than in other healthy children.

165. The answer is D. *(Psychiatry—Child and Adolescent)*

The physical findings and mention about weight should make you think about the possibility of bulimia nervosa. The described knuckle scraping and enamel erosion can occur with a person who repeatedly sticks her fingers into her throat to induce vomiting. These patients may be thin, normal weight, or overweight (in contrast with patients who have anorexia, in which underweight status is required to make a diagnosis). Asking about brushing one's teeth could be considered a part of good health maintenance, but given the scenario described, choice **D** is the preferred answer.

166. The answer is C. *(Psychiatry—General)*

Adjustment disorder describes a person who does not handle a fairly normal event in life well, such as a breakup, job loss, or moving. In this case, the girl has a depressed mood associated with it. She does not meet the criteria for a more serious psychiatric disorder, such as major depression or bipolar disorder. Dysthymia is depressed mood for more days than not for a period of 2 or more years without an episode of major depression. Cyclothymia is mild depression (not major depression) alternating with hypomania without an episode of full-blown mania (think of it as a mild bipolar disorder).

167. The answer is C. *(Biostatistics)*

Whether intentional or not, most people do an experiment to try to prove something. If the experimenter knows which group patients are in, he or she may take the same comment or outcome and call it *no effect* in the placebo group versus *some effect* in the treatment group. This is known as interviewer bias and can be eliminated by blinding the experimenter as to which group the patient is in.

Unacceptability bias occurs when a patient does not admit to embarrassing behavior or, for example, claims to exercise more than he or she does or take a medication he or she doesn't to please the interviewer. Recall bias occurs with retrospective studies and defines the differential recall that may occur based on the outcome (e.g., a woman remembers her husband drinking more than he did if he died of alcoholism, less than he did if he died in church of a heart attack). Lead-time bias is classically described in cancer screening tests that improve cancer survival. The question is whether the increased survival is due to improved treatment and cure or just earlier detection. Nonresponse bias happens during a telephone or other survey when people do not respond.

168. The answer is C. *(Biostatistics)*

People who take more pills have more diseases or more severe disease and probably die of their diseases, not the medications. Disease would be the confounding variable in this case. If a researcher measures the number of ashtrays owned and mortality and concludes that ashtrays cause death, smoking would be the confounding factor. Interviewer bias is not likely when the outcome is death and the measurement is so objective (number of pills). The large number of subjects in the study makes a type II error much less likely.

169. The answer is C. *(Biostatistics)*

The purpose of screening is to identify conditions that would benefit from earlier intervention. Using screening to identify a condition that cannot be treated costs money and provides little or no benefit. Highly sensitive tests are preferred for screening, which carries the risk of a higher false-positive rate. Highly specific tests are preferred for confirmation of disease (ideally, these tests need to be sensitive and specific so that there is not an unacceptable level of false-negatives). When a disease is rare, the likelihood of a false-positive result increases, and the positive predictive value decreases. Increasing sensitivity often decreases specificity, as the number of false-positive results increases.

170. The answer is D. *(Preventive Medicine)*

Immunocompromised patients should not receive this live vaccine with the exception of HIV-positive patients, who should receive the vaccine because the benefits seem to outweigh the risks, unless patients are severely immunocompromised. Health care workers should receive the vaccine to prevent them from transmitting rubella to pregnant women. Pregnant women should not receive the vaccine because of concerns over rubella in pregnancy. This vaccine should be avoided in individuals with an anaphylactic reaction to eggs or neomycin.

171. The answer is B. *(Preventive Medicine)*

Influenza vaccine is indicated for all adults age 50 and older as well as for adults with chronic medical conditions who are younger than age 50. Influenza vaccine is given to children on aspirin therapy to *prevent* Reye's syndrome, as children taking aspirin who have or develop influenza are at an increased risk for Reye's syndrome. The pneumococcal vaccine is indicated in all newborn children (before the age of 20) and is especially important in those children not previously vaccinated with certain disorders (e.g., sickle cell disease, immunocompromised conditions, lung or cardiovascular disorders) and is indicated in all adults 65 and older regardless of health status (earlier in those with significant health problems). Tetanus boosters are recommended every 10 years in all adults, even in the absence of current or recent wounds. The toxicity of the tetanus booster is minimal. Most of the toxicity associated with the childhood vaccine is from the pertussis component (DPT = diphtheria, pertussis, tetanus), which is not part of the tetanus booster vaccine. Patient desire is a perfectly valid indication for the hepatitis B vaccine in those not vaccinated at birth, and all young adults as well as any high-risk older adults should be offered the vaccine.

172. The answer is B. *(Medicine—Geriatrics)*

In 2000, there were an estimated 35 million persons age 65 or older in the United States, accounting for almost 13 percent of the total population, and this number is increasing. Approximately 5% live in nursing homes. About 15% of people older than 65 suffer from some form of dementia; this percentage increases with increasing age (e.g., <5% from 65-69 years of age, but closer to 30% in those over age 85). People in this age group are more likely to commit suicide than younger persons. Sundowning, or confusion or worsening delirium or dementia at night, is not normal in healthy persons of any age.

173. The answer is B. *(Medicine—Infectious Disease)*

This man most likely has acquired immunodeficiency syndrome (AIDS) from human immunodeficiency virus (HIV) infection. The sexual history is relevant because the leading cause of HIV is still homosexual sex, although heterosexual transmission has increased significantly. He has most likely developed *Pneumocystis carinii* pneumonia given the diffuse bilateral interstitial infiltrates (wouldn't be expected with pneumococcal pneumonia) and fairly marked hypoxia. Breath sounds may be normal in this condition (and with any pneumonia). Because of a depletion of CD4 white cells and immune dysfunction, these patients often have normal or decreased white blood cell counts with an infection. The preferred treatment is trimethoprim-sulfamethoxazole (Bactrim).

174. The answer is B. *(Medicine—Infectious Disease)*

HIV should be in the differential diagnosis if infectious mononucleosis is considered. When the CD4 count drops to less than $200/mm^3$, patients are considered to have AIDS even if asymptomatic. HIV antibodies may take 1–3 months (rarely longer) to develop, which becomes important when someone requests testing based on recent risk-taking behavior. HIV patients should receive the inactivated polio vaccine if not already vaccinated, but the oral poliovirus vaccine should be avoided. The HIV ELISA test is a screening test, which must be confirmed with a Western blot HIV test before the diagnosis is made (and before the patient is told the test results).

175. The answer is E. *(Medicine—Immunology)*

Type II hypersensitivity is due to preformed antibodies (IgG or IgM) that cause tissue damage. All are good examples of this type of reaction except the PPD skin test, which is a classic example of type IV (or cell-mediated) hypersensitivity caused by sensitized T lymphocytes that release inflammatory mediators.

176. The answer is C. *(Emergency Medicine)*

Remember the ABCs. This patient may need pharmacologic treatment for anaphylaxis but has lost his airway and needs one quickly or he will die. Intravenous fluids and epinephrine are useful adjuncts, but neither are the first step. Antihistamines and corticosteroids are not useful for anaphylaxis, though they are useful for milder cutaneous reactions or prolonged reactions, respectively.

177. The answer is B. *(Medicine—Neurology)*

Creatine phosphokinase levels normally are markedly elevated when the diagnosis is made because of muscle deterioration. Muscular dystrophy usually is seen first in boys between the ages of 3 and 7 and is an X-linked recessive disorder of dystrophin. Muscle biopsy can confirm a suspected diagnosis. A new blood test called Single Condition Amplification/Internal Primer sequencing (SCAIP) now allows sequencing of the entire dystrophin gene to find mutations that can confirm Duchenne muscular dystrophy (and the carrier status) in 95% of cases, averting the need for biopsy.

178. The answer is A. *(Medicine—Neurology)*

This woman most likely has myasthenia gravis, a disorder of neuromuscular transmission secondary to anti–acetylcholine receptor antibodies that attack these receptors in the muscle. Diagnosis can be made by administering the anticholinesterase drug edrophonium (the Tensilon test) or by nerve conduction studies and electromyography. Muscle biopsy would show only nonspecific denervation effects on the muscle. Immediate corticosteroids are not required because the patient is stable, and treatment should be withheld until the diagnosis is made. Treatment involves medicine and surgery. Most patients are advised to have a thymectomy, which improves symptoms and treats or prevents thymomas (common in these patients). Long-acting acetylcholinesterase inhibitors, such as pyridostigmine, commonly are used for treatment.

179. The answer is D. *(Medicine—Neurology)*

This man has symptoms of parkinsonism, which may be caused by medications that block dopamine receptors, such as antipsychotics. Idiopathic parkinsonism increases the risk of suicide (as do most chronic, debilitating diseases) as well as dementia. Medications that increase dopamine in the basal ganglia (levodopa and carbidopa, bromocriptine, amantadine, selegiline) often improve symptoms, as may anticholinergic medications and possibly surgery.

180. The answer is A. *(Preventive Medicine)*

Annual Pap smears should be initiated by age 18 or 3 years after first sexual intercourse, whichever is sooner. Monthly (not annual) breast self-examinations in women are recommended starting around the age of 20. In many cases, women are the first to detect their own breast cancers. Lung cancer screening currently is not recommended even in high-risk patients. Clinical trials with CT scans of the chest in high-risk persons are ongoing. Prostate cancer screening generally is advised to begin at 40 (African Americans) or 50 (other races) years of age, as prostate cancer is rare prior to age 40.

181. The answer is D. *(Medicine—General)*

This woman most likely has Graves' disease with atrial fibrillation and pretibial myxedema, a specific finding of hyperthyroidism caused by Graves' disease (not seen with other causes of hyperthyroidism). Radioactive ablation, antithyroid medications, and/or surgery may be used to treat this condition, though medications are not curative and are typically used as temporizing therapies only. Although viral thyroiditis is a potential cause of hyperthyroidism, it does not cause pretibial myxedema and is not as common as Graves' disease. Thymectomy often is a part of myasthenia gravis treatment, and markedly elevated catecholamine breakdown products in the urine suggest a pheochromocytoma. Alprazolam sometimes is used in generalized anxiety disorder, which this woman probably does not have.

182. The answer is B. *(Medicine—Gastroenterology)*

This patient most likely has celiac sprue or gluten sensitivity with a classic case of dermatitis herpetiformis. Steatorrhea may occur with small bowel diseases, owing to malabsorption. Choice **A** describes a normal small bowel mucosa, which would not be expected. In gluten insensitivity, the villi become markedly atrophic, and small bowel biopsy often is used to confirm the disease, although a trial of a gluten-free diet can be prescribed to see if it works if the patient is not a good biopsy candidate. Avoidance of gluten often causes resolution of symptoms, including the dermatitis herpetiformis.

Antibiotics do not help, although they can help with tropical sprue, a bacterial disease usually seen outside the United States with similar symptoms that does not cause dermatitis herpetiformis. Crohn disease is in the differential diagnosis and may cause strictures but does not cause dermatitis herpetiformis (with its fairly characteristic appearance and IgA deposits) and usually results a significant history of abdominal pain by the time it produces a stricture.

183. The answer is E. (Medicine—General)

The figure reveals pyoderma gangrenosum, a painful ulcerative disorder that is commonly associated with systemic conditions, particularly inflammatory bowel disease, rheumatoid arthritis and monoclonal gammopathy. Other less commonly associated conditions include sarcoidosis, lupus, HIV infection, Wegener's granulomatosis, and Behcet's syndrome. The bilateral hilar lymphadenopathy with bilateral interstitial lung infiltrates is highly suggestive of sarcoidosis, which commonly affects reproductive-age black women. Tuberculosis is highly unlikely to cause this type of x-ray pattern, usually preferring the upper lobes when reactivated. Paragonimiasis is rare in the United States, usually affecting those in the Far East. Although it may be confused with tuberculosis, it generally would not cause the given chest film findings. Goodpasture's syndrome is more common in men, doesn't generally cause bilateral hilar adenopathy, and most likely would affect the kidney and cause hemoptysis. Leukemia wouldn't cause the chest x-ray findings described in the case either.

184. The answer is A. (Pharmacology)

Tetracyclines (particularly doxycycline) and the antipsychotic chlorpromazine are the classic agents for photosensitivity. Patients should be counseled on avoidance of the sun or use of heavy sunscreen to avoid severe sunburns. Sulfa drugs, oral contraceptives, NSAIDs (e.g., piroxicam, ibuprofen), digoxin and amiodarone also may cause photosensitivity.

185. The answer is E. (Emergency Medicine)

Cat bites on the hand have a fairly high infection rate, often with *Pasteurella multocida*. Amoxicillin with clavulanate and ampicillin with sulbactam commonly are used to prevent infection in this setting. Wounds should be cleaned thoroughly with soap and bandaged, but suturing and cauterization should be avoided initially because of infection concerns, especially with a delayed presentation, as in this case (if you're wondering why it took the parents two days to bring the child in, you get a gold star!). Rabies generally is not seen in the United States from cat or dog bites, and prophylaxis is not indicated.

186. The answer is D. (Pediatrics—Infectious Disease)

This child most likely has bronchiolitis, which tends to occur in 0- to 18-month-old infants in the fall and winter. Treatment is largely supportive because the cause usually is the respiratory syncytial virus. Ribavirin or anti-RSV immune globulin can be used in severe cases or when the child has other serious health problems but is not used in routine cases. Other less common causes of bronchiolitis are the influenza and parainfluenza viruses. Chest radiograph usually shows hyperinflation, not diffuse infiltrates.

187. The answer is A. (Medicine—Infectious Disease)

This patient most likely has an infection with *Rickettsia rickettsii*, the cause of Rocky Mountain spotted fever, which is transmitted by a tick bite. The characteristic rash, which starts on the distal extremities then spreads toward the trunk, is the most important diagnostic clue. The disease is most common on the East coast (despite its name), especially the southeastern states. Immediate intravenous antibiotics, usually doxycycline or chloramphenicol, are indicated.

188. The answer is D. (Medicine—Infectious Disease)

This patient most likely has infectious mononucleosis from an Epstein-Barr virus infection. All of the choices except **D** would not be unusual with infectious mononucleosis. Auer rods, which are intracellular inclusion bodies that resemble tennis rackets, are seen in certain subtypes (particularly the M3 subtype) of acute myelocytic leukemia.

189. The answer is D. *(Dermatology)*

The patient has grade I or mild cervical intraepithelial neoplasia due to human papillomavirus (HPV) infection, as evidenced by koilocytosis (labeled "K"), which describes a prominent clear cytoplasmic halo around the nucleus. Additionally, binucleate cells (labeled "D") and dyskeratotic cells (labeled "D"; describes individual cell keratinization) can be seen, which are also indicative of HPV infection. The degree of dysplastic change is quite mild, as evidenced by a fairly normal nuclear-to-cytoplasm ratio and lack of involvement of many cells. PID is not diagnosable on Pap smear – it is a clinical diagnosis, though inflammatory changes can be seen when PID is present.

190. The answer is D. *(Dermatology)*

This child has developed a keloid, which is in essence, a significantly hypertrophic scarring reaction, often to minor trauma such as ear piercing. It is most commonly seen in African Americans and unlikely to spontaneously regress. Fortunately, it is a benign lesion that is of primarily cosmetic concern and has no propensity to metastasize. Attempts at excision may meet with recurrence that is worse than the original lesion.

191–196. *(Psychiatry—General)*

The answers are the following: **191. J**   **192. D**   **193. I**   **194. B**   **195. H**   **196. G.**

The personality disorders are characterized by onset in childhood or adolescence, are difficult to treat, and describe a way of interacting with the world that causes the person recurrent problems when attempting to relate to others. There are 10 main personality disorders:

1. *Paranoid*—paranoid; think everyone out to get them (friends, too); often start lawsuits

2. *Schizoid*—the classic loner; no friends and no interest in having friends

3. *Schizotypal*—bizarre beliefs (ESP, cults, superstition, illusions) and manner of speaking but no psychosis

4. *Avoidant*—no friends but wants them; scared of criticism and rejection, so avoids others (inferiority complex)

5. *Histrionic*—overly dramatic and attention-seeking; inappropriately seductive; must be center of attention

6. *Narcissistic*—egocentric, lack empathy, use others for their own gain, sense of entitlement

7. *Antisocial*—most frequently tested; long criminal record (con men), torture animals and set fires in childhood (history of pediatric conduct disorder required for this diagnosis), aggressive, don't pay bills or support children, liar, no remorse or conscience; strong association with alcoholism and drug abuse and somatization disorder; usually male

8. *Borderline*—have unstable mood, behavior, relationships (many bisexual), and self-image; look for splitting (people are all good or all bad and frequently may change categories), suicide attempts, micropsychotic episodes (2 minutes of psychosis), impulsiveness, and constant crisis

9. *Dependent*—cannot be (or do anything) alone; wife will stay with abusive husband; very dependent on others

10. *Obsessive-compulsive*—anal-retentive, stubborn, rules more important than objectives, restricted affect, cheap

197–200. *(Medicine—Neurology)*

The answers are the following: **197. C**   **198. D**   **199. A**   **200. B.**

The first patient has pseudotumor cerebri, characterized by a markedly elevated opening pressure but otherwise normal CSF. The second patient has a subarachnoid hemorrhage, characterized by a grossly bloody CSF and slightly increased pressure. The third patient has bacterial meningitis, characterized by high cell count with mostly neutrophils, decreased glucose, and mildly increased protein and opening pressure. The last patient has multiple sclerosis, characterized by mildly elevated cell count with mostly lymphocytes and mildly elevated protein. Choice **E** could describe a patient with tuberculous or fungal meningitis, where the glucose is low and protein high (as in bacterial meningitis), but the cell count elevation is less dramatic and characterized by a higher percentage of lymphocytes (not like bacterial meningitis).

ANSWERS AND EXPLANATIONS

201. The answer is B. *(Neurosurgery)*

Early detection coupled with minimal delay in treatment is associated with the best outcome in the setting of spinal cord compression. Delays in treatment worsen the pretreatment function, which is well correlated with the patient's eventual outcome. The longer treatment is delayed, the more likely it is that increasing, irreversible neurologic damage will occur. In severe injury, there often is little hope for meaningful recovery.

202. The answer is E. *(Medicine—Infectious Disease)*

This is the classic description of sporotrichosis, which is treated with long-term (i.e., ≥ 3–6 months) itraconazole, fluconazole, amphotericin B, or oral potassium iodide. *Streptococcus* and *Staphylococcus* infections, although possible, are likely to cause pain and fever.

203. The answer is D. *(Medicine—Infectious Disease)*

Sepsis from encapsulated organisms, such as *Streptococcus pneumoniae*, *Neisseria meningitidis*, and *Haemophilus influenzae*, becomes much more likely after a splenectomy. All persons should receive the *S. pneumoniae* vaccine after a splenectomy.

204. The answer is C. *(Medicine—Infectious Disease)*

Haemophilus often produces a pneumonia that is indistinguishable from pneumococcal, also known as classic or typical, pneumonia. Typical pneumonia tends to have a short prodrome, productive cough, high fever, and a lobar consolidation pattern on chest radiograph. *Haemophilus* is probably the most common cause of typical pneumonia in children and the second most common cause in adults, after *S. pneumoniae*. The other choices all tend to cause an "atypical" (i.e., not like typical or pneumococcal pneumonia) pneumonia, with a longer prodrome, patchy and/or multilobe lung involvement on chest radiograph, low-grade fever, and nonproductive cough.

205. The answer is C. *(Medicine—Oncology)*

Human chorionic gonadotropin is commonly followed during choriocarcinoma treatment. Liver and certain testicular tumors may be followed with alpha fetoprotein (alpha-fetoprotein), and epithelial ovarian cancer is most commonly associated with CA-125 antigen, although other tumor markers may be used with ovarian germ cell tumors. Pancreatic cancer most commonly is followed with CA 19-9 and CEA antigens. Breast cancer may be followed with CA 15-3 or CA 29-9. Acid phosphatase rarely is used but becomes elevated with prostate cancer that has extended outside the outer prostatic capsule.

Tumor Marker	Cancer(s)
Alpha fetoprotein (AFP)	Liver (hepatocellular carcinoma), gonad (yolk-sac tumors)
Carcinoembryonic antigen (CEA)	Colon, pancreas, other gastrointestinal tumors
Prostate-specific antigen (PSA)	Prostate (early)
Acid phosphatase	Prostate (only with extension outside the capsule)
Human chorionic gonadotropin (HCG)	Hydatiform moles, choriocarcinoma
CA-125	Ovary
S-100	Melanoma, central nervous system and nerve tumors
CA 19-9	Pancreas
CA 15-3, CA 27-29	Breast

206. The answer is B. *(General Knowledge and Principles)*

Anyone who is competent can refuse care, and their wishes should be respected in the absence of depression or other factors that may render them incompetent. A physician should be capable of determining competence at the bedside, with psychiatric or court evaluation reserved for difficult or special situations.

207. The answer is E. *(Ear, Nose, and Throat Surgery)*

Hairy leukoplakia is a manifestation of Epstein-Barr virus infection in those who are immunocompromised (particularly HIV/AIDS patient) and generally is not associated with oral cancer. Tobacco in all forms and alcohol are the classic causative agents of most oral/head and neck malignancies (usually squamous cell), and erythroplakia is a classic description of carcinoma in situ or early cancer in the mouth. Erythroplastic lesions are inflamed, erythematous, and granular or slightly abraded in appearance.

208. The answer is D. *(Dermatology)*

This is most likely a basal cell skin cancer and should be removed entirely. If you are wrong, there is no harm done other than a small scar, and given the classic description in a person older than age 70 with occupational sun exposure, you are much more likely to be right. Doing only a partial biopsy would not afford the patient a cosmetic benefit and may require him to have a second biopsy.

209. The answer is A. *(Medicine—Oncology)*

When carcinoid tumors metastasize to the liver, the serotoninergic products released are no longer broken down before they reach the systemic circulation and thus the carcinoid syndrome begins. The most bothersome symptoms to patients usually are cutaneous flushing, abdominal cramping, and diarrhea. Right-sided heart valve fibrosis may develop, but left-sided valve lesions usually are not seen because the lung breaks down the serotonin products. With a primary bronchial carcinoid, left-sided valvular lesions may be seen, though this is quite rare because bronchial carcinoids rarely produce significant amounts of active seritonergic products. Elevated urinary 5-hydroxyindoleacetic acid, a serotonin breakdown product, is a valuable diagnostic aid.

210. The answer is C. *(Medicine—Hematology)*

Factor XI deficiency is rare but would result in a bleeding tendency. The others are well-established causes of an increased tendency to form thrombi. Factor V Leiden mutation, which is caused by a single point mutation, is thought to be the cause of as many as 25% of cases of idiopathic recurrent deep venous thrombi and pulmonary emboli.

211. The answer is D. *(Medicine—Rheumatology)*

The lupus anticoagulant causes a prolonged partial thromboplastin time test but paradoxically causes an increased tendency for thrombosis. It also is associated with a false-positive VDRL syphilis test and recurrent first-trimester abortions. Given the presence of all of these things in the history, this is the most likely cause.

212. The answer is C. *(Medicine—Hematology)*

This patient most likely has disseminated intravascular coagulation secondary to an underlying malignancy. Patients may present with bleeding or clotting symptoms. The pattern of coagulation pathology includes all three tests (prothrombin time, partial thromboplastin time, and bleeding time), which cannot be explained by warfarin ingestion, fibrin deficiency, or von Willebrand disease. In disseminated intravascular coagulation, low platelets and low fibrin levels usually are seen secondary to being used up during the widespread intravascular coagulation. Hepatic necrosis could conceivably explain this pattern of coagulation abnormalities but tends to present suddenly and dramatically (i.e., no 40-lb weight loss, which takes time to develop) and there is no mention of risk factors for this rare condition.

213. The answer is B. *(Medicine—Rheumatology)*

This patient most likely has fibromyalgia, a poorly understood benign disorder that often is aggravated by stress. The hallmarks are negative inflammation markers (e.g., sedimentation rate, C-reactive protein), normal creatine phosphokinase (CPK) levels, and normal electromyography and muscle biopsy. Patients have point tenderness in affected muscles, typically in the distribution shown below.

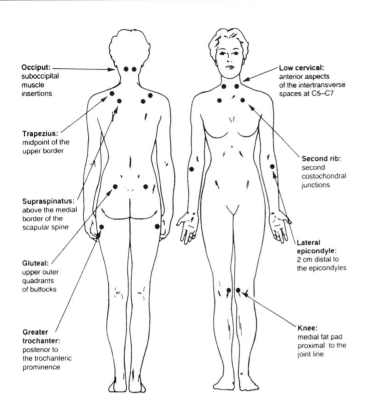

Occiput:
suboccipital
muscle
insertions

Trapezius:
midpoint of the
upper border

Supraspinatus:
above the medial
border of the
scapular spine

Gluteal:
upper outer
quadrants
of buttocks

Greater
trochanter:
posterior to
the trochanteric
prominence

Low cervical:
anterior aspects
of the intertransverse
spaces at C5–C7

Second rib:
second
costochondral
junctions

Lateral
epicondyle:
2 cm distal to
the epicondyles

Knee:
medial fat pad
proximal to the
joint line

Location of the 18 (9 pairs) specific tender points in patients with fibromyalgia. (From Freundlich B, Leventhal L: The fibromyalgia syndrome. In Schumacher HR Jr, Kippel JH, Koopman WJ (eds): Primer on the Rheumatic Diseases, 10th ed. Atlanta, Arthritis Foundation, 1993, pp 247–249, with permission.)

Fibromyalgia also tends to occur in younger women who are often anxious or under stress. Treatment includes aspirin and other nonsteroidal anti-inflammatory medications, antidepressants, and rest. Polymyositis would cause an elevated creatine phosphokinase level and tends to affect women older than age 35, and polymyalgia rheumatica usually has a markedly elevated sedimentation rate and affects older women, usually older than 50. Both of these conditions also generally involve primarily proximal muscles, whereas fibromyalgia may involve any muscle group. Dermatomyositis should have skin findings, classically a heliotrope (i.e. purplish) rash around the eyelids, but is otherwise similar to polymyositis. Polyarteritis nodosa is a vasculitis that tends to affect the visceral organs (e.g., kidneys, bowel) and should also cause an elevated sedimentation rate and positive P-ANCA titer.

214. The answer is A. *(Medicine—Rheumatology)*

This patient most likely has Buerger's disease, or thromboangiitis obliterans, which is a severe Raynaud's-type phenomenon that occurs in men between the ages of 20 and 40 who smoke, often heavily. Patients must quit smoking, or the condition may progress to severe ischemia and gangrene in the extremities. The disorder does not occur in non-smokers, and only 5% of patients are women. The disease may remit completely when smoking is stopped, although not always. Continued smoking makes all other treatments ineffective.

215. The answer is C. *(Medicine—Infectious Disease)*

This patient most likely has Lyme disease and developed erythema chronicum migrans, the classic skin rash seen in up to 75% of affected persons. If asked, the patient may recall being bitten by a tick, but the description of the rash after a camping trip in Wisconsin should be enough to make a presumptive diagnosis while awaiting confirmatory results. Although aspirin may be an important adjunct for symptom relief, *Borrelia burgdorferi*, the responsible spirochete, should be treated with doxycycline, ceftriaxone or amoxicillin. The patient's headache and photophobia may represent an aseptic meningitis, which can occur with Lyme disease.

216. The answer is B. *(Medicine—Rheumatology)*

The presence of crystals in an inflamed joint should make you think of gout and pseudogout. Gout has **n**eedle-shaped crystals that have **n**egative birefringence, and pseudogout has rhomboid crystals that have weakly positive birefringence (**p** in pseudogout equals **p**ositive birefringence—helps some to remember). An elevated uric acid level does not automatically mean gout, and a normal uric acid level does not exclude gout. Septic arthritis should cause more white blood cells with greater than 75% neutrophils and no crystals. Podagra is gout involving the big toe.

217. The answer is A. *(Surgery—General)*

The most common cause of a postoperative fever in the first 24 hours is atelectasis, which this patient most likely has. Early ambulation, incentive spirometry, and minimal use of narcotics to control pain all help to minimize this condition. By suppressing the cough reflex, narcotics increase the chances of developing atelectasis. Because of intrinsic hypoventilation, obesity also increases the likelihood of developing atelectasis. Atelectasis may lead to pneumonia. Antibiotics are inappropriate at this point in time because there is no evidence of infection. On examination, crackles sometimes can be heard with atelectasis.

218. The answer is B. *(Medicine—General)*

Pseudotumor cerebri is the most likely diagnosis in a young, otherwise healthy, obese woman with papilledema, negative brain imaging, and little to no loss of vision. A lumbar puncture in these patients is normal other than an increased opening pressure. A posterior fossa brain tumor, although possible and sometimes missed by a CT scan if early in its course, is rare in this age group and often has accompanying neurologic signs. Optic neuritis should cause a decrease in visual acuity, although the optic disks often appear swollen. A subarachnoid hemorrhage by itself does not usually cause papilledema and would be visualized on CT scan in most instances. It also tends to have a more dramatic, sudden presentation. Leukemia should cause other historical or physical findings, such as lymphadenopathy, weight loss, or infections.

Treatment for pseudotumor cerebri often is supportive, and weight loss for obese patients may be all that is needed. Therapeutic, repeated lumbar punctures or placement of a lumbar shunt can be used to lower the pressure. Loss of vision, although fairly uncommon in this condition, is the major complication.

219. The answer is C. *(Medicine—Hematology)*

This woman has beta-thalassemia minor. Iron overload can occur with these patients, who have an excess of iron, and iron therapy should not be given in this condition. Although reticulocytosis does occur with iron therapy and a 3- to 6-month course of therapy generally is indicated, this woman has beta-thalassemia, not iron deficiency. The diagnosis is clinched by a combination of Mediterranean descent and a microcytic, hypochromic anemia with reticulocytosis and an elevated hemoglobin A_2 level, which is quite specific for beta-thalassemia (and is not seen in vitamin or mineral deficiency–induced anemias). The miscarriage could be related to a genetic fetal anemia but not due to beta-thalassemia minor, which does not cause symptoms until a few months after birth. Miscarriage may occur with alpha-thalassemia, in which a four-gene mutation can lead to fetal hydrops.

Given the three other healthy children, it is unlikely that the husband is a carrier for beta-thalassemia. The woman requires no treatment for the mild, self-limiting anemia or the history of miscarriage because she had subsequent deliveries without difficulty. A trigger number for the level of hemoglobin that requires a transfusion should be avoided. The decision to transfuse should be based on clinical grounds (i.e., symptoms, coexisting medical problems), not on a laboratory value. Constipation is a common complaint in individuals taking iron supplements and does not warrant a work-up in someone this age.

220. The answer is D. *(Medicine—Nephrology)*

Thiazide diuretics absorb calcium, preventing more of it from going into the urine, where it may precipitate out and form a calcium stone. Anything that increases calcium or oxalate excretion into the urine increases the risk of calcium stones. Hyperoxaluria is an uncommon condition usually caused by small bowel disease (e.g., Crohn disease) or resection.

221. The answer is D. *(Urology)*

This patient most likely has urolithiasis, or a urinary tract stone, which should be observed to see if it passes spontaneously. Narcotics can be given for pain, which is often severe, and high levels of fluid intake or intravenous fluids should be given to help in trying to get the stone to pass. While you are waiting, it is appropriate to try to determine the composition of the stone and the underlying cause, if possible. Urinalysis with laboratory analysis of any crystals or stones found is important, and a calcium level is reasonable as an initial test because calcium stones are the most common type (roughly 75% of cases). Surgical intervention is reserved for large, impacted stones that fail to pass. As a rough rule of thumb, stones 5 mm or less will generally pass with conservative management.

222. The answer is C. *(Pediatrics—General)*

Keeping the different hematologic and kidney disorders straight can be difficult. Hemolytic-uremic syndrome is similar to thrombotic thrombocytopenic purpura in that both have anemia and thrombocytopenia thought to be due to intravascular-mediated destruction in inflamed vessels. Hemolytic-uremic syndrome affects young children (usually < 4 years old) and classically occurs after a bout of infectious diarrhea, often *Escherichia coli* type O157:H7, and primarily involves the kidney. Thrombotic thrombocytopenic purpura affects adults, often has no associated infection, and presents with neurologic symptoms and signs in addition to kidney and other organ manifestations. Idiopathic thrombocytopenic purpura is a pure platelet problem caused by antiplatelet antibodies with no kidney involvement or anemia. Henoch-Schönlein purpura affects the kidney but does not cause anemia or thrombocytopenia and classically produces a skin rash on the lower extremities.

223. The answer is C. *(General Knowledge and Principles)*

The kidneys, adrenal glands, aorta, vena cava, most of the duodenum, and most of the pancreas are retroperitoneal structures. The anal canal is in the pelvis. The other choices are intraperitoneal structures.

224. The answer is C. *(Medicine—Infectious Disease)*

This woman most likely has a urinary tract infection based on the symptoms and the result of a good urinalysis sample (the lack of epithelial cells indicates a good urinary sample). *E. coli* causes roughly 80% of urinary tract infections. *Trichomonas* and *Chlamydia* spp. generally cause vaginal or cevical/pelvic infections, respectively. S*taphylococcus saprophyticus* and *Streptococcus bovis* are less common causes of urinary tract infections, though most strains of staph and strep do not reduce nitrates to nitrites (i.e. would cause nitrites to be negative in a urinalysis).

225. The answer is B. *(Laboratory Medicine)*

This is a contaminated urine sample as evidenced by the presence of large numbers of epithelial cells. The most likely cause of the blood in a woman would be the vagina (e.g., menstrual bleeding). A clean-catch specimen should not have epithelial cells in it. The bacteria may or may not be from the urinary tract in this setting. If there is concern regarding urinary tract pathology, a new specimen should be obtained.

226. The answer is D. *(Medicine—Nephrology)*

Magnesium, potassium, and phosphorus levels become elevated with renal failure, and supplementation can be dangerous. Calcium supplements may prevent bone loss and act as a phosphate binder. Water-soluble vitamins are removed in dialysis. Patients are counseled regarding avoidance of potassium-rich foods, such as bananas and orange juice.

227. The answer is A. *(Preventive Medicine)*

Obesity increases the risk of type II diabetes; overall mortality (at any age); hypertension; hypertriglyceridemia (also weakly associated with hypercholesterolemia); heart disease and coronary artery disease; gallstones (cholesterol stones); hypoventilation, Pickwickian syndrome, and sleep apnea; symptomatic osteoarthritis; cancer (especially endometrial cancer); thromboembolism; and varicose veins. A thin body habitus makes osteoporosis more likely; obesity increases the level of endogenous estrogen and actually decreases the risk of osteoporosis.

228. The answer is D. *(Medicine—General)*

This patient has most likely developed the syndrome of inappropriate antidiuretic hormone (SIADH) secondary to pain and narcotic administration. She needs the intravenous fluids turned off and free water restricted. Hypertonic saline should not be ordered on the boards unless the patient has seizures resulting from hyponatremia (may cause brainstem damage from central pontine myelinolysis). Increasing the fluid rate worsens the hyponatremia. Demeclocycline is used for refractory cases of SIADH to induce mild nephrogenic diabetes insipidus (counteracts the SIADH) and is not appropriate at this time. Small cell lung cancers are not amenable to resection, and the patient had normal electrolytes when she came into the hospital, making the lung cancer less likely as the cause.

229. The answer is A. *(Medicine—Endocrinology)*

ACTH disappears when the pituitary gland is removed, causing cortisol to decrease because its release is not stimulated. CRH should rise because the feedback inhibition from ACTH and cortisol is missing.

230. The answer is A. *(Medicine—Endocrinology)*

Excess thyroxine intake would cause increased thyroxine, resulting in feedback inhibition of TRH and TSH. This same pattern of abnormality would occur with an intrinsic thyroid disorder that caused too much thyroid hormone to be produced (e.g., Graves disease, toxic thyroid adenoma, toxic multinodular goiter). A history, physical exam, and/or nuclear medicine thyroid scan would be able to distinguish these conditions even though the serum lab values are similar. The derangements listed in choice **B** would occur with a TSH-secreting pituitary adenoma.

231. The answer is A. *(Pediatrics—Neonates)*

Physiologic jaundice affects as many as 50% of term newborns and even more premature infants, usually starting on day 2 to 4 of life. It rarely causes kernicterus and is thought to be due to immaturity of the liver with decreased metabolic capacity. *Any jaundice present at birth is pathologic, not physiologic.*

232. The answer is A. *(Pediatrics—Neonates)*

This is the normal physiologic jaundice of the newborn. Total bilirubin levels reach a peak on day 3 to 5 of life that is normally less than 9 to 10 mg/dL. In this otherwise healthy infant, only routine follow-up is required. If the total bilirubin peaks at less than 9 to 10 mg/dL in an otherwise healthy term infant, no further evaluation or treatment generally is required. If the jaundice deepens or the child develops symptoms, repeat serum bilirubin levels should be drawn.

233. The answer is A. *(Pediatrics—General)*

Especially in children, any febrile or infectious illness can result in systemic complaints related to the gastrointestinal tract, such as nausea, vomiting, and diarrhea. The odds of there being two coexisting diseases are much less likely than having one disease explain both conditions. The frank otitis media seen on physical examination coupled with a fairly high fever is enough to cause the gastrointestinal symptoms.

234. The answer is C. *(Medicine—Gastroenterology)*

Chronic reflux esophagitis can lead to Barrett's metaplasia of the distal esophagus, which carries a risk of malignant transformation into an esophageal adenocarcinoma. Adenocarcinoma of the esophagus is the most common subtype of esophageal carcinoma for this reason. The other conditions are not associated with reflux.

235. The answer is C. *(Medicine—Gastroenterology)*

Pancreatitis is not due to an infection (other than rare cases of viral pancreatitis), and antibiotics are not indicated. The other measures are standard in the management of acute pancreatitis. Narcotics are appropriate for pain, which can be severe, once the diagnosis is made. Normally, meperidine is preferred over morphine because of the latter's potential for causing sphincter of Oddi spasm and possibly worsening pain.

236. The answer is B. *(Medicine—Gastroenterology)*

Chronic pancreatitis, though an inflammatory condition, does not respond to corticosteroid treatment to any significant degree. Most cases of chronic pancreatitis in the United States are due to alcoholism. Gallstones and gallbladder disease do not cause chronic pancreatitis, which is primarily due to the fact that cholecystectomy is routinely performed after a single episode of gallstone pancreatitis. The other choices are important therapeutic measures in chronic pancreatitis.

237. The answer is E. *(Medicine—Gastroenterology)*

The barium swallow and symptoms are classic for achalasia, which is caused by a hypertensive lower esophageal sphincter that does not relax well and an esophagus with abnormal peristalsis. Unlike patients with scleroderma, patients with achalasia do not get reflux, which cannot occur through the tightly closed sphincter. Gastrointestinal cancer is rare in this age group and normally would not cause severe chest pain. Barrett's esophagus results from reflux (heartburn symptoms usually present).

238. The answer is B. *(Medicine—Gastroenterology)*

Liver disease or inflammation tends to cause a mixed hyperbilirubinemia and normally does not cause clay-colored stools (although it may cause darkened urine). With a biliary obstruction, bilirubin cannot be excreted into the gut, and the stools become clay or gray colored. Conjugated bilirubin appears in the urine and causes a darkening of the urine, in contrast with unconjugated bilirubin, which is tightly bound to albumin and thus not filtered into the urine.

239. The answer is D. *(Pediatrics—Neonates)*

The physical findings and chest radiograph are classic for infant respiratory distress syndrome (i.e. hyaline membrane disease), which is more common in premature infants and infants born to diabetic mothers. The cause is a lack of pulmonary surfactant. Chlamydial pneumonia and cystic fibrosis do not tend to cause respiratory symptoms at birth. Carbon monoxide poisoning is unlikely without a history of unusual environmental exposure, and pulmonary hypoplasia is rare and not a good explanation for the chest radiograph findings.

240. The answer is E. *(Dermatology)*

The diagnosis of acne vulgaris, or acne, can be made on appearance alone in most cases. Acne has not been shown to be caused by diet, sex (including masturbation), or exercise. It is not thought to be an autoimmune phenomenon. First-line therapy is topical agents, such as benzoyl peroxide and salicylic acid, which often are available in over-the-counter preparations. Topical antibiotics can be tried, such as clindamycin or tetracycline. These are thought to be effective because of *Propionibacterium acnes* involvement in the pathogenesis. Oral antibiotics and oral contraceptives in women can be tried. Topical isotretinoin can be tried for resistant cases. As a last resort, oral isotretinoin can be tried. This drug often is effective, but because it is teratogenic and can cause liver damage and joint pain, it is not a first-line agent. Remember to discuss the risks, get a negative pregnancy test, and advise birth control for women before starting oral isotretinoin.

241. The answer is B. *(Dermatology)*

The white patches shown are most characteristic of tinea versicolor, also called pityriasis versicolor, a fungal infection. This condition often is noticed in Caucasians after sun exposure because the lesions fail to tan and become more noticeable. Treatment with selenium sulfide lotion or topical antifungals often is effective. The other choices all tend to cause pigmented lesions.

242. The answer is D. *(Pediatrics—General)*

An aspirated foreign body is most likely to go down the right side and lodge in a right middle or lower lobe bronchus. A congenital pulmonary anomaly should have caused infections sooner, and the other choices should present with other infections or symptoms in other parts of the body (and lung). The phrase "otherwise healthy" is meant to steer you away from cystic fibrosis, congenital immunodeficiency and HIV infection.

243–250. *(General Knowledge and Principles)*

The answers are the following: 243. D   244. C   245. D   246. B   247. A   248. A   249. D   250. A.

This is straight memorization and regurgitation, which is less prevalent on USMLE exams than it used to be, but can never completely disappear given the vast amount of ever increasing knowledge medical school graduates must accumulate. The figure for question 249 depicts a myelomeningocele, one of the more severe forms of spina bifida, which is a polygenic/multifactorial disorder.

ANSWERS AND EXPLANATIONS

251. The answer is C. *(Medicine—Infectious Disease)*

Moraxella and *Haemophilus* are gram-negative coccobacilli that can cause bronchitis, especially in patients with chronic obstructive pulmonary disease. Although a gram-negative diplococcus, *Neisseria* is an unlikely cause of bronchitis. *Streptococcus* species are gram-positive, whereas *Mycoplasma* lacks a true cell wall and thus does not show up well with Gram staining.

252. The answer is D. *(Medicine—Infectious Disease)*

This organism usually affects patients with immunosuppression or patients who smoke and drink alcohol excessively. The classic reservoir of infection is an environmental water source, such as an air-conditioning unit. *Chlamydia psittaci* is associated with exposure to birds, and the other choices are transmitted through contact with an infected person.

253. The answer is D. *(Medicine—Infectious Disease)*

See the following chart for classic differences between typical (i.e., caused by or similar to the pneumonia caused by *S. pneumoniae*) versus atypical pneumonia:

	Typical Pneumonia	Atypical Pneumonia
Prodrome	Short (< 2 days)	Long (> 3 days)—headaches, malaise, arthralgias
Fever	High (> 102°F)	Low (< 102°F)
Age	> 40	< 40
Chest film	One distinct lobe involved	Diffuse or multilobe involvement
Organism	*S. pneumoniae, H. influenzae*	Many (*H. influenzae, Mycoplasma, Chlamydia*)
Best empirical antibiotic	Third-generation cephalosporin or broad-spectrum fluoroquinolone (e.g., levofloxacin)	Azithromycin

Blood cultures are more likely to be positive with *S. pneumoniae* than with atypical pneumonias.

254. The answer is B. *(Pediatrics—Neonates)*

Prostaglandin production is shut off, not stimulated by increased oxygen, which is why indomethacin sometimes is used in an attempt to close a patent ductus arteriosus and intravenous prostaglandins can be given to keep the ductus patent, as in a complicated cyanotic heart disease in which closure of the ductus could worsen the child's condition. The other choices are correct.

255. The answer is B. *(Medicine—Cardiology)*

Medications that slow the heart down and allow for increased filling time, such as beta blockers or centrally acting calcium channel blockers, are thought to help diastolic dysfunction. This condition usually is due to a thickened, stiff ventricle, as seen in hypertension and hypertrophic cardiomyopathy. The other choices may worsen the condition, especially if they cause a reflex tachycardia. Digoxin worsens hypertrophic cardiomyopathy and does not help diastolic dysfunction caused by hypertension.

256. The answer is B. *(Obstetrics)*

Although maternal smoking has not been linked to definite structural abnormalities in the fetus, it has been linked to premature rupture of the membranes, placental abruption, intrauterine fetal death, intrauterine growth retardation, increased neonatal mortality, and increased risk of sudden infant death syndrome.

257. The answer is A. *(Pediatrics—Cardiology)*

Most ventricular septal defects are small, resolve spontaneously, and require only observation. Larger and more hemodynamically significant defects may require surgical closure. Prostaglandin and prostaglandin inhibitors, such as indomethacin, are used for patent ductus arteriosus management, not ventricular septal defects.

258. The answer is C. *(Pediatrics—Hematology)*

This child could have hemophilia A (factor VIII deficiency) or B (factor IX deficiency), but type A is much more common. Idiopathic thrombocytopenia does not affect the partial thromboplastin time but can cause a prolonged bleeding time. Henoch-Schönlein purpura does not affect standard clotting tests. Von Willebrand's disease causes primarily a prolonged bleeding time, but also may prolong the partial thromboplastin time slightly.

259. The answer is D. *(Orthopedics)*

A severe compound (open) fracture with absent pulses distally is an orthopedic (and vascular) emergency requiring immediate operation for open reduction and exploration of the wound to attempt to re-establish blood flow before tissue necrosis occurs. As a general rule of thumb, open fractures (e.g., overlying skin breakdown/laceration) require open operative reduction and antibiotics, while many closed fractures (obverlying skin intact) can be treated with closed reduction (i.e., casting). Of course, there are exceptions.

260. The answer is D. *(Medicine—Cardiology)*

This woman has the murmur of mitral stenosis, which is a common valve affected by rheumatic heart disease. Mitral stenosis prevents large amounts of blood flow or increased pressure from reaching the left ventricle. The left atrium frequently enlarges and hypertrophies secondary to having to generate higher pressures to overcome the stenotic valve. Blood also backs up into the pulmonary circulation, which can cause pulmonary hypertension and right ventricular pathology.

261. The answer is D. *(General Knowledge and Principles)*

This patient is oxygenating adequately with 3 L nasal cannula and probably does not require a change in respiratory care. She has failed a more than adequate fluid challenge (did it make things worse?) and should not be given more fluids in light of her distended neck veins. Invasive hemodynamic monitoring is indicated to determine the exact cause of the patient's hypotension. Discussing code status with a patient who has an altered mental status is inappropriate. Heparin should not be given in the absence of a clear indication.

262. The answer is A. *(Surgery—Trauma)*

The patient had some response to the initial fluid with an improvement in blood pressure and pulse and should be given another liter of Ringer's lactate, the intravenous fluid of choice in the setting of trauma. Dextrose and water solutions are not appropriate in this setting because the patient needs volume expansion. CT scan of the head is not indicated at this time because no head injury was described and the patient needs to be stabilized first. The patient's examination is fairly benign, and laparotomy would be premature. CT scan of the abdomen and pelvis with oral and IV contrast would be a better first step if there is suspicion of internal injuries (which is appropriate given the abdominal bruise, tenderness and altered mental status, which makes physical exam less relaible).

263. The answer is D. *(Pediatrics—Hematology)*

The presence of pancytopenia in a child without a history of medication use should make you think of acute lymphocytic leukemia. The peak age for this disorder is 3 to 5 years old, and it is more common in children with Down syndrome. Lymphoma is unlikely to cause pancytopenia at presentation. Parvovirus B19 can cause severe anemia (red cell aplasia) in patients with immunodeficiency or high-turnover anemias, classically in sickle cell disease, but rarely causes significant symptoms in those without high-turnover anemias. Parvovirus infection does not generally cause pancytopenia. Although aplastic anemia from toxin exposure is possible, the history is not suggestive, and this is uncommon in the United States. Benzene and insecticides are the classic toxins that can cause aplastic anemia.

264. The answer is B. *(Neurosurgery)*

Epidural hematomas usually are due to meningeal artery (classically the middle meningeal artery) bleeding and frequently occur in the setting of a temporal bone skull fracture. Patients commonly lose consciousness from the blow to the head or brisk nature of the bleeding with resultant severe intracranial hypertension. Rapid, dramatic onset of symptoms is common with epidural hematomas because arterial bleeding often is brisk and causes increased pressure within the crowded intracranial space rapidly. Epidural hematomas most commonly are lenticular shaped (in the shape of a biconvex lens) on CT scan. Choices **A**, **C**, and **D** describe subdural hematomas. The classic history of epidural hematomas is initial loss of consciousness followed by a brief lucid interval, then rapid deterioration. Like most classic presentations, it is not very common to see clinically (many are comatose from the time of initial injury).

265. The answer is D. *(Medicine—Pulmonology)*

An exudate is seen when the pleural fluid is purulent, as from a severe bacterial lung infection or empyema. The glucose level should be low, a positive Gram stain would be expected (although not always present), the pleural-to-serum lactate dehydrogenase ratio should be greater than 0.6, and the pleural-to-serum protein ratio should be greater than 0.5. The fluid usually appears turbid and has a high white count consisting mostly of neutrophils.

266. The answer is A. *(Pharmacology)*

Phenylephrine is primarily an alpha$_1$-agonist and has little direct action on the heart's contractility. With the exception of milrinone, the other agents all cause increased contractility through their beta$_1$-agonist effects and to some degree through beta$_2$ effects. Milrinone is a phosphodiesterase inhibitor that increases contractility by increasing the level of cyclic adenosine monophosphate (c-AMP) in heart muscle.

267. The answer is E. *(Medicine—General)*

Almost all of the complications of type II diabetes are seen in type I diabetes, and they usually occur more quickly in type I diabetes. A hyperosmolar state is more typical of type II diabetes, with diabetic ketoacidosis typically seen in type I diabetes. Obesity, although not technically a complication of type II diabetes (more of a cause), is not seen commonly in persons with type I diabetes.

268. The answer is E. *(Medicine—General)*

Angiotensin-converting enzyme inhibitors should be first-line agents in diabetics that can tolerate them because of their protective effects on the kidneys. Angiotensin-converting enzyme inhibitors should not be used in pregnant women because of concerns over possible teratogenic effects. These agents may precipitate renal failure in patients with renal artery stenosis and may aggravate hyperkalemia. A patient with atrial fibrillation and episodes of a rapid ventricular response probably would be served better by an agent that slows the atrioventricular node, such as a beta blocker or centrally acting calcium channel blocker.

269. The answer is D. *(Medicine—General)*

The coarctation usually is just distal to the left subclavian artery. The right subclavian artery comes of the innominate, or brachiocephalic artery and is not related to the aorta. The other choices are true. Rib notching occurs on the inferior portions of the ribs because this is where the neurovascular bundle lies. The enlarged intercostal arteries in this condition can erode the lower parts of the ribs. The upper extremity hypertension can cause aneurysmal dilation of the circle of Willis, and aneurysmal rupture is not uncommon in untreated patients (rarely seen today, as most patients are fixed before this complication can occur).

270. The answer is C. *(Medicine—Infectious Disease)*

Macrolide antibiotics or extended-spectrum fluoroquinolones are the treatments of choice for *Legionella* pneumonia. The other choices are unlikely to treat the infections at all. *Chlamydia* has no cell wall and thus cannot be treated with any of the penicillins. Aztreonam is used to treat serious infections with gram-negative rods but has no activity against anaerobes or gram-positive organisms. Metronidazole is the agent of choice to treat *C. difficile* colitis, with oral vancomycin an alternative choice. Oral agents are used to treat this condition, and the aminoglycosides are given parenterally. Tetracycline is not effective in treating group A streptococcus, the most common cause of streptococcal pharyngitis. Oral penicillins are the agents of choice, with erythromycin usually preferred in patients who are penicillin allergic.

271. The answer is E. *(Medicine—General)*

There are many different complications of long-standing diabetes. Cranial nerve palsies are common and can cause sudden onset of double vision and unilateral gaze paresis that depends on the specific cranial nerve involved (often cranial nerve VI). This condition usually goes away within 2 months and is self-limiting. Autonomic neuropathy can cause orthostatic hypotension and gastroparesis, which can result in early satiety and nausea and vomiting shortly after eating. Shortness of breath can be due to uncontrolled diabetes with acidosis or dehydration or secondary to a coronary event from diabetes-accelerated atherosclerosis.

272. The answer is C. *(Medicine—General)*

The thinking regarding beta blockers has changed. The benefits are now thought to outweigh the risks in certain patients who formerly were not given beta blockers. In the setting of a heart attack, a large increase in survival has been shown in patients who receive beta-blocker therapy. Severe asthma is a relatively strong contraindication to beta-blocker therapy, but stable chronic obstructive pulmonary disease is not. Use of beta blockers in diabetics and patients with stable congestive heart failure is encouraged in the setting of a myocardial infarction. Patients with unstable congestive heart failure (i.e., pulmonary edema) first should be stabilized before starting on a low dose of beta blocker. Beta blockade can mask the sympathetic activation signs and symptoms of hypoglycemia (e.g., sweating, tachycardia) in diabetics on drug therapy, thus patient education is important. Claudication may get worse in the setting of $beta_2$-receptor blockade, but this risk is small and outweighed easily by the survival benefit in the setting of a heart attack. $Beta_1$-specific antagonists also can be used to reduce this largely theoretical risk.

273. The answer is D. *(Surgery-General)*

This patient was hypokalemic 2 days ago and started to develop the classic symptoms of hypokalemia—worsening muscular weakness and ileus. There was no mention of potassium replacement, and the patient continued to receive high-volume maintenance fluid without potassium while not eating. The potassium level is most likely below 3 at this point, when life-threatening cardiac arrhythmias may occur. Decreased or absent tendon reflexes are common with severe hypokalemia. The patient most likely is on the verge of respiratory muscle paralysis, thus her shortness of breath from "weakness." The other items usually do not occur with hypokalemia. If the patient had renal insufficiency, distended neck veins may occur from iatrogenic hypervolemia, but with normal kidney function (evidenced by normal creatinine and BUN), this would not occur.

274. The answer is C. *(Medicine—General)*

Neuropathy usually takes many years to develop and would be unexpected in new-onset diabetes, especially to the extent described in choice C. Blurry vision is a common complaint because of swelling of the lenses, which resolves within a few weeks of good blood glucose control. Orthostatic hypotension is common and is due to dehydration. It goes away after rehydration, although after many years of diabetes, it could be due to autonomic neuropathy, in which case it would not go away with rehydration. Polydipsia, polyphagia (frequent eating), and polyuria (including nocturia) are the classic symptoms of diabetes.

275. The answer is D. *(Medicine—Rheumatology)*

This patient most likely has depression or fibromyalgia. In a 29-year-old with a normal sedimentation rate, creatine phosphokinase level, and complete blood count, a serious muscle disorder is unlikely. Polymyositis and polymyalgia rheumatica tend to occur in people older than age 40. Polymyositis most likely would cause an elevated creatine phosphokinase, and polymyalgia should cause an elevated sedimentation rate. Electromyography, nerve conduction study, and muscle biopsy may be possible diagnostic considerations in the future; however, they are unlikely to be useful. For board purposes, always get more history whenever it is an option unless the patient is unstable and needs an immediate life-saving intervention. More history is cheaper, less invasive, and often more useful than "fancy" tests for initial work-up of most conditions.

276. The answer is B. *(Medicine—General)*

You may be asked to implement the current cholesterol management and treatment values in a patient on Step 2. This patient has four primary atherosclerosis risk factors: smoking, diabetes, hypertension and positive family history. He also has a low HDL, which is an additional independent risk factor, as is elevated cholesterol. Elevated cholesterol, however, is not counted as a risk factor when deciding on the total number of risk factors to determine the optimal treatment option for elevated cholesterol. The only risk factor this patient lacks is age (men>45 and women>55 are at increased risk)! The current guidelines are as follows:

No CHD Risk Factors	Two or More CHD Risk Factors	Intervention
Total cholesterol < 200	Total cholesterol < 200	Remeasure in 5 years*
Total cholesterol 200–239		Counsel and recheck in 1–2 years*
Total cholesterol > 239	Total cholesterol > 200	Do fasting lipoprotein analysis (gives LDL)
LDL < 160	LDL < 130	Remeasure in 1 year to determine whether patient meets goals
LDL 160–189	LDL 130–159	Diet
LDL > 189	LDL > 159	Medications

CHD = coronary heart disease, LDL = low-density lipoproteins.
*Unless HDL < 35 mg/dl, in which case do a full fasting lipoprotein analysis to measure LDL.
Note: With evidence of CHD (which includes known coronary artery disease or peripheral vascular disease), use medications when LDL ≥ 130, with a target LDL < 100.

277. The answer is B. *(Medicine—Oncology)*

Although breast cancer is the most common cancer in women, lung cancer is the number one cause of cancer deaths in women (and men) in the United States. Breast cancer is the second leading cause of death in women, with colon cancer third.

278. The answer is D. *(Medicine—Oncology)*

All of the choices result in an increased risk of cancer. Only xeroderma pigmentosa is primarily inherited in an autosomal recessive fashion, however. This condition results in an increased risk of skin cancers because of a faulty DNA repair mechanism. The presence of familial polyposis coli is a virtual guarantee of colon cancer if the colon and rectum are not removed surgically but is inherited in an autosomal dominant manner in most cases. The multiple endocrine neoplasia syndromes are inherited in an autosomal dominant fashion as well and cause a variety of endocrine neoplasms depending on the specific multiple endocrine neoplasia subtype. Neurofibromatosis usually is autosomal dominant and can result in skin, nervous system, and other tumors. Down syndrome increases the risk of leukemia but is caused by trisomy 21, not inherited in an autosomal fashion.

279. The answer is C. *(General Knowledge and Principles)*

It is important to take control of the interview with a patient. Gentle redirection back to the problem is the most appropriate course of action at this point. Although old medical records always are helpful, a patient who brings in a thick stack of records and demands you to read them should cause the *psychiatry* flag to be raised in the back of your mind. Going too quickly to a psychiatric slant may offend the patient, however, and prevent you from building trust and gaining the confidence of the patient. Going along with the patient's wishes in this setting may lead to further demands (which are quite likely to be inappropriate also).

280. The answer is B. *(Medicine—Nephrology)*

The other choices all would be expected in someone with chronic renal failure. A metabolic acidosis with compensatory respiratory alkalosis would be more typical of renal failure, however.

281. The answer is A. *(Medicine—Nephrology)*

Removing one kidney leaves 50% of the baseline glomerular filtration rate and would not be expected to cause acute renal failure, provided that no previous kidney disease is present. The same is true of unilateral nephrolithiasis. The other choices are common causes of acute renal failure. Dehydration and congestive heart failure cause prerenal renal failure, rhabdomyolysis plugs up the renal filtration system causing intrarenal renal failure, and benign prostatic hypertrophy (BPH) causes postrenal renal failure.

282. The answer is E. *(General Knowledge and Principles)*

This patient is probably tired because of taking on a second full-time job. There is no particular reason to suspect HIV or depression without clues to their presence. The elevated total thyroid hormone level most likely is related to the elevated thyroid-binding globulin levels that can occur with contraceptive use. If Graves' disease or surreptitious ingestion of thyroxine were present, the thyroid-stimulating hormone levels should be low, not normal. There are no findings on physical examination to make hyperthyroidism likely either. If clinical suspicion was high, a free thyroxine level could be obtained, which measures the biologically active unbound thyroxine, and would control for the increased levels of thyroid-binding globulin that commonly occur with oral contraceptive use (and pregnancy).

283. The answer is C. *(Medicine—General)*

Hypothyroidism is one of the causes of carpal tunnel syndrome and can cause fatigue and constipation. Tinel's and Phalen's signs are physical examination maneuvers that strongly suggest a diagnosis of carpal tunnel syndrome, but the diagnosis already has been made with nerve conduction studies. Occult blood in the stool is not associated particularly with carpal tunnel syndrome (nor is colon cancer), and antiacetylcholine receptor antibodies, which occur with myasthenia gravis, are not associated with carpal tunnel syndrome.

284. The answer is E. *(Medicine—Endocrinology)*

The patient most likely has subacute (de Quervain's) thyroiditis, a viral infection of the thyroid gland that often is preceded by upper respiratory infection symptoms. Acutely the patient may become hyperthyroid, owing to inflammation of the gland and release of follicular colloid. Hypothyroidism sometimes may occur after several weeks, when the thyroid gland becomes *spent*, but normal thyroid function often returns within a few months. The treatment is nonsteroidal anti-inflammatory drugs. Corticosteroids sometimes are used for severe disease, but nonsteroidal anti-inflammatory drugs are the appropriate first choice. Bacterial thyroiditis is much less common as a cause for a similar presentation and fungal infection of the thyroid gland is rare. Elevated thyroid-stimulating immunoglobulin and antibody levels are seen in Graves' disease, which would not be expected to cause a tender thyroid gland. Because of the acute nature of the symptoms and gland tenderness, neoplasm is very unlikely.

285. The answer is A. *(Medicine—Gastroenterology)*

The figure reveals cirrhosis, with broad fibrous bands (labeled "F" in the figure) disrupting the lobular architecture. No inflammation / inflammatory cells are seen to suggest chronic active hepatitis. Hepatocellular carcinoma and hepatic adenoma would not have regular fibrous bands through them and the cells are not grossly dysplastic, though the figure is a low-power view. The patient is certainly at risk for hepatocellular carcinoma. Hepatic adenoma also tends to occur in younger women on birth control pills. As a rule of thumb, when you're stuck, try to answer all questions that have figures without using the figure. If you pick the best answer, then look at the figure based on the information in the passage alone, you can then use the figure to confirm your answer (or ignore the figure if you have no idea what it shows). This is primarily useful when you're not sure what the figure shows—if you know what the figure shows, then use the information it gives you! Although this approach does not always work, it might have worked in this question, since the firm, nodular, nonenlarged liver, splenomegaly, and gradually increasing ascites/abdominal girth are all typical for cirrhosis and not the other conditions listed.

286. The answer is A. *(General Knowledge and Principles)*

Crigler-Najjar syndrome causes an unconjugated hyperbilirubinemia, whereas the others cause a mixed or primarily conjugated hyperbilirubinemia. Only conjugated bilirubin shows up in the urine because unconjugated bilirubin is bound tightly to albumin and not filtered through the glomeruli into the urine.

287. The answer is C. *(Medicine—Pathology)*

The passage is supposed to describe the *owl-eyed* Reed-Sternberg cell, which is a diagnostic characteristic of Hodgkin lymphoma. The peak incidence is in young persons 15 to 34 years old, and cervical lymphadenopathy, night sweats, and weight loss are the classic presentation. The other choices would not cause the presence of binucleated cells and/or the extent of the constitutional symptoms mentioned.

288. The answer is D. *(Medicine—Infectious Disease)*

The man has pharyngeal and esophageal candidiasis, which means he is likely immunocompromised. Testing for HIV and/or other immunosuppression work-up is indicated. The figure reveals numerous organisms with both hyphal (labeled "H" in the figure) and yeast (labeled "Y") forms. *Candida* spp. (typically *Candida albicans*) exist as normal flora on the skin and in the mouth and genital tract. Overgrowth can occur in the mouth of healthy infants (thrush) and the genital tract of healthy women treated with antibiotics, but in most other patients, a *Candida* infection indicates diabetes or immunodeficiency. In this patient, downward growth of *Candida* occurred from the mouth, not the hematogenous route. The treatment of choice is antifungals (e.g., fluconazole). There is no particular association with esophageal reflux. Odynophagia in immunocompromised patients can be due to various infections, but is most commonly due to *Candida*. Others include herpes, CMV, and HIV, all of which can cause ulceration and severe symptoms (may prevent patients from eating).

289. The answer is C. *(Orthopedics)*

This infant likely has congenital hip dysplasia (formerly called *congenital hip dislocation*). Medical (nonsurgical) treatment is preferred, using splints, slings, harnesses, or special diapers to hold the affected hip in abduction and external rotation, allowing the acetabulum to form properly as the child grows. The other choices are all true (i.e. incorrect answers to the question). Females and infants with a breech presentation are more likely to develop this condition, and a family history can sometimes be elicited. The infant has a positive Ortolani's sign (palpable or audible click with thigh abduction when the hips and knees are flexed). Ultrasound is preferable to radiographs in younger infants because the epiphyses are not visualized on radiographs due to lack of ossification.

290. The answer is A. *(Surgery—General)*

This patient most likely has acute cholecystitis. Ultrasound is the initial imaging study of choice in most suspected cases because it is accurate, inexpensive, does not require contrast material or radiation exposure, and is usually readily available in a hospital setting. The presence of gallstones and inflammation around the gallbladder are highly suggestive of cholecystitis. If necessary, a nuclear hepatobiliary scan (e.g., a HIDA scan) can be used to confirm the diagnosis (nonvisualization of the gallbladder generally means an obstructed cystic duct from cholecystitis). Given the patient's demographics (remember the **4 Fs**—**f**at, **f**orty, **f**ertile, and **f**latulent) and history of painful attacks that sound like typical biliary pain, cholecystitis should be high on the differential diagnosis list.

Hepatitis seems unlikely, given the normal liver enzymes and lack of mentioned risk factors (if the boards want you to chase a diagnosis, they usually give you one or more clues). 5′-Nucleotidase can be used to confirm that an elevated alkaline phosphatase is due to bile duct inflammation (because alkaline phosphatase also can come from bone or placenta) but is not really required in this classic scenario. Although the patient's blood pressure is elevated, the elevation is mild and would not prevent acute/immediate surgical intervention (the treatment of choice for acute cholecystitis that is severe or does not respond to conservative management).

291. The answer is D. *(Emergency Medicine)*

The patient has meningitis, probably with meningococcus (given the skin petechiae), and is bacteremic and about to go into septic shock. Antibiotics and intravenous fluids need to be started immediately to treat this medical emergency. Although you may want to do a lumbar puncture or MRI first, these are diagnostic, not therapeutic, modalities. While you are trying to arrive at a correct diagnosis, the patient may die. Acute bacterial meningitis can be rapidly fatal, and immediate therapy should not be delayed. This is one of the exceptions to the rule of obtaining a diagnosis before starting treatment.

With modern agglutination assays to detect antigens in the cerebrospinal fluid, pretreatment with antibiotics for 10–30 minutes while the patient is being prepared for a lumbar puncture probably would not affect your ability to identify a specific organism. Although ordering a complete metabolic profile is acceptable, it is not the best answer because antibiotics and lumbar puncture are more important actions. Prophylactic anticonvulsants are not indicated in meningitis.

292. The answer is A. *(Medicine—General)*

This patient is obese and on metformin, so it can be presumed that he is a type II diabetic. His positive Babinski sign on the left means that he has an upper motor neuron lesion, probably from a lacunar infarct (small or mini stroke) owing to hypertension and almost certain atherosclerosis, given his multiple risk factors. The S$_4$ heart sound comes from a stiff, non-compliant ventricle that is seen most commonly in the setting of left ventricular hypertrophy. There is no evidence to suggest a lower motor neuron lesion (causes areflexia and would not cause a positive Babinski sign). Although diabetics commonly have peripheral neuropathy, it is usually sensory in nature.

293. The answer is C. *(Medicine—General)*

The patient most likely has Klinefelter's syndrome, or a 47 XXY chromosome anomaly, which results in the presence of Barr bodies. Almost all of these patients are infertile with underdeveloped and poorly or nonfunctioning testicles. The classic body habitus is described in the question, although the phenotype can vary. Although some patients may have subtle deficiencies in language skills, only a small percentage are considered to be truly mentally retarded. Patients with Klinefelter's syndrome are no more likely to be homosexual than the general population, giving the patient a 90% to 95% chance of being heterosexual.

294. The answer is E. *(Gynecology)*

This question describes a woman with Turner's syndrome, or 45 XO chromosome anomaly. The lack of a second X chromosome would cause an absence of Barr bodies. In this condition, primary amenorrhea and lack of secondary sexual characteristics occur because of a failure of normal ovarian development (i.e., the ovaries are nonfunctional). These patients tend to have normal or above-average verbal IQ but often have mathematical deficiencies. There is nothing in the question to suggest a pituitary neoplasm.

295–300. *(Pharmacology)*

The answers are the following: 295. G   296. C   297. A   298. E   299. I   300. G.

Thiazides can cause allergic reaction in individuals who are allergic to sulfa as well as cause or worsen hyperuricemia and hypercalcemia. Loop diuretics cause calcium excretion (opposite effect) and commonly are used to treat hypercalcemia, although they also may cause allergic reactions in individuals allergic to sulfa. Many of these are straight memorize and regurgitate questions. Stevens-Johnson syndrome is the most severe form of the spectrum of allergic reactions that includes erythema multiforme and is commonly associated with the use of sulfa drugs. HMG-CoA reductase inhibitors can cause liver and muscle damage, and periodic monitoring of liver function tests is required with this class of agents. Tricyclic antidepressants, now considered second-line agents in the management of depression and other related conditions due to the betterr side effect profile of serotonin-specific reuptake inhibitors (SSRIs) used to be the most common cause of prescription drug overdose due to their cardiac toxicity. Aminoglycosides can potentiate the effects of neuromuscular blockade, in addition to their nephrotoxic and ototoxic effects.

ANSWERS AND
EXPLANATIONS

301. The answer is D. *(Pediatrics—Neonates)*

The umbilical vein carries blood from the maternal circulation and has the highest oxygen saturation in the fetal circulation. This blood then goes up to the heart, into the aorta, and up into the carotid arteries. The upper body receives more oxygen-rich blood than the lower extremities. This is because blood from the pulmonary artery, which is more desaturated because of being composed mainly of venous return from the upper and lower extremity veins, passes through the ductus arteriosus into the descending aorta to mix with the higher saturation blood from the left ventricle. The umbilical artery arises from the iliac arteries and thus would be expected to have roughly the same oxygen saturation as the iliac and femoral arteries. The femoral vein would have the lowest oxygen saturation of the named vessels after draining the lower extremity.

302. The answer is C. *(Medicine—General)*

This patient has probable pancreatitis (could confirm with a lipase level, as this should also be elevated) and needs medical management in a hospital setting. There is no current indication for esophagogastroduodenoscoy (i.e., EGD), surgery or blood transfusion with the limited information given. Sending the patient home is inappropriate because pancreatitis is associated with significant morbidity and mortality. CT scan (or MRI) with contrast is increasingly being used to determine severity and/or the cause (if not known) at initial presentation, but is most helpful in the detection and follow-up of pancreatitis complications (e.g., pseudocyst, abscess), which take days to develop.

303. The answer is D. *(Medicine—Hematology)*

Emphysema (and COPD in general) often causes secondary polycythemia. Menstrual-age women, pregnant women, premature infants, and children in rapid stages of growth are at increased risk for anemia, especially if their diets are inadequate (e.g., a vegan can develop vitamin B_{12} deficiency). Peptic ulcer disease can lead to gastrointestinal bleeding and subsequent anemia.

304. The answer is B. *(Medicine—Cardiology)*

Renal failure results in hyperkalemia. Azotemia, hyperkalemia, hyperphosphatemia, hypermagnesemia, hypocalcemia, and acidosis can also occur. Significant renal involvement with lupus has a strong negative impact on prognosis.

305. The answer is A. *(Medicine—Cardiology)*

The electrocardiogram shows first-degree heart block and bradycardia (heart rate < 50), a potential side effect of antihypertensives that slow conduction through the atrioventricular node, including beta blockers and centrally acting calcium channel blockers (verapamil and diltiazem).

306. The answer is B. *(Radiology)*

The barium enema shows a classic "apple core" lesion from an adenocarcinoma, which has resulted in GI bleeding (melena). Colonic adenocarcinoma is a common cause of lower GI bleeding in adults (rare in adolescents and young adults; those affected at this age likely have some sort of familial tendency [e.g., familial polyposis]). Testing for such bleeding is currently one of the cornerstones of colon cancer screening. Taking all cases of colon cancer, 5-year survival is at least 50%. The modified Dukes classification is commonly used for staging (a TNM classification also exists):

Dukes Stage	Description
A	Limited to mucosa
B	Extension into (B1) or through (B2) muscularis propria, no nodal spread
C	Limited to (C1) or extension through (C2) the bowel wall with nodal metastases
D	Distant metastases

As with many cancers, the "ballpark it if you have to guess" 90/60/30/10 rule (i.e., stage I [in TNM classification] or stage A [Dukes] has roughly a 90% survival rate, stage II/B = 60%, stage III/C = 30%, stage IV/D = 10%) fits for the 5-year survival rates in colon carcinoma. Also similar to many other malignancies, stage A (or I) is treated with surgery alone and the primary treatment for stage D/IV is chemotherapy. A mixture of treatments (e.g., surgery and adjuvant therapies) is typically employed for stages B/II and C/III.

307. The answer is A. *(Psychiatry—General)*

Flight of ideas describes when a person's thoughts shift rapidly from one topic to another. It is seen classically in mania, along with pressured speech and other symptoms. Flight of ideas also can be seen in psychosis but usually is not associated with the other choices.

308. The answer is A. *(Obstetrics)*

Because the woman is pregnant, heparin or a low molecular weight heparin is the treatment of choice because warfarin is teratogenic. There are also regimens in use that involve giving some form of heparin for the 1st trimester (heparins don't cross the placenta and thus are not teratogenic) and after the 35th week (to prevent drug-related maternal and perinatal hemorrhage, since warfarin crosses the placenta and has a longer half-life), with warfarin used for the 2nd trimester and first part of the 3rd trimester (no longer significantly teratogenic and patients prefer pills to shots). Aspirin and no treatment are inadequate forms of therapy.

309. The answer is D. *(Medicine—Neurology)*

Huntington's disease is an autosomal dominant condition that results in movement, psychiatric, and neurologic dysfunctions. Personality changes, dementia, and psychosis in the late stages are common. There is no cure for this condition, and early diagnosis is not crucial for prognosis. The only advantage of early diagnosis is genetic counseling because individuals with the disease may decide not to have children. CT scan or MRI often reveals characteristic atrophy of the caudate nucleus.

310. The answer is A. *(Psychiatry—General)*

Venlafaxine is an antidepressant (non-tricyclic inhibitor of serotonin and norepinephrine), which may help treat depression, but also may trigger mania and would be inappropriate monotherapy for long-term management of bipolar disorder. The classic mood stabilizer is lithium, with valproic acid gaining acceptance as a first-line agent. Carbamazepine generally is considered a second-line agent for mania. Lamotrigine, another antiepileptic drug, has been shown to be useful in patients with treatment-resistant bipolar disorder. Similar to carbamazepine, it is not considered a first-line agent.

311. The answer is B. *(Medicine—Rheumatology)*

All of the other choices are caused by systemic lupus erythematosus (SLE). Hair loss sometimes is seen in SLE, but hirsutism is not. The American College of Rheumatology has devised 11 diagnostic criteria to be used for the diagnosis of SLE. To have an official diagnosis of SLE, a person must meet at least 4 of the criteria at some point during the illness. Besides the other choices in the question (*note:* serositis usually implies pleuritis or pericarditis), the other 7 criteria are discoid rash, photosensitivity, renal disorder (e.g., proteinuria), neurologic disorder (e.g., seizures, psychosis), hematologic disorder (e.g., anemia, leukopenia), immunologic disorder (e.g., anti-DNA or anti-Smith antibody titer, false-positive rapid plasma reagin or VDRL syphilis test), and a positive antinuclear antibody titer. Women being treated for SLE may develop hirsutism, but it is typically related to long-term corticosteroid use.

312. The answer is C. *(Medicine—General)*

Felty's syndrome describes the triad of rheumatoid arthritis, splenomegaly, and neutropenia. It is a classic board-type of question regarding rheumatoid arthritis, although rarely seen. Many frustratingly rare syndromes are asked about on boards, but fortunately, these questions are in the minority and only ask for recognition of the classic triad or other basic facts about the condition.

313. The answer is D. *(Medicine—Oncology)*

All of these choices often present when metastases already are present. Choriocarcinoma, classically occurring in women after pregnancy (or an abortion; both types known as gestational choriocarcinoma), is highly sensitive to chemotherapy in most cases, even when metastases are present. Additionally, the location in the uterus and secretion of β-HCG allow earlier onset of symptoms and detection in many cases. Methotrexate is the classic agent that results in a high percentage of cure with gestational choriocarcinoma, even with widespread metastases. Interestingly, ovarian and testicular choriocarcinoma (not gestation related), which are extremely rare as "pure" germ cell tumors (more commonly seen in mixed germ cell tumors with more than one histologic cell type), are resistant to methotrexate and have a poorer prognosis. The other choices tend to have a poor prognosis at the time of presentation due to later stage by the time symptoms develop and/or a poor response to treatment.

314. The answer is A. *(Pharmacology)*

Infliximab is an antitumor necrosis factor-alpha agent that has shown promise in treating inflammatory, autoimmune-like conditions such as rheumatoid arthritis. The other agents are all used to reduce estrogenic stimulation of the breast in the setting of breast cancer, thus suppressing the growth and recurrence of tumors. These agents are primarily useful in the setting of tumors that demonstrate estrogen and/or progesterone receptors on their surface (common). Aromatase inhibitors (e.g., anastrozole, letrozole) keep androgen from being converted to estrogen. Selective-estrogen receptor modulators (e.g., tamoxifen, raloxifene) occupy the estrogen receptors in some tissues, such as breast, but cause much less stimulation of the receptor in breast tissue compared to circulating estrogen (versus increased estrogenic-like activity in bones, thus can also be used in osteoporosis treatment). Gonadotropin-releasing hormone agonists (e.g., goserelin, leuprolide) cause a "chemical castration" by inhibiting release of follicle-stimulating hormone (FSH) and luteinizing hormone (LH) via feedback inhibition when given in a continuous manner. Estrogen receptor antagonists/downregulators (e.g., fulvestrant) occupy the estrogen receptor and have no agonist properties. This agent also downregulates estrogen receptor expression.

Traditional chemotherapeutic agents (e.g., cyclophosphamide, methotrexate, paclitaxel) are also used in breast cancer, and are especially important in breast cancers that do not express hormone receptors. Trastuzumab is a monoclonal antibody (i.e. immunotherapy) that attaches to the HER2/neu protein, present in roughly 25% of breast cancers, and has been effectively used for breast cancers that are HER2 positive.

315. The answer is A. *(Pharmacology)*

Aztreonam has a spectrum of antimicrobial activity limited to gram-negative organisms, which cause most urinary tract infections (e.g., *E. coli*, *Serratia*, *Pseudomonas*, *Proteus*, *Klebsiella*). Aztreonam is not effective against anaerobic, atypical, or gram-positive organisms, which are the most likely causes of the other choices.

316. The answer is A. *(Medicine—Infectious Disease)*

Macrolide antibiotics (e.g., azithromycin, clarithromycin, erythromycin) are one of the treatments of choice for *Chlamydia* and other atypical pneumonias. The other choices are not thought to have good activity against *Chlamydia*.

317. The answer is E. *(General Knowledge and Principles)*

The spleen acts as a center of hematopoiesis during fetal life and can return to this role if needed, such as during myelofibrosis or conditions with high red cell turnover, such as thalassemia major. The other choices are well-known functions of the spleen. The spleen can release up to 100 ml of blood into the circulation when needed. This can be important in times of hemorrhage to prevent death. Senescent, or old, red blood cells are destroyed and broken down by the spleen.

318. The answer is A. *(Medicine—Oncology)*

Basal cell is the most common type of skin cancer and the least likely to cause metastatic disease and death. It usually is found on sun-exposed areas, as are squamous cell skin cancers. Skin cancer is the most common cancer in humans but rarely life-threatening. Melanomas are the most worrisome type of skin cancer because they metastasize commonly and frequently cause death. The treatment of choice for nonmelanoma skin cancers is local excision or destruction. Metastatic cancer and cutaneous T-cell lymphoma are diagnostic considerations when a skin lesion is present but are much less common.

319. The answer is B. *(Biostatistics)*

Sensitivity is calculated by dividing the number of true positives of the test by the total number of people with the disease. The gold standard number of 5000 should be used as the total number of people with the disease (even though the gold standard is almost never 100% accurate). The number of true positives in this case is 3000 because 1000 of the 4000 people who tested positive were culture negative. 3000/5000 = 0.6 = 60%. The positive predictive value is calculated by dividing the number of true positives by the total number of people with a positive test (i.e., true positives plus false positives) and thus would be 3000/4000 = 75%.

320. The answer is D. *(Preventive Medicine)*

At this age, heart disease would be the most likely cause of death, followed by cancer.

321. The answer is B. *(Preventive Medicine)*

Accidents are the most common cause of death in whites aged 15 to 19, with suicide and homicide the second and third leading causes of death in this group, respectively.

322. The answer is B. *(Obstetrics)*

The 3rd through 8th weeks after conception are the time of organogenesis, when a fetus is most susceptible to teratogenic agents. Before this time, the fetus either aborts or is unaffected by a teratogenic agent. After 8 weeks, teratogenesis is less likely and often is less severe because the major organ systems already have been established/formed.

323. The answer is A. *(General Knowledge and Principles)*

Although a patient's wishes should be respected, open communication to help understand the patient's wishes is important. The patient may not want to know the diagnosis because she is afraid she will be unable to pay for treatment or for some other reason that can be addressed. Whenever you can get more history on Step 2, unless the patient is crashing in front of you, choose to get it. Questions like this can be frustrating, since they deal with style and bedside manner, but are commonly asked on USMLE exams. When patients' actions puzzle you, the first step is to ask why they do what they do or think the way they think. Try to avoid being paternalistic (i.e., avoid telling patients you know what is best for them).

324. The answer is A. *(Pharmacology)*

Sucralfate forms a polymer in the acidic environment of the stomach. This polymer binds directly to injured tissue and can form a protective coating over an area of ulceration. The other agents have their primary actions after being absorbed into the bloodstream, with the exception of magnesium hydroxide, an antacid. Magnesium hydroxide reacts with the protons in gastric acid to neutralize them and, similar to sucralfate, is not absorbed to any significant degree from the bowel.

325. The answer is C. *(Pharmacology)*

Although rarely needed, glucagon can be used for its cardiac inotropic effects when beta-blocker overdose occurs. It increases cyclic-AMP (i.e., c-AMP) without affecting sympathetic beta receptors. Glucagon is also useful for hypoglycemia when glucose is not available and to inhibit the bowel, such as during an imaging study of the bowel.

326. The answer is C. *(Obstetrics)*

A choriocarcinoma and molar pregnancy in general may occur after any pregnancy, whether it results in the birth of a child or not. Most cases (50%) derive from a complete molar pregnancy, but others occur after an abortion/miscarriage

(25%), term delivery (20%), or ectopic pregnancy (5%). Metastatic choriocarcinoma and invasive mole are responsive to chemotherapy, and often can be cured with treatment (usually methotrexate or dactinomycin). The first two choices are classic presentation data for gestational trophoblastic disease. Most cases can be treated and cured with dilation and curettage, unless invasion or metastasis has occurred, which is less common than a *contained* mole.

327. The answer is A. *(Gynecology)*

Although syphilis (i.e., condyloma lata) should be considered in this patient, condylomata acuminata (venereal or genital warts) are much more common and fit the given description better. The lesions are classically described as cauliflowerlike in appearance and are often pedunculated (unlike condyloma lata). The cause is human papillomavirus. Squamous cell vaginal cancer in a 33-year-old woman is unlikely, especially in a question that fails to mention bleeding, ulceration, or severe pruritus, possible clues of malignancy. The fact that the lesions are painless and not ulcerated should steer you away from herpes, which does not cause exophytic or pedunculated lesions. Chancroid, resulting from *Haemophilus ducreyi*, classically causes painful genital ulcers and impressive inguinal lymphadenopathy.

328. The answer is D. *(General Knowledge and Principles)*

In septic shock, the pulmonary artery wedge pressure tends to be normal to low. Congestive heart failure and cardiogenic shock are the classic examples of conditions resulting in an elevated pulmonary artery wedge pressure, which correlates roughly with the right atrial pressure. Severe mitral valve disease increases right atrial pressure, and the pressure backs up into the pulmonary veins to increase the wedge pressure as well. Renal failure can increase the wedge pressure through hypervolemia.

329. The answer is C. *(General Knowledge and Principles)*

The peripheral vasculature *clamps down* (i.e., constricts) when severe hypovolemia is present, causing an elevation of systemic vascular resistance, in an attempt to maintain blood pressure and thus perfusion to vital organs. Cardiac output and pulmonary wedge pressure both are likely to be low secondary to the intravascular volume depletion. Urine output decreases, and the specific gravity of the urine increases. The person may develop a decrease in orthostatic blood pressure (i.e., orthostatic hypotension) or frank hypotension. The skin is characteristically cold and clammy.

330. The answer is B. *(Medicine—Cardiology)*

Although the other choices are classic symptoms for right-sided heart failure, which often is secondary to lung disease (cor pulmonale) or left heart failure, pulsus alternans is a classic symptom of left-sided heart failure. Pulsus alternans describes a pulse that is regular in time but alternates between strong and weak beats because of severe left ventricular dysfunction. The right side of the heart would not be expected to affect the pulse in this way.

331. The answer is E. *(Surgery—General)*

In a postmenopausal woman with a new, hard breast mass and a family history of breast cancer, you should assume immediately that the woman has breast cancer until you prove otherwise. A delay in management (i.e., follow-up exam in 1–2 months) is not appropriate. Imaging of the breast itself in this case will be primarily useful as a baseline for future comparison. Stereotactic biopsy is typically reserved for suspicious calcifications that are difficult to sample using other techniques. An ultrasound- or clinically guided percutaneous biopsy could be used to confirm the diagnosis, but these are not listed choices. If imaging or percutaneous biopsy revealed noncancerous results, an excisional biopsy would most likely still be needed in such a patient, who has clinical findings and risk factors that make her breast lesion highly suspicious for cancer. A needle biopsy can miss cancers because of sampling error. A CT scan to look for metastatic disease should be postponed until a tissue diagnosis of cancer is made and positive lymph nodes are found in the axilla. MRI is a tool that is increasingly being utilized for breast lesion evaluation, but mammography and ultrasound would be the initial imaging modalities of choice in this patient.

332. The answer is A. *(Psychiatry—Child and Adolescent)*

In contrast to individuals with anorexia nervosa, people with bulimia often are normal weight and commonly are overweight. Although individuals who have bulimia and coexisting anorexia (which is common) are underweight, it would be unusual for an individual with "pure" bulimia to be pathologically underweight. By definition, individuals with anorexia fail to maintain 85% of their ideal weight. Most individuals with anorexia or bulimia are women. In bulimia, binge eating is followed by purging behavior, which may include exercise, fasting, intentional vomiting, or laxative or diuretic abuse.

333. The answer is A. *(Pediatrics—Urology)*

Vesicoureteral reflux is a common cause of recurrent urinary tract infections in children. Hypospadias, exstrophy of the bladder, and prune-belly syndrome all would result in abnormal physical examination findings. Prune-belly syndrome (Eagle-Barrett syndrome) is a triad that consists of absent abdominal wall musculature, hydronephrosis and urinary tract abnormalities, and cryptorchidism. A ureterocolic fistula would be expected to cause a history of stool seen in the urine and would be much less common than vesicoureteral reflux. Posterior urethral valves are another consideration in boys (not seen in girls), but often present shortly after birth with signs of bladder outlet obstruction (i.e. bilateral hydronephrosis).

334. The answer is E. *(Pediatrics—General)*

Hemolytic-uremic syndrome is characterized by the triad of acute renal failure (one of the most common causes of acute renal failure requiring dialysis in children), microangiopathic hemolytic anemia, and thrombocytopenia (secondary to the microangiopathy with platelet activation and consumption). Most cases follow a gastroenteritis type of illness, classically from *E. coli* O157:H7, *Shigella*, *Salmonella*, or *Campylobacter*. Antiplatelet antibodies are not responsible for thrombocytopenia in hemolytic-uremic syndrome.

335. The answer is E. *(Pediatrics—Oncology)*

Osteogenic sarcoma has a peak incidence in the 10- to 20-year-old age group. It is much less common than the other choices in a 3-year-old. Leukemia is the most common malignancy in 3-year-old children, followed by central nervous system tumors, which usually are in the posterior fossa. Neuroblastoma and Wilms' tumor are two of the most common solid tumors in 3-year-old children.

336. The answer is A. *(Pediatrics—Oncology)*

Neuroblastoma is seen in children less than 5 years old in approximately 90% of cases. It would be extremely unlikely in a 13-year-old. Leukemia, lymphoma, and primary bone tumors (osteogenic sarcoma and Ewing's sarcoma) are probably the top three malignancies in adolescents. Soft tissue sarcomas, such as rhabdomyosarcomas, are fairly common malignancies in this age group as well.

337. The answer is D. *(Medicine—Hematology)*

Knowing obscure syndromes rarely adds many points to one's board scores, but there are often a couple of questions about them. When one of these syndromes is asked about, generally only a classic presentation or definition is used. The X-linked Wiskott-Aldrich syndrome is defined by a triad—thrombocytopenia, immunodeficiency, and eczema. Glanzmann's thrombasthenia, idiopathic thrombocytopenic purpura, and the Bernard-Soulier syndrome are all platelet disorders but are not particularly associated with eczema or immunodeficiency. The Kasabach-Merritt syndrome is said to occur when thrombocytopenia results from giant hemangiomas, secondary to platelet clumping and consumption within the hemangiomas.

338. The answer is A. *(Surgery—General)*

Patients do not always admit to their alcohol habits, even when asked directly. A patient who had not had a drink since surgery classically would develop delirium tremens around postoperative day 2 or 3. This also is the best choice because the others are unlikely. Hypoadrenalism is unlikely in the setting of hypertension and normal electrolytes. Normal electrolytes rule out hyponatremia, and occult hyponatremia is a made-up entity. A pulmonary embolus large enough to cause delirium is likely to result in some drop in the pulse oximetry reading, tachypnea, tachycardia, pain, or hypotension. Sepsis is a possibility, and blood cultures would not be unreasonable, but the man has been afebrile and has a normal physical examination and no pain. Unless a patient is at the extremes of age or seriously immunosuppressed from disease or immunosuppressant drugs, patients should have a fever or localizing symptoms in the setting of infection.

339–344. *(Obstetrics)*

The answers are the following: 339. C   340. D   341. H   342. A   343. B   344. G.

Third-trimester bleeding is high yield for Step 2. Always do an ultrasound before a pelvic examination in this setting. The differential diagnosis can be intimidating at first.

The predisposing factors for *placenta previa* include multiparity, increasing age, multiple gestation, and prior previa. This condition is why you always do an ultrasound before a pelvic examination. Bleeding is painless and may be profuse. Ultrasound is 95% to 100% accurate in diagnosis. A cesarean section is required for delivery, but you may try to admit affected women with bed or pelvic rest and tocolysis if woman is preterm, stable, and the bleeding stops.

The predisposing factors for *abruptio placentae* include hypertension (with or without preeclampsia), trauma, polyhydramnios with rapid decompression after membrane rupture, cocaine or tobacco use, and preterm premature rupture of the membranes. A woman can have this condition without visible bleeding (blood contained behind placenta). Affected patients usually have pain, uterine tenderness, and increased uterine tone with hyperactive contraction pattern, and there is fetal distress. This condition may cause disseminated intravascular coagulation if fetal products enter the maternal circulation. Ultrasound detects a minority of cases (unreliable). Treat with intravenous fluids (and blood if needed) and rapid delivery (vaginal preferred when possible).

Risk factors for *uterine rupture* include previous uterine surgery (especially classic is cesarean sections with a vertical incision in the past), trauma, oxytocin, grand multiparity (several previous deliveries), excessive uterine distention (multiple gestation, polyhydramnios), abnormal fetal lie, cephalopelvic disproportion, and shoulder dystocia. This condition is extremely painful, has a sudden onset, and often causes maternal hypotension or shock. Fetal parts can be felt in the abdomen, or the woman's abdominal contour may change. Treat with immediate laparotomy and usually hysterectomy after delivery.

Isolated fetal bleeding is usually from *vasa previa* or *velamentous insertion of the cord*. The biggest risk factor is multiple gestation (higher the number of fetuses, higher the risk). Bleeding is painless, and the mother is completely stable, while the fetus shows worsening distress (tachycardia initially, then bradycardia as fetus decompensates). Apt test is positive on uterine blood (differentiates fetal from maternal blood). Treat with immediate cesarean section.

Other causes of third-trimester bleeding include cervical or vaginal lesions from herpes, gonorrhea, or *Chlamydia*; *Candida*; cervical or vaginal trauma, usually from intercourse; bleeding disorders, which rarely present antepartum (more common postpartum or known history from childhood); and cervical cancer.

A *bloody show* describes what happens with cervical effacement—a blood-tinged mucous plug may be released from the cervical canal, heralding the onset of labor (this is normal and a diagnosis of exclusion).

345–349. *(Psychiatry—General)*

The answers are the following: 345. H   346. E   347. A   348. B   349. D.

With the so-called somatoform disorders, patients do not behave the way they do on purpose. They have an underlying unconscious problem that drives their symptoms. In somatization disorder, the patient has multiple different complaints in multiple different organ systems over many years and has had extensive workups in the past. The focus is on symptoms. In conversion disorder, patients have an obvious precipitating factor (fight with boyfriend), then have unexplainable neurologic symptoms (go blind, have paralysis, stocking/glove numbness). With hypochondriasis, the patient often keeps believing he or she has the same disease, despite extensive negative workup. The focus often is on the disease. In body dysmorphic disorder, there is a preoccupation with an imagined physical defect (teenager thinks his or her nose is too big when it is normal sized). These patients commonly request plastic surgery, which does not cure their disorder any more than losing weight cures an anorexic. Treat all of these disorders with frequent return clinic visits, psychotherapy, or both.

With a factitious disorder, patients intentionally create their illness or symptoms (e.g., shoot themselves up with insulin to get hypoglycemia) and subject themselves to procedures to assume the role of a patient, also called the *sick role* (there is no financial or other secondary gain). This is different from somatoform disorders because the symptoms are created intentionally, whereas in somatoform disorders, the patient believes the symptoms and does not create them on purpose.

Malingering occurs when a patient intentionally creates his or her illness for secondary gain (to get money, to get out of work, to get narcotics). The difference between malingering and factitious disorder is what the patient gets out of making up symptoms. Malingerers do not want to undergo procedures because they do not want to assume the sick role (e.g., "Forget the x-ray, doc; just give me a prescription for those codeine pills and a note to get out of work.").

Dissociative fugue or psychogenic fugue occurs when a patient has amnesia and travels, assuming a new identity. Dissociative identity disorder (i.e., multiple personality disorder) is an illness probably more commonly seen in the movies than in real life, but this disorder is the one most likely to be associated with childhood sexual abuse.

350. The answer is C. *(Medicine—General)*

The figure demonstrates fissuring and erythema at the angle of the lips, known as angular cheilosis. This finding is associated with various B-vitamin deficiencies, including riboflavin (vitamin B_2), niacin (vitamin B_3), pyridoxine (vitamin B_6), and cyanocobalamin (vitamin B_{12}). It may also be seen in some cases of iron deficiency. Additionally, this finding can be due to dental problems (e.g., dentures), dry mouth (i.e., abnormally decreased salivation) or *Candida* infection. Angular cheilosis has not been associated with thiamine (vitamin B_1) deficiency or the other listed choices.

ANSWERS AND EXPLANATIONS

351. The answer is A. *(Medicine—General)*

Marfan's syndrome is thought to be related to a mutation in microfibrillin, a connective tissue protein. Inheritance is autosomal dominant, not X-linked. Arachnodactyly, or long, thin digits, is classic, as is joint hyperextensibility. Affected persons usually are tall, and their arm span exceeds their height. Joint hyperextensibility; sternum deformities; dislocation of the lens (ectopia lentis); myopia (near-sightedness); retinal detachments; and aortic dilation, dissection, and regurgitation at a young age are common.

352. The answer is A. *(Pediatrics—General)*

Bowleggedness (genu varus) is common in toddlers. Most cases resolve spontaneously by 18 months. Mild cases with no other skeletal deformities (such as evidence of rickets or other skeletal dysplasia) require only observation. Severe cases that fail to resolve may cause osteoarthritis of the knees in adults. Splints may be used in these more severe cases if the deformity fails to resolve spontaneously. Referral to a specialist is indicated in these cases. The important thing to know is that mild cases do not require treatment or referral at this young age, especially with a normal radiograph. If evidence of rickets was present on radiograph, oral calcium might be a therapeutic option depending on the specific type of rickets.

353. The answer is B. *(Medicine—Nutrition)*

Kwashiorkor is due to protein deficiency, although total caloric intake, which usually comes from starches, may be normal. Marasmus is due to a lack of calories or, put more simply, starvation. Children with kwashiorkor often have anemia, diffuse edema, an enlarged fatty liver, a flaky dermatitis, and an apathetic appearance and demeanor. Children with marasmus often have anemia, subcutaneous and muscular wasting, a normal liver, lack of edema, loose hanging skin, and an alert demeanor with excessive hunger. Mixed forms of these disorders are seen more commonly than pure types.

354. The answer is D. *(Medicine—Nutrition)*

In starvation, weight loss occurs; the body tries to compensate by decreasing the basal metabolic rate. The decreased metabolic rate comes from various changes in the body's physiology, such as bradycardia, decreased cardiac output and blood pressure, and a decreased respiratory rate and body temperature. Apathy, lack of energy, and a decreased work capacity are the end results. Insulin levels are decreased and glucagon levels are increased because gluconeogenesis is important to maintain a glucose supply. Loss of libido, gonadal atrophy, and amenorrhea in women are common. Diarrhea commonly develops and may cause death. Mucosal atrophy in the bowel and immunodeficiency contribute to the development of diarrhea.

355. The answer is D. *(Medicine—Nutrition)*

Individuals who are vegans not only avoid meat, but also avoid animal products, such as eggs, milk, and cheese. Vitamin B_1, B_3, and B_6 all can be found in vegetables and many enriched cereal products. Vitamin D is acquired mainly from sunlight in individuals who do not eat animal products. Deficiency of this vitamin is rare in adults unless they have inadequate intake *and* a lack of sunlight exposure. Vitamin B_{12} comes entirely from animal sources. Vitamin B_{12} can be found in nonanimal foods and water only if bacterial contamination has occurred because certain microorganisms produce vitamin B_{12}. Strict vegans are thus at risk for vitamin B_{12} deficiency.

356. The answer is A. *(General Knowledge and Principles)*

Courvoisier's sign describes a nontender, palpable gallbladder, usually caused by pancreatic cancer. Courvoisier postulated that a fibrotic gallbladder wall, which would be expected with cholelithiasis and chronic cholecystitis owing to chronic inflammation, would not be able to distend readily and would not be palpable. If a malignancy, such as pancreatic cancer or a bile duct malignancy, occluded the cystic duct of a healthy gallbladder (acutely or subacutely), the gallbladder would be more likely to distend to the point of being palpable. Acute cholecystitis and cholangitis cause tenderness in the region of the gallbladder, although the gallbladder usually is not palpable.

357. The answer is A. *(Medicine—Oncology)*

Smoking is the most potent pancreatic cancer risk factor of the choices given (and the strongest modifiable risk factor identified to date), with the risk increased 2- to 3-fold in heavy smokers. Age also is a potent risk factor, with most cases occurring in persons older than age 50. Blacks have a higher risk than whites, and males are affected more commonly than females. Alcohol, cholelithiasis, and diabetes have not been established firmly (i.e., controversial) as risk factors for pancreatic cancer. Most believe chronic pancreatitis is a risk factor, but the evidence is not particularly strong. When in doubt, smoking is always a good guess for cancer causation.

358. The answer is A. *(Medicine—General)*

Acute pancreatitis may be caused by hypercalcemia but generally is not caused by hypocalcemia. The other choices are known causes of pancreatitis. Hypocalcemia is related to pancreatitis, however, because its presence during a bout of acute pancreatitis is a marker for a poorer prognosis (one of Ranson's prognostic criteria).

359. The answer is E. *(Laboratory Medicine)*

Although amylase levels have been noted to increase in some cases of diabetic ketoacidosis, there is no particular causative association between hypoglycemia and elevated amylase levels. The point of this question is to make you remember that every elevated amylase level is not pancreatitis. The most important one to remember is damaged or perforated bowel, such as a perforated ulcer and intestinal obstruction, perforation, or infarction, because each of these can cause epigastric pain and elevated amylase levels. Other conditions associated with elevated amylase include pregnancy and alcoholism (without pancreatitis), due to an increase in salivary gland amylase, other causes of an acute surgical abdomen (e.g., appendicitis), and ectopic pregnancy (especially with rupture). The lipase level is rarely as elevated in these conditions as it is in pancreatitis, which may help distinguish them from each other in some cases. Mumps and other causes of parotid gland inflammation can elevate amylase levels but do not affect lipase levels or cause abdominal pain. Renal failure elevates amylase levels because of failure of clearance, although other electrolyte disturbances and elevated creatinine levels usually make this diagnosis easier to make.

360. The answer is A. *(Medicine—Oncology)*

Hematuria is the most common presenting sign of renal cell carcinoma and is usually microscopic but may gross. In an adult, hematuria should not be ignored, and may be due to any type of urinary tract malignancy (in most cases, we worry about a renal cell carcinoma or a transitional cell carcinoma of the bladder or collecting system/ureter). When microscopic hematuria occurs, a repeat urinalysis is the best way to proceed because bladder catheter trauma, myoglobin, or menstrual bleeding in women can all cause a spurious result. Next a microscopic examination of the urine can be done to ensure a positive dipstick result is not due to myoglobin. Gross hematuria in an adult in the absence of obvious trauma usually warrants an endoscopic or radiographic evaluation.

Although renal failure would be unexpected unless bilateral, diffuse involvement of the cancer occurred, the other choices in this question could be presenting signs of renal cell carcinoma. They are less common than hematuria, however. Hypertension can occur, often secondary to renovascular compression resulting in activation of the renin-angiotensin axis or segmental renal ischemia. Spread to the inferior vena cava and lung metastases are fairly common modes of spread. Most renal cell carcinomas are now discovered at an earlier stage, thus a palpable flank mass is now an uncommon physical exam finding (though known as one of the classic presenting findings).

361. The answer is B. *(Medicine—Oncology)*

Chronic infestation with *Schistosoma haematobium* primarily increases the risk of squamous cell carcinoma of the bladder, not transitional cell neoplasms. The other choices all increase the risk of transitional cell neoplasms of the bladder. Phenacetin is a prodrug formulation of acetaminophen that is no longer available in the United States but is used in other countries. The most important risk factor in the United States is smoking because industrial regulations and awareness and avoidance of prolonged cyclophosphamide therapy have decreased the importance of these risk factors.

362. The answer is D. *(Urology)*

Priapism describes a prolonged, typically painful penile erection in the absence of sexual stimulus or desire. It is generally a urologic emergency because prolonged cases commonly result in permanent impotence. Needle decompression or surgery often is needed in an effort to preserve future erectile function. Most cases are thought to be due to pelvic vascular thrombosis, such as that from sickle cell disease or a blood dyscrasia. Trazodone and certain antipsychotics, such as chlorpromazine, also are suspected of causing priapism by unknown mechanisms. Estrogen or other hormonal therapy, such as with stilbestrol, is useful in patients with sickle cell disease to prevent recurrent episodes.

363. The answer is A. *(Gynecology)*

Stress incontinence is the most common type of urinary incontinence in women and usually is associated with aging, multiparity, and pelvic relaxation. Urine may be lost whenever intra-abdominal pressure increases, such as from lifting, straining, sneezing, or coughing—these are the classic symptoms. Urge incontinence is described by patients as a sudden urge to urinate followed by incontinence—there often is no relation to activity. Overflow incontinence occurs when the bladder is chronically overdistended and eventually overcomes the urinary sphincter resistance. Patients usually complain of abdominal fullness, inability to initiate or maintain a urinary stream, and random dribbling of urine. A neurogenic bladder may cause the bladder to be hypotonic or hypertonic. Hypertonic bladders usually cause frequent urination and may overlap with urge incontinence symptoms. Hypotonic bladders may cause urinary retention and overlap with overflow incontinence symptoms. Psychogenic incontinence is a diagnosis of exclusion and is more common in children—look for clues of underlying psychiatric problems.

364. The answer is D. *(Urology)*

This patient most likely has epididymitis, which in younger patients is most commonly due to sexually transmitted pathogens, primarily *Chlamydia trachomatis* and *Neisseria gonorrhoeae*. Chlamydia is more likely to be asymptomatic and to present with no history of sexually transmitted disease. Gonorrhea is a less common cause of epididymitis and is more likely to be symptomatic. Doxycycline is the treatment of choice for chlamydia, although it is not effective for gonorrhea. The only other choice is penicillin, however, which does not cover either organism effectively (many gonococcoal strains are now resistant and penicillin has no activity against *Chlamydia* spp., which lack a cell wall). In persons older than age 50, epididymitis is usually due to urinary tract infection–causing organisms, and fluoroquinolones commonly are used for treatment.

Testicular torsion would be in the differential diagnosis but is uncommon after age 25. Ultrasound also shows increased testicular blood flow in epididymitis versus absent blood flow in torsion. A positive Prehn's sign, or decreased pain with testicular elevation, is classic in epididymitis. In torsion, elevation of the affected testicle usually has no effect or makes the pain worse. Treatment for torsion is surgical exploration with orchiopexy of both testicles. Orchiectomy may be needed if the testicle is necrotic.

365. The answer is E. *(Psychiatry—General)*

This woman has developed tardive dyskinesia, a potentially disabling side effect that classically occurs with long-term antipsychotic use. Although seemingly less common with newer antipsychotic agents, it appears to occur with all antipsychotics and seems to be partly a product of dopamine blockade. Stopping the antipsychotic is advised if possible, and switching to a newer agent may help if symptoms require use of an antipsychotic. There is no effective treatment for this condition, which has been said to appear in up to 50% of chronically medicated, institutionalized patients. If the medication can be stopped, symptoms eventually may lessen somewhat but often do not disappear completely except in mild cases. Older women and individuals on long-term antipsychotic therapy are most likely to develop this condition.

366. The answer is D. *(Medicine—Oncology)*

Although adjuvant radiation therapy may improve survival slightly, the mainstay of treatment for small cell lung cancer is chemotherapy. Clinically, the main division of lung cancer is into small cell and non–small cell, which encompasses squamous cell, adenocarcinoma, large cell, and bronchioloalveolar types. Small cell cancer is treated with chemotherapy because of early metastases, whereas the mainstay of non–small cell cancers detected early enough is surgery with the possible addition of chemotherapy, radiotherapy, or both. Late stage (IIIb and IV) non–small cell cancers generally are treated only with radiotherapy and chemotherapy because surgery increases morbidity and offers no hope for cure. Hormonal therapy has little role in lung cancer treatment at this time.

367. The answer is D. *(Medicine—Pulmonology)*

This patient most likely has obstructive sleep apnea (OSA), a more common condition than previously thought. Studies have documented an association of OSA with a 4-fold increased risk of car accidents and an increased risk of hypertension, heart disease, neuropsychiatric impairment (including depression, memory problems, irritability, and reduced libido), and increased medical care usage. Although obesity is the classic risk factor for OSA, drugs (e.g., sedatives, alcohol) and upper airway variants or acquired blockages that impede air flow also can cause OSA. The mainstay of treatment is continuous positive airway pressure breathing devices worn at night. Oral appliances are a possibility. The goal of both of these devices is to splint the airway open because collapse of the airway during sleep is thought to be responsible for the condition. Patients who are obese also should be counseled and helped to lose weight. Surgical therapy is controversial, except in patients who have a specific correctable lesion identified, and is variable in effectiveness. It is not typically a first-line treatment.

368. The answer is A. *(Medicine—General)*

The formula for body mass index (BMI), which is fair game for the boards, is ([weight in kilograms]/[height in meters]^2), or for those who refuse to think in metrics: ([weight in pounds ∞ 705]/[height in inches]^2). This woman has a BMI of 50 kg/m^2. Individuals with a BMI greater than 40 kg/m^2 have an extremely high health risk from obesity, regardless of age or sex, and need treatment. Black and Hispanic women are disproportionately affected by the health risks of obesity. Patients with a BMI greater than 40, if conservative management fails, are considered for gastric bypass procedures in an attempt to reduce weight. A BMI greater than 25 is defined as overweight, with a BMI greater than 27.5 defined as obese. A BMI of greater than or equal to 40 is considered morbid obesity.

This woman needs a Pap smear in addition to anticipatory guidance. She also needs blood pressure and, most would argue, cholesterol and diabetes screening. She should be advised to begin an exercise and diet program to lose weight. If this fails to produce results, only then would referral for bariatric (i.e., weight reduction) surgery be appropriate. People do "outgrow" childhood asthma fairly commonly, and an inhaler is not needed in the absence of symptoms.

369. The answer is D. *(Medicine—General)*

Although this question may seem a little picky, it is more helpful on the boards to be well versed in common diseases than to know every obscure disease. The National Cholesterol Education Program (NCEP) Adult Treatment Panel is the gold standard and should be learned. The risk factors defined by the NCEP (to be used when deciding whether or not to treat cholesterol and what the goals of treatment should be) include the following:

- Age: men 45 or older, women 55 or older or with premature menopause that are not on hormone replacement therapy

- Family history: premature coronary heart disease (definite myocardial infarction or sudden death) in first-degree (i.e., aunts do not count) male relative before age 55 or first-degree female relative before age 65

- *Current* cigarette smoking

- Hypertension (140/90 mmHg cutoff) or currently on antihypertensive therapy

- Diabetes mellitus

- Low level of high-density lipoprotein cholesterol (< 35 mg/dL)

370. The answer is A. *(Medicine—Infectious Disease)*

Both hepatitis A and E are acquired by contaminated food and water. Hepatitis E is rare in the United States other than in travelers to other parts of the world, whereas hepatitis A is fairly common and occurs in local epidemics from a common source. Hepatitis B, C, and D are all acquired by the parenteral route—the absent risk factors listed in the question cause most acute cases in adults.

371. The answer is E. *(Medicine—Hematology)*

Type O negative blood can be used in an emergency setting with minimal risk of a major transfusion reaction. People with type O blood are said to be *universal donors* because they can donate to people with type O, A, B, or AB blood. People with type AB blood are said to be *universal recipients* because they can receive blood from type O, A, B, or AB donors. The converse of these statements is not true. People with type AB blood can donate only to others with type AB blood, and people with type O blood can receive only from others with type O blood. Type A can receive from type A or O, whereas type B can receive from type B or O. People with Rh-negative blood can receive blood only from Rh-negative donors, but Rh-positive recipients can receive blood from Rh-positive and Rh-negative donors.

372. The answer is A. *(Gynecology)*

Intrauterine devices are most suited for older, monogamous women. The risk of pelvic inflammatory disease, infertility, and ectopic pregnancy are increased with the use of this form of contraception, and most physicians hesitate to use this form of birth control in a young, nulliparous, promiscuous woman with eventual plans to have children. The other methods would be appropriate, although only a diaphragm with spermicide would provide some protection against sexually transmitted diseases. Oral, implantable, and injectable hormonal contraceptives seem to reduce the risk of pelvic inflammatory disease. Smoking is an absolute contraindication for hormonal birth control only after age 35.

373. The answer is A. *(Gynecology)*

This woman most likely has primary dysmenorrhea, or menstrual cramps. Nonsteroidal anti-inflammatory drugs are the first-line agent for this condition, which is thought to be partially due to excessive prostaglandin ($PGF_{2-\alpha}$) production by the endometrium. The type of pain and the timing described in the question are classic. Birth control pills or medroxyprogesterone depot injections can be used and are highly effective if a woman does not desire pregnancy and can tolerate the side effects.

374. The answer is E. *(Pediatrics—General)*

The infant displays a normal pattern of crying and needs no further workup. First-time parents often are amazed at how much an infant can cry and have no basis for comparison. A 2-week-old infant cries approximately 2 hours a day on average. Crying tends to increase to a maximum of roughly 3 hours a day at 6 weeks of age, then decreases to roughly 1 hour per day by 3 months of age. At 7 months of age, 0.5 hour a day or less is not abnormal, unless markedly different from previous patterns.

Although it may be appropriate to ask about the mother's frustration level, directly asking about child abuse at this early stage in the physician-family relationship without any evidence or reason to suspect it might be interpreted as callous. Most parents would not take the implied accusation lightly. Anticipatory guidance is important at every pediatric visit and simply means that you alert parents to common pitfalls and conditions that may occur in their child and how to deal with them. Several routine vaccines are indicated at around 6 months of age.

375. The answer is B. *(Preventive Medicine)*

Young, inexperienced drivers are the most likely group to be involved in a fatal car accident. Males, probably owing to increased risk taking and aggressiveness while driving, have a higher death risk than females. Individuals older than age 65 have an increased risk of fatal accidents as well because of deteriorating physical health and skills, but their risk is still much lower than that of adolescents and young adults. The lowest risk is in middle-aged individuals (35 to 55 years old).

376. The answer is A. *(Pediatrics—Adolescent)*

Pregnancy rates are higher among U.S. teens than in almost every other developed country that maintains such data. There are approximately 1 million teen pregnancies per year, and at least 1 in 10 adolescent girls aged 15 to 19 gets pregnant every year. Roughly 40% of these pregnancies are terminated by elective abortion (roughly 15% terminate by miscarriage and 45% result in live births). Black teens have a pregnancy rate roughly double that of white teens and a lower abortion rate, resulting in a birth rate more than double that of whites. Only around 10% of teen pregnancies are intentional, and most occur out of wedlock. Teen birth and pregnancy rates are higher among the poor in any ethnicity.

377. The answer is B. *(Pediatrics—Adolescent)*

Intrauterine devices do not protect against any form of STD and increase the risk of pelvic inflammatory disease. Intrauterine devices are not recommended for use in teens. The other statements are all true. The most common viral STD is thought to be human papillomavirus, the cause of genital warts and condylomata acuminata (and anogenital cancers).

378. The answer is E. *(Pediatrics—Adolescent)*

Annual gonorrhea and chlamydia screening is widely accepted in sexually active girls, given the high prevalence of these diseases in sexually active teens and the possible consequences of pelvic inflammatory disease and infertility. Many also recommend screening boys annually with cultures or a urine leukocyte esterase test (and culture if positive). A fasting lipid profile screen may be appropriate in adolescents with a strong family history but not annually. A tuberculosis skin test would be appropriate on an annual basis only in extremely high-risk individuals (in prison, AIDS, very high community prevalence). A one-time screen around age 15 is recommended. Complete blood counts or hemoglobin and hematocrit determination is not generally advised annually in adolescent boys; it may be more appropriate in adolescent girls, especially those with a history of heavy periods or athletic activity. Annual prostate examinations are not needed until the 40s or 50s.

379. The answer is E. *(Psychiatry—Child and Adolescent)*

Although isolated cases have been associated with the congenital rubella syndrome, autistic disorder, or autism, is usually idiopathic and thought to have a fairly strong genetic component. Concordance rate in monozygotic twins was 64% in one commonly quoted study versus 9% in dizygotic twins. Males are affected more often than females by at least a 2:1 ratio. About two thirds of affected children are mentally retarded with standard IQ testing.

Using the standard DSM (*Diagnostic and Statistical Manual of Mental Disorders*) IV-R criteria, symptoms must begin by 3 years of age. The three hallmarks of the disorder are impaired social interaction, impaired communication and language, and marked restriction in activity and interests. Repetitive, stereotypic motor activity and behavior (and interests) constitute one of the major DSM IV-R criteria.

380. The answer is B. *(Pediatrics—Neonates)*

A milky white discharge, sometimes stained with blood, is usually normal in the first week after birth and is thought to be due to the withdrawal of maternal hormones. The umbilical cord should have two arteries and one vein—the presence of one artery and one vein should raise concern over possible congenital urinary tract (usually renal) abnormalities. Gastroschisis presents lateral to the midline (on the right side in almost all cases), has no true sac, and typically contains only small bowel, all helping to differentiate it from omphalocele (midline, true hernia sac, often contains bowel and/or liver). The normal heart rate in a newborn is 95 to 180 beats/min. A rate less than 70 beats/min or greater than 200 beats/min should prompt an order for an electrocardiogram to determine the type of arrhythmia present. The pupillary light reflex should be present consistently by around 32 weeks' gestation and thus in a term newborn would be present at birth.

381. The answer is E. *(Pediatrics—Neonates)*

Apnea is a respiratory pause lasting several seconds (usually at least long enough to cause desaturation and often bradycardia). In a preterm infant, there are many possible causes of apnea, including each of the choices as well as seizures, hypothermia, airway obstruction, and drug withdrawal.

382. The answer is E. *(Pediatrics—Neonates)*

Although birth injury may occur during a cesarean section, this procedure reduces the incidence of birth injury and perinatal death rate in most cases. Cesarean sections increase the risk of maternal morbidity and mortality, however, and should be performed only after an assessment of maternal and infant risk. The other choices are all associated with subarachnoid hemorrhage, especially very-low-birth-weight status, which generally occurs in premature children.

383. The answer is E. *(Pediatrics—General)*

The fragile X syndrome is probably second only to Down syndrome as a diagnosable cause of mental retardation. The most common cause of mental retardation overall, however, is probably idiopathic. The cause of fragile X syndrome is an excessive repetition of a specific trinucleotide sequence, allowing prenatal diagnosis. Because the number of repeats has a threshold effect on severity, the severity can be predicted fairly accurately before birth. This threshold effect makes genetic counseling and prenatal evaluation for couples at risk even more important and helpful. Female carriers are often affected by the syndrome (roughly 50% of female carriers have mental retardation or learning disabilities). Sterility is not usually present.

384. The answer is B. *(Psychiatry—Addiction Psychiatry)*

Insomnia is one of many common symptoms in heroin withdrawal. Withdrawal often produces opposite effects of intoxication. Heroin causes apathy, drowsiness, psychomotor retardation, respiratory depression, miosis, constipation, and analgesia. Withdrawal causes many opposite symptoms: agitation, insomnia, mydriasis, diarrhea, nausea, and heightened pain sensitivity. Isolated heroin withdrawal is not life-threatening, although patients may feel as though they want to or are going to die.

385. The answer is A. *(Psychiatry—General)*

Antisocial persons can be extremely charming, especially when they are trying to manipulate someone or stand to gain from a more pleasant approach. Should "turning on the charm" fail, the charm has a tendency to evaporate quickly, being replaced by hostility. The other choices are true and represent paraphrased DSM IV-R criteria for the named disorders.

386. The answer is D. *(Urology)*

With a history of benign prostatic hypertrophy (BPH) and evidence of an obstruction distal to the bladder in a male, BPH should be the prime (most common) consideration. The obstruction must be below the bladder because the bladder and both ureters are dilated. This type of obstruction is unlikely to be related to urolithiasis unless the stone is in the bladder neck obstructing urine outflow. Nephrolithiasis, or a renal calculus, would not produce a distal obstruction (unless the stone moved). A distal obstruction is not consistent with medical (versus surgical or obstructive) renal disease.

The patient needs a Foley catheter placed to drain the bladder. If a Foley catheter cannot be placed because of BPH, a suprapubic catheter needs to be placed. Retrograde urethrogram is unnecessary in this setting, although it is indicated before Foley catheter placement in the trauma setting when evidence of possible urethral injury is present. Ultimately the patient probably will need a transurethral resection of the prostate or prostatectomy because medical management has failed. Terazosin is not a first-line drug for hypertension, and studies have shown an increased risk of heart failure in patients treated with terazosin compared with standard first-line agents (e.g., beta blockers, thiazide diuretics, angiotensin-converting enzyme inhibitors). However, in a patient with BPH, one drug can "kill two birds with one stone" and is likely to increase compliance, thus this is an appropriate antihypertensive therapy for this patient.

387. The answer is C. *(Pediatrics—General)*

Most infants cannot build a tower of 2 blocks until around 15 months. Most infants reach for familiar objects around the age of 3 months, sit unsupported and babble incoherently at around 6 months, and feed themselves with a bottle at 9 months. At 1 year, infants often are walking with minimal or no help, saying a few words ("mama," "dada"), throwing objects, and imitating actions. At this age, most infants understand the word *no* as well.

388. The answer is E. *(Pediatrics—General)*

This infant has been abused and manifests the classic presentation for the *shaken baby syndrome*. Retinal hemorrhages are present in many abused younger children, who are generally less than 1 year old. Subdural hematomas also are common and the second classic manifestation of the shaken baby syndrome. The injuries are due to violent shaking of the infant, who may be thrown against a soft surface, such as a bed. The infants may or may not have bruises, depending on the other types of abuse sustained. A *skeletal survey* is commonly used to document old fractures, which give further proof of abuse. The local agency that handles child abuse should be called, based only on suspicion—definite proof or a parental confession is not required (many parents deny abuse). The parents generally should be confronted and told that social services are being alerted.

Pulse oximetry is reasonable in the setting of tachypnea, which is likely due to the subdural hematoma. Neurosurgical consultation is advised in the setting of a subdural hematoma, especially with lethargy, which should be considered evidence of neurologic deterioration. Although the child is tachypneic, the examination gives no clues to the presence of a foreign body in the trachea, which classically produces stridor. A chest radiograph usually is obtained rather than a lateral neck film when a tracheobronchial foreign body is suspected because the lower airways and the lungs also can be imaged (unless there are specific findings to suggest an upper airway obstruction, which this child lacks).

389. The answer is B. *(Obstetrics)*

This woman has a size-dates discrepancy and needs a fetal ultrasound to evaluate the cause, which may be as simple as incorrect dates or may be more serious. Between 20 and 35 weeks gestation, the measurement from the symphysis pubis to the top of the uterine fundus in centimeters should equal the numer of weeks gestation. More than 2–3 cm discrepancy is considered significant (i.e., a size-dates discrepancy). Mild ankle edema and heartburn are common complaints in pregnancy, especially in the third trimester, and are not a cause for concern. Severe edema or edema elsewhere (e.g., hands, face) should make you think of possible preeclampsia. Symptomatic treatment for heartburn with antacids can be given. There is no current indication for bed rest or hospital admission.

390. The answer is D. *(Obstetrics)*

A transverse cervical os means trauma to the cervix has occurred and is presumptive evidence of a previous vaginal delivery but does not suggest current pregnancy. Amenorrhea is the most common symptom of pregnancy. Hegar's sign is softening and compressibility of the lower uterine segment and is suggestive of pregnancy. Chadwick's sign is a dark discoloration of the vulva and vaginal walls and also is suggestive of pregnancy. Other possible signs of pregnancy are linea nigra (a pigmented vertical line in the center of the skin of the abdominal wall that represents a pigmentation of the linea alba), chloasma (facial erythema or the *mask* of pregnancy), weight gain, an abdominal mass and auscultation of a fetal heart beat.

391. The answer is A. *(Gynecology)*

Always rule out pregnancy as the first step in working up primary or secondary amenorrhea. The other causes are less common. Diabetes does not cause amenorrhea, but may be associated with obesity and the polycystic ovary syndrome.

392. The answer is E. *(Pediatrics—Gynecology)*

This is straight word association for a rare malignant tumor of childhood. Hydatiform mole and choriocarcinoma tend to affect reproductive-age women who become pregnant. Physiologic discharge generally occurs only in neonates. Nonspecific vaginitis is probably the most frequent cause of a pediatric vaginal discharge, but the discharge does not resemble a "bunch of grapes," which is the classic gross description of sarcoma botryoides, a specific subtype of rhabdomyosarcoma.

393. The answer is A. *(Pediatrics—General)*

This child does not have precocious puberty because by definition onset of secondary sex characteristics must occur before age 9 (age 8 in girls) to be considered premature. Normal onset of puberty occurs between the ages of 9 and 14 for boys and the ages of 8 and 13 for girls. MRI may be appropriate in the setting of precocious puberty because intracranial neoplasms or malformation may be a cause, although true precocious puberty usually is idiopathic. Gonadotropin-releasing hormone agonists are given in untreatable forms of precocious puberty to arrest sexual development and help prevent premature epiphyseal closure. Adrenal neoplasms do not cause true precocious puberty but may cause virilization and secondary sexual characteristics to develop. Growth hormone is not indicated in this setting.

394–398. (*Medicine—Oncology*)

The answers are the following: 394. A   395. H   396. F   397. E   398. C.

Acute lymphocytic leukemia is most common in children, with a mean age of onset around 4 years old. It tends to present with symptoms of pancytopenia and is the most likely disorder of those listed to be cured with treatment. Multiple myeloma tends to present with renal insufficiency, bone pain, and pneumococcal pneumonia. Bence-Jones proteinuria and a monoclonal spike of IgG or IgA also are present in most cases. Waldenström's macroglobulinemia classically causes hyperviscosity syndrome symptoms (e.g., headache, visual disturbances) and Raynaud's phenomenon. Chronic lymphocytic leukemia patients often live for many years after the diagnosis without treatment. Because cure is rare, it is important not to overtreat this disease given its indolent course. Polycythemia vera tends to cause facial rubor (*plethoric* appearance or facies is a buzzword), hyperviscosity syndrome symptoms, and a bleeding tendency. The classic symptom is pruritus after a hot bath or shower (may be due to histamine release). The hemoglobin, white blood cell count, and platelet count are all classically elevated. Mycosis fungoides is a T-cell lymphoma classically described as a skin rash, which often is plaquelike, that will not go away after multiple treatments are tried.

Chronic myelocytic leukemia tends to present in middle-aged adults with a high white blood cell count and the Philadelphia chromosome translocation. Acute myelogenous leukemia tends to present in middle-aged adults with pancytopenia symptoms, and patients may have Auer rods (intracellular bodies that resemble tennis rackets) or disseminated intravascular coagulation. Hodgkin disease classically occurs in young adults with fever, night sweats, weight loss (the 3 B-type symptoms), and localized adenopathy in the neck or chest. The diagnosis can be made if Reed-Sternberg cells (owl-eyed binucleated cells) are seen in a biopsy specimen. Hairy cell leukemia tends to cause massive splenomegaly and the malignant cells demonstrate the classic hair-like projections on peripheral smear.

399. The answer is A. (*Pediatrics—Neonates*)

With bowel sounds heard in the left hemithorax and tubular collections of air in the left thorax on chest x-ray, the diagnosis is a left-sided congenital diaphragmatic hernia. As is typical in affected neonates, the presentation is related to respiratory distress rather than gastrointestinal problems. The herniation of bowel loops in the thorax (large majority of cases occur on the left side and reflect the more common Bochdalek type of hernia) compresses the developing lung on that side and may shift the heart and mediastinum to the opposite side, as in this child, and cause compression of the opposite lung as well. The end result of this compression is poor lung development (i.e., pulmonary hypoplasia) and prognosis is most closely related to the pulmonary function/degree of hypoplasia, as surgical repair is fairly easy to accomplish from a technical standpoint. Extracorporeal membrane oxygenation (i.e., ECMO) and other heroic measures may be needed to keep such infants alive due to the respiratory insufficiency.

As part of initial management, a nasogastric tube is commonly placed (did you notice its presence in the center of the x-ray?) to keep the bowel loops decompressed. Remember that the loops of bowel contain no air until a child is born and starts swallowing air/breathing. This can result in distension of bowel loops in the thorax and worsen respiratory distress from local mass effect on the lungs, thus a nasogastric tube is used to keep these loops decompressed.

400. The answer is C. (*Dermatology*)

The history, physical exam and figure are most compatible with a diagnosis of vitiligo, a disorder that is likely at least in part an autoimmune condition. A genetic/familial predisposition has been noted, but the disorder is acquired, with skin changes typically first appearing between 10 and 30 years of age. Coalescing areas of nonpalpable depigmentation are noted, often about the head, neck, chest, hand and/or wrist areas. The underlying pathophysiologic process is destruction of melanocytes, resulting in a paucity or absence of these melanin-producing cells in a biopsy specimen of affected areas. Patients have an increased risk for other autoimmune disorders, such as pernicious anemia, Hashimoto thyroiditis, Addison disease and diabetes mellitus.

Treatment is sometimes successful but only needed for cosmetic reasons. Photochemotherapy (i.e., give topical or systemic agents that are activated when exposed to UV light), corticosteroids and avoidance of tanning of nonaffected areas (makes affected areas stand out more) are commonly used. Nonaffected areas can also be depigmented to match the areas of vitiligo-induced depigmentation. Because treatment is not required and corticosteroids have numerous serious side effects, a careful assessment of the risks, benefits, and patient needs would be required before corticosteroids would be recommended. Vitiligo is not normally associated with an elevated sedimentation rate.

ANSWERS AND EXPLANATIONS

401. The answer is E. *(Emergency Medicine)*

All of the statements given are true. Most episodes of drowning in younger children occur in private swimming pools, where supervision may be less than optimal. Cold-water submersion is thought to increase the chance of survival by lowering metabolism and oxygen consumption. The classic phrase, "they're not dead until they're warm and dead," arises from such amazing case reports as the one in which 30 to 45 minutes of CPR and advanced cardiac life support in a hypothermic patient resulted in sudden resuscitation without permanent neurologic sequelae once the patient was properly warmed. In adolescents and adults, alcohol and other drug use are partially to blame for many different preventable deaths, including automobile accidents, drowning, homicide, suicide, and death by fires.

402. The answer is D. *(Psychiatry—General)*

An acutely psychotic person, especially if violent or threatening violence, represents a psychiatric emergency. These patients commonly are hospitalized, against their will if needed, and given tranquilizers, benzodiazepines, and/or other drugs to calm them. Restraints should be used if there is a risk of violence or the staff's safety is at risk. Cocaine and other stimulants cause mydriasis, not miosis. Patients with psychosis secondary to mania may become agitated and violent similar to any other psychotic patient. Because young males are most commonly affected by acute dystonias when given antipsychotics, diphenhydramine, benztropine, or another anticholinergics commonly are needed and even given prophylactically by some clinicians. Although anticholinergics may cause hyperpyrexia (high fever) in rare instances (usually overdose), the risk is low, and these agents should be used without hesitation if signs of dystonia occur.

403. The answer is E. *(Psychiatry—General)*

Although the other choices are correct, the global assessment of functioning is a measure of the highest functioning level achieved during the past year, given as a number between 1 and 90, with 90 representing the highest level of functioning. Some psychiatrists use two values, the first being the highest level achieved in the last year and the second being the current level (at the time of the interview).

404. The answer is A. *(Psychiatry—General)*

Defense mechanisms are used to protect the ego from unacceptable thoughts or feelings. They can be healthy in some cases, but more frequently they hamper personal development.

Projection is the attribution of unacceptable impulses to others (e.g., a man who cannot handle his homosexual urges who thinks everyone else is a homosexual, while ignoring his own sexual impulses).

Splitting (choice **B**) is classically seen in borderline personality disorder and involves categorizing things or people as "all good" or "all bad." Chaos is caused in interpersonal relationships when a person is switched from one category to the other, which may happen frequently.

Sublimation is a healthy defense mechanism in which unacceptable drives are used to perform socially acceptable actions (an angry, violent person becomes a successful boxer).

Doing/undoing (choice **C**) describes when unacceptable actions are acted out in reverse in an attempt to "atone for one's sins."

Intellectualization occurs when emotions and impulses are controlled by talking and thinking about them rather than experiencing them.

Rationalization (choice **D**) involves assigning improper logic to an unacceptable action or impulse to make it seem more acceptable.

Dissociation involves modifying one's character or sense of identity to avoid emotional distress. It is seen in fugue, hysterical conversion reactions, and most dramatically in dissociative identity disorder (i.e., multiple personality disorder).

Regression (choice **E**) is returning to an earlier stage of development or functioning, which is seen commonly in sick persons.

Denial is an avoidance of reality involving a refusal to accept what one sees and hears.

405. The answer is C. *(Preventive Medicine)*

Primary prevention involves preventing a disease from occurring. An example is an antismoking program to prevent the myriad of diseases that can occur in those who smoke. The goal of secondary prevention is to detect and treat disease at the earliest possible stage to reduce the prevalence of the disease. Cancer screening measures are examples of secondary prevention. Tertiary prevention involves trying to reduce the morbidity and disability of disease through rehabilitation and other supportive services. In psychiatry, this prevention commonly involves helping people reach the highest level of mental and social functioning possible.

406. The answer is B. *(Psychiatry—General)*

Behavior learned with a fixed-interval reinforcement is more likely to become extinct, or go away, when the reinforcement is stopped than variable reinforcement. Variable reinforcement is the underlying principle of slot machines, when the payoff may occur at any time. If a reward is received every time an action is performed (fixed-interval continuous reinforcement), the behavior is often rapidly learned, but quickly goes away when the expected reward fails to materialize. In behavior learned with variable reinforcement, the person is used to continuing the behavior without an immediate reward.

The closer the reward is to the behavior one is trying to reinforce, the more likely it is to be effective. If the reward or punishment is delayed, the person (or the dog that keeps peeing on the carpet) may not associate the behavior with the consequence or reinforcement. Positive reinforcement is desired (food, drugs), whereas as negative reinforcement prevents an undesired consequence (avoid getting yelled at, avoid a painful shock). Both can be very effective in causing a desired behavior.

Shaping involves gradually getting the subject to perform a task by rewarding activity that resembles the task. Someone being trained to talk may get a reward first for opening the mouth, then for making any sound, then for saying individual words, then for speaking in complete sentences. The behavior is shaped gradually by rewarding each successive step that resembles more closely the desired behavior. For parents, scolding a child may unintentionally be a form of positive reinforcement and actually increase the undesired behavior. This is especially true when unaffectionate and inattentive parents are always nagging or scolding a child because this may be the only attention the child gets from the parents. Performing an undesired activity may get the child what he or she needs—attention.

407. The answer is B. *(Medicine—Infectious Disease)*

The screening tests for syphilis include the RPR and VDRL tests. These are nonspecific, nontreponemal tests that should be confirmed with a specific treponemal antigen test, such as the fluorescent treponemal antibody-absorbed test (FTA-ABS) or microtiter hemagglutination assay for *Treponema pallidum* (MHA-TP). The nonspecific tests can be falsely positive in many conditions (classically lupus), including older age, and often become negative after treatment of syphilis (may be followed to confirm successful treatment). The treponemal antigen (specific) tests often remain positive for life, with or without treatment, and usually are unreliable in the setting of reinfection. Spirochetes can be found in primary chancres and secondary skin lesions but would not generally be recovered from a urethral swab. Spirochetes are also seen rarely once the disease has progressed into the latent or tertiary stage.

408. The answer is D. *(Pharmacology)*

Gemfibrozil is used primarily for its effects on hypertriglyceridemia and has little effect on low-density lipoproteins. The other choices are correct. Niacin often is tolerated poorly because of flushing, which can be reduced by pretreatment with aspirin and gradually increasing the dose over time. Liver function tests should be ordered before HMG-CoA reductase agents such as simvastatin are used. Monitoring of liver function tests generally is done at least every 6 months.

409. The answer is E. *(Obstetrics)*

Breech presentation means that the child is sacrum first instead of skull first in relation to the birth canal. This increases the risk for birth injury. An increased incidence of breech presentation is seen with congenital anomalies, including anencephaly and hydrocephalus. Uterine anomalies or fibroids and multiple gestation increase the risk of breech presentation. Toward the end of the second trimester, approximately one third of infants have a breech presentation, but this number gradually decreases to around 5% by term. In this question, the fetus probably has more than an 80% likelihood of converting to a normal presentation.

The most common type of breech presentation is the frank breech (50% to 75%), which involves flexion of the thighs with the knees straight so that the feet of the fetus are near its head. The illustrated renderings of breech presentations have shown up on the boards in the past. The phrase "Frank kisses his own feet" may help you remember the difference between complete and frank breech. Complete, the least common type of breech presentation (5% to 10%), refers to flexed thighs and knees. A footling breech (20% to 25% of cases) is flexed thighs and knees, but at least one foot extends below the buttocks (the child goes foot or feet first).

External cephalic version is often attempted to manually try to convert the child to a vertex presentation. If this fails, vaginal delivery is sometimes attempted if restrictive criteria are met. Footling breeches should not be delivered vaginally, and prematurity and low birth weight are other common reasons to avoid a trial of vaginal delivery. It is common for obstetricians to perform a cesarean section routinely on any breech presentation because vaginal delivery is fraught with hazards (such as cord compression and head entrapment) even in experienced hands.

410. The answer is A. *(Gynecology)*

Leiomyomas of the uterus (i.e., fibroids) are one of the most common tumors in women and a common indication for a cesarean section. They develop in approximately 20% of women by age 40. They can cause menorrhagia, dysmenorrhea, pelvic pain, infertility, and other problems. The chance of a leiomyosarcoma arising from within a fibroid tumor is low (1 in 1000), but not zero. The tumors are hormonally responsive so that birth control pills and pregnancy can cause rapid enlargement, whereas gonadotropin-releasing hormone analogues taken regularly and menopause usually *shrink* the tumors. Gonadotropin-releasing hormone can be used clinically for this effect in the management of fibroids. Rapid enlargement of a fibroid tumor after menopause should make one suspicious for malignant transformation.

411. The answer is D. *(Gynecology)*

Pelvic relaxation becomes more common with age, especially after menopause, because hormone withdrawal promotes atrophy of pelvic tissues, including support structures. The other choices generally are hormone-sensitive or hormone-related conditions that decrease significantly in incidence after menopause.

412. The answer is A. *(Obstetrics)*

Roughly 50% to 80% of women experience postpartum blues or *dysphoria*. Symptoms include sleep disturbances, emotional lability, and difficulty concentrating. Symptoms generally go away within 2 weeks after birth, and reassurance usually is all that is needed. Postpartum depression is essentially major depression that occurs after pregnancy—hospitalization and antidepressants may be needed. It occurs in roughly 10% of women during the postpartum period. Postpartum psychosis occurs less than 1% of women and may cause women to harm themselves, their infant, or both. Antipsychotics given in an inpatient setting generally are needed. Endomyometritis is a possible cause for a postpartum fever and should cause uterine tenderness.

413. The answer is A. *(Ethics)*

In these circumstances, full medical and surgical interventions should be performed. Always treat the patient as you see fit if you lack a reason to do otherwise (e.g., living will asks you not to, etc.) and no one is available to make decisions. You do not need the courts, ethics committee, or an attorney's permission to initiate treatment.

414–423. *(General Knowledge and Principles)*

The answers are the following: 414. O 415. E 416. S 417. D 418. G 419. P
420. H 421. K 422. A 423. C.

See the following table for a description of these classic signs and syndromes.

Sign/Syndrome	What the Sign or Syndrome Means
Beck's triad	Jugular venous distention, muffled heart sounds, and hypotension in cardiac tamponade
Brudzinski's sign	Pain on neck flexion with meningeal irritation (meningitis)
Charcot's triad	Fever or chills, jaundice, and right upper quadrant pain with cholangitis
Chvostek's sign	Tapping on the facial nerve elicits tetany in hypocalcemia
Courvoisier's sign	A painless, palpable gallbladder plus jaundice equals pancreatic cancer
Cullen's sign	Bluish discoloration of periumbilical area from retroperitoneal hemorrhage (pancreatitis)
Cushing's reflex	Hypertension, bradycardia, and irregular respirations with high intracranial pressure
Grey Turner's sign	Bluish discoloration of flank from retroperitoneal hemorrhage (think pancreatitis)
Homan's sign	Calf pain on forced dorsiflexion of the foot with deep venous thrombosis
Kehr's sign	Pain in the left shoulder with a ruptured spleen
Leriche's syndrome	Claudication and atrophy of the buttocks with impotence (aortoiliac occlusive disease)
McBurney's sign	Tenderness at McBurney's point with appendicitis
Murphy's sign	Arrest of inspiration when palpating under the rib cage on the right with cholecystitis
Ortolani's sign/test	Palpable or audible click in congenital hip dysplasia caused by abducting infant's flexed hips
Prehn's sign	Elevation of a painful testicle that relieves pain in epididymitis (versus testicular torsion)
Rovsing's sign	Pain at McBurney's point in appendicitis that is caused by pushing on left lower quadrant
Tinel's sign	Paresthesias in carpal tunnel syndrome elicited by tapping on the volar surface of the wrist
Trousseau's sign	Carpopedal spasm (tetany) in hypocalcemia caused by pumping up a blood pressure cuff
Virchow's triad	Stasis, endothelial damage, and hypercoagulability (deep venous thrombosis risk factors)

424. The answer is C. *(Pediatrics—Gastroenterology)*

This type of history could be compatible with anal atresia as well, but you would not be able to perform a rectal examination, and this condition usually is detected in the well-baby newborn examination in the nursery (or by mom at home) shortly after birth. Duodenal atresia would present in the first week of life and would not cause abdominal distention. Strangulated hernia and necrotizing enterocolitis would not generally cause obstipation from birth. In Hirschsprung's disease, a rectal biopsy would reveal the absence of nerve ganglia, and the treatment is surgical resection of the denervated bowel.

425. The answer is B. *(Orthopedic Surgery)*

Although the other choices are possible causes, osteoporosis is the most common cause of pathologic fractures, especially involving the spine and hips in elderly adults. Primary bone tumors are rare in adults. Metastatic causes are an important cause that should be excluded but are not as common as osteoporosis.

426. The answer is A. *(Pediatrics—Neonates)*

The three classic causes of neonatal conjunctivitis are chemical agents, *Chlamydia*, and gonorrhea, though others certainly occur (e.g., viral, other bacteria). Chemical conjunctivitis occurs in the *first 24 hours* of life and is due to the topical silver nitrate or erythromycin that is put in the neonate's eyes prophylactically to reduce the incidence of gonorrheal conjunctivitis. Chemical conjunctivitis normally resolves within 48 hours and requires no treatment. Gonorrheal conjunctivitis usually occurs between the *second and fifth days* of life, generally in children who did not receive ocular chemoprophylaxis, and is likely if the question mentions a mother who had a purulent cervical discharge. It tends to be quite purulent and is treated with systemic antibiotics (e.g., ceftriaxone) as well as topical therapies. Chlamydial conjunctivitis (also called *inclusion conjunctivitis*) begins on the *5th to 14th days* of life, is not prevented effectively by chemoprophylaxis, and not uncommonly comes from an asymptomatic mother. Treatment is with oral and topical antibiotics. Oral antibiotics (usually erythromycin) are used to help prevent the development of chlamydial pneumonia, a relatively common complication.

427. The answer is B. *(Surgery—Trauma)*

By definition, tamponade means cardiac compression caused by a critical volume of fluid in the pericardial sac resulting in decreased cardiac output. You would therefore not expect a patient with tamponade to have an increased blood pressure, and often these patients are hypotensive. This is especially true in trauma because of the implied rapid onset without time for the body to develop compensatory mechanisms (as may occur in pericarditis or malignancy). The other choices, in addition to pulsus paradoxus (an exaggerated fall in blood pressure during inspiration), are all classic in cardiac tamponade. If a patient is markedly hypovolemic, distended neck veins may be absent. Treatment of tamponade, if unstable, involves emergent pericardiocentesis. If stable, echocardiography normally is performed to confirm the diagnosis first, and the patient can be taken to the operating room or cardiac catheterization suite for an open or an ultrasound-guided procedure, which is less likely to result in complications.

428. The answer is C. (Obstetrics)

The other choices are associated with premature delivery. It is not known why anencephaly is associated with prolonged gestation, but some suspect it may be due to a lack of normal stimulatory fetal hormone production because of abnormal central nervous system development.

429. The answer is C. (Obstetrics)

A biophysical profile is an easy, relatively inexpensive, and noninvasive means to monitor the fetus in high-risk pregnancies, such as those involving maternal diabetes, mild preeclampsia, or intrauterine growth retardation. The components of a biophysical profile include a nonstress test (20-minute fetal heart tracing to look for normal variability) and a fetal ultrasound for amniotic fluid volume estimation and to check fetal breathing and body movements.

430. The answer is A. (Psychiatry—Addiction Psychiatry)

The patient has most likely overdosed on heroin or some other opiate. The scabs on his forearms are most likely from repeated intravenous injection. These patients are at high risk for HIV because of needle sharing, although they may also acquire HIV from sexual intercourse with other intravenous drug users. Although opiate abuse may result in impotence, this is not universal. Miosis (pinpoint pupils) is characteristic of intoxication and respiratory depression and death may result from opiate overdose. Intoxicated patients are often docile; violent behavior is classic with phencyclidine (PCP) or stimulants (e.g., amphetamines, cocaine). Withdrawal from opiates is not life-threatening (although patients often feel and act as though they are going to die). Withdrawal symptoms include diarrhea, pain and hypersensitivity to painful stimuli, insomnia, and "gooseflesh" or goose bumps. Naloxone can reverse dramatically the effects of opioids on the central nervous and respiratory systems and can precipitate acute withdrawal in those who are addicted.

431. The answer is C. (Psychiatry—Child and Adolescent)

This is a classic age and description for separation anxiety disorder. Perhaps in part because of his father's death, the child fears what will happen to his mother if they are separated. Conduct disorder describes the pediatric equivalent of antisocial personality disorder, which is not suggested by the case scenario. Oppositional-defiant disorder might be a consideration if the child always argued with mom, but because they have a good relationship outside of the school issue, this is unlikely. Child abuse is always something to think about and could be occurring at the school, but there are no special reasons to suspect it in this scenario. Attention-deficit hyperactivity disorder results in hyper kids with short attention spans.

432. The answer is A. (Psychiatry—Child and Adolescent)

This child is most likely experiencing side effects from dextroamphetamine use, which may include abdominal pain, anorexia, insomnia, weight loss, and growth suppression. It is important to weigh the risks against the benefits when prescribing these powerful stimulants to patients, especially children. Although malingering and somatization disorder are possibilities, these are diagnoses of exclusion in most cases, and there is no suggestive history. Henoch-Schönlein purpura may cause abdominal pain, but there is little to support this diagnosis (e.g., no skin rash) given in the question. Urgent psychiatric referral is not indicated.

433. The answer is C. (Obstetrics)

This woman has a hydatiform mole. Although preeclampsia can occur in the second trimester (less common than in the third), a hydatiform mole should be suspected when a woman gets preeclampsia before 20 weeks' gestation. The condition often results in a virtually pathognomonic snowstorm pattern on ultrasound with no fetal visualization. There is no fetus in the setting of a complete mole.

434. The answer is A. *(Gynecology)*

Although theoretically implants and oral contraceptive pills should be equally efficacious, pills require daily patient compliance, which is rarely 100%. The other methods are less effective, but of the choices listed, only condoms have been shown to be fairly effective at reducing spread of sexually transmitted diseases.

435. The answer is D. *(Gynecology)*

Pelvic relaxation is common in women who have had many children. The "location of the bulge" is a classic giveaway in combination with the symptoms. Urethroceles are located in the lower anterior vaginal wall and cause urinary symptoms; cystoceles are located in the upper anterior vaginal wall and cause urinary symptoms. Rectoceles are located in the lower posterior vaginal wall and cause difficulty with defecation. Enteroceles are located in the upper posterior vaginal wall. Ectopic ureteroceles may or may not cause incontinence, but would present shortly after birth, since these are congenital anomalies.

436. The answer is B. *(Biostatistics)*

The p-value tells you how likely it is that the data are different simply because of random chance. The p-value tells you the likelihood of making a type I error (rejecting the null hypothesis when it is true). A type II error describes accepting the null hypothesis when it is false. Power describes the ability of a study to detect a type II eror and can be increased by increasing the sample size. You cannot say that surgery alone is better with certainty, as in choice **E**, with the limited amount of information given. In other words, a study that shows statistical significance may have serious design flaws (e.g., bias, no randomization) that invalidate (or at least tarnish) its results.

437. The answer is D. *(Biostatistics)*

The chi-squared test is used to compare two percentages or proportions (nonnumeric or nominal data), whereas the t-test and ANOVA are used to compare means (numeric or continuous data).

438. The answer is A. *(Dermatology)*

The figure and history of weight loss are highly suspicious for malignancy-related acanthosis nigricans, which is typically due to a visceral adenocarcinoma (e.g., lung, GI). The lesions are described as areas of skin thickening and increased pigmentation with associated warty excrescences and a velvet-like feel on palpation. The axillary and groin regions are commonly affected areas, but widespread involvement can also occur. A benign form with similar, though often milder, skin changes can be seen in obese individuals and/or those with endocrine disturbances. Hidradenitis suppurativa is a painful condition that has a predilection for the axilla, but causes inflamed nodules and pustules that often break down to form abscesses, sinuses, and scarring. Pemphigoid vulgaris and pemphigoid are both blistering disorders (blisters and/or large bullae should be present). Dermatitis herpetiformis is associated with celiac sprue and gluten insensitivity and would not typically develop suddenly in an older adult. This condition also typically causes intense pruritis and is not usually found in the axilla (favors knees, elbows, scalp and buttocks).

439. The answer is C. *(Gynecology)*

The history, description and figure are consistent with an intraductal papilloma, a benign papillary tumor of the lactiferous ducts that most often occurs in major ducts close to the nipple. The lack of cellular atypia should steer you away from invasive lobular carcinoma, which arises from the lobule, not the duct. Likewise, fibroadenomas and phyllodes tumor are not intraductal tumors and thus also do not typically cause a bloody nipple discharge. A unilateral clear or bloody nipple discharge should always make you worry about invasive ductal carcinoma (though both can also be caused by intraductal papillomas and other conditions), which does come from the ducts but is associated with cellular atypia and invasion.

440. The answer is D. *(Surgery—General)*

Intussusception can occur, but is a rare cause of large bowel obstruction and more commonly causes small bowel obstruction (from ileocolic intussusception). The other choices are some of the most common causes of large bowel obstruction in adults.

441. The answer is D. *(Surgery—General)*

Indirect hernias are the most common type of hernias in any age group and both sexes. In this type, the hernia sac travels through the inner and outer inguinal rings (protrusion begins lateral to the inferior epigastric vessels) and into the scrotum or labial region as as result of a patent processus vaginalis (congenital defect). Direct hernias lack a true sac and protrude medial to the inferior epigastric vessels because of weakness in the abdominal musculature (of Hesselbach's triangle). Femoral hernias are more common in women, and the hernia (also no true sac) goes through the femoral ring onto the anterior thigh (located below the inguinal ring). These hernias are quite susceptible to incarceration or strangulation. Incisional hernias can occur after a wound (classically a surgical incision).

Strangulation and incarceration are not types of hernias but rather describe complications of hernias. Incarceration is when herniated organs get trapped and become swollen and edematous. Strangulation occurs when the entrapment becomes so severe that the blood supply is cut off (can lead to necrosis) and is a surgical emergency. The patient may present with small bowel obstruction symptoms and shock.

442. The answer is D. *(Medicine—Cardiology)*

Synchronized cardioversion may be attempted, but unsynchronized cardioversion generally is reserved for ventricular tachycardia or fibrillation. Treatment depends on symptoms, however, and cardioversion is initially reserved for unstable patients. Amiodarone, quinidine, procainamide, and ibutilide have all been used for attempted chemical cardioversion with some success. Slowing the ventricular rate with β-blockers, digoxin, or centrally acting calcium channel blockers (i.e., verapamil or diltiazem) is important to prevent cardiovascular decompensation in those with a rapid ventricular rate/response. Anticoagulation is used to prevent clot formation in the fibrillating atrium and warfarin (heparins more for acute use due to parenteral formulation) is one of the primary treatments for chronic atrial fibrillation due to structural and/or ischemic heart damage.

443. The answer is B. *(Medicine—Cardiology)*

Amyloidosis may cause a restrictive cardiomyopathy but is not generally associated with dilated cardiomyopathy. The other choices are classic causes of a dilated cardiomyopathy, though technically, coronary artery disease is supposed to be excluded from the definition of a cardiomyopathy. This precise definition is, however, often of little use clinically, as the generally irreversible nature of the condition merits similar congestive heart failure-type treatments regardless of the cause.

444. The answer is A. *(Dermatology)*

This girl had an allergic reaction to the material in the earrings (most likely nickel) and developed a contact dermatitis. This type IV hypersensitivity reaction is also seen with poison ivy exposure and is exploited by the purified protein derivative (PPD) skin test for tuberculosis. The only required treatment is removal of the earrings and future avoidance of the material. Although this is an allergic reaction, there is no particular reason to suspect that the child is asthmatic. If infection occurred, it would likely be cellulitis (which is often caused by gram positive staphylococci or streptococci), but the bilateral symmetric nature of the process, lack of tenderness and pruritis are not typical for cellulitis.

445. The answer is B. *(Pediatrics—Infectious Disease)*

Group A streptococcus, usually *S. pyogenes*, may cause scarlet fever if the infecting species produces erythrogenic toxin. Treating streptococcal pharyngitis can reduce the incidence of this now rarely seen condition.

446. The answer is B. *(Pediatrics—General)*

This child most likely has glomerulonephritis, which is most frequently poststreptococcal glomerulonephritis in this age group. Treatment is largely supportive, and prognosis is good. Red blood cell casts are fairly specific for glomerulonephritis. Minimal change disease causes loss of podocyte foot processes, nephrotic syndrome (4+ or heavy proteinuria), lipiduria, and hyperlipidemia. Proteinuria is common with poststreptococcal glomerulonephritis, but is characteristically mild (i.e., not in the nephrotic range)

447. The answer is E. *(Pediatrics—Infectious Disease)*

This child most likely has erythema infectiosum. The other choices accurately describe the condition, which is caused by parvovirus B19. The "slapped-cheek" facial rash is a clue that you'll need to be able to specifically suspect this condition. Aplastic crisis can occur when this virus infects patients with shortened red blood cell life span or bone marrow problems, classically sickle cell or HIV patients.

448. The answer is A. *(Orthopedics)*

Osteosarcoma has a peak incidence in individuals 10 to 30 years old. The other statements are correct. Approximately half of all cases occur around the knee (proximal tibia and distal femur).

449. The answer is B. *(Medicine—Oncology)*

A clear link between aspirin use and gastric cancer has not been established. In Japan, gastric cancer is one of the most common overall malignancies and in the 1930s was the most common overall malignancy in the United States. Elimination of dietary carcinogens with better food preservation is thought to play a role in the marked worldwide decline in gastric cancer. The marked consumption of smoked foods (e.g., smoked fish) is thought to play a role in the higher incidence of gastric cancer in Japan. *Helicobacter pylori* has been linked to gastric cancer as well (considered a carcinogen), thought to be a result of chronic inflammation.

450. The answer is C. *(Medicine—Oncology)*

At least 30% to 40% of neuroblastomas are thought to arise from the adrenal gland, although other areas in the sympathetic chain may be sites of origin. Paragangliomas are essentially pheochromocytomas that arise outside of the adrenal gland. Nephroblastoma and Wilms' tumor are synonyms, and this tumor comes from the kidney. Carcinoids usually arise from the small bowel, appendix, bronchus or rectum.

ANSWERS AND EXPLANATIONS

451. The answer is D. *(Ethics)*

This situation is difficult. Although adults can make their own decisions, children are protected by the state. In most instances, the parents' wishes should be respected, but if they refuse a simple, life-saving intervention, the courts should be involved. It would be appropriate to involve the hospital ethics committee, although this was not an option. Always try to reason with the parents first in this setting, but if this fails, you should attempt to gain permission to do what you believe is right for the child.

452. The answer is E. *(Pediatrics—General)*

Boys younger than age 6 who develop a urinary tract infection or girls younger than age 6 with two or more urinary tract infections need to be screened for congenital renal disease (more aggressive guidelines exist that recommend screening girls after their first urinary tract infection). Often these patients have vesicoureteral reflux or posterior urethral valves (boys). These conditions are important to detect because treatment can prevent progression to serious renal disease and kidney failure. The screening tests of choice are a renal ultrasound and a voiding cystourethrogram.

453. The answer is D. *(Pediatrics—Gastroenterology)*

Hypertrophic pyloric stenosis commonly presents in the first three months of life with increasing nonbilious vomiting after feeding that classically becomes projectile as time goes on. The child is characteristically quite hungry, lacks abdominal distention, and has the classic olive-shaped mass in the epigastrium representing the hypertrophied pylorus. Treatment usually is surgical, and the prognosis is excellent. Upper gastrointestinal tract atresias present within the first week of life and do not cause a mass. Hirschsprung's disease causes feculent and bilious vomiting and abdominal distention. Splenic hematoma would be uncommon in the absence of a blunt trauma history and would be unlikely to cause a mass in the epigastrium.

454. The answer is A. *(Orthopedic Surgery)*

Metastatic bone disease in adults is more common than all the primary bone malignancies combined.

455. The answer is C. *(Ophthalmology)*

The most common form of glaucoma is open-angle glaucoma (85–90% of cases), which slowly causes visual loss as a result of a chronic, often mild elevation of intraocular pressure. Patients do not experience pain or other symptoms, and medications generally are used in the early stages of the disease. Choices **A**, **B**, **D**, and **E** describe closed-angle glaucoma, the rarer but more infamous and dramatic form of glaucoma that can cause acute painful attacks (which may be brought on by the use of anticholinergic medications) with nausea and vomiting and acute visual disturbances. With closed-angle glaucoma, a peripheral iridectomy (usually done with a laser to burn a hole into the peripheral iris) usually is performed to prevent future attacks of markedly increased intraocular pressure.

456. The answer is C. *(Ophthalmology)*

Conjunctivitis does not cause decreased visual acuity, other than transient blurriness from debris in the tear film that resolves with eye blinking. Decreased visual acuity should prompt the search for other, more serious conditions. The other statements are true. Hand washing can help prevent spread of viral conjunctivitis, which usually is the result of an adenovirus infection.

457. The answer is B. *(Surgery—Trauma)*

Tension pneumothorax is associated with a hyperresonant or tympanic percussion sound on the affected side. A dull percussion note would be expected with a pleural effusion, which may coexist with a pneumothorax. The other choices are consistent with a tension pneumothorax. You should be able to recognize the appearance of a simple pneumothorax on chest radiograph as well as a tension pneumothorax, which describes a pneumothorax plus mediastinal shift away from the side of the injury because of a buildup of trapped air. A tension pneumothorax often occurs after blunt trauma but also is possible in the setting of penetrating trauma. Treatment is with needle thoracentesis followed by chest tube placement.

458. The answer is C. *(Obstetrics)*

Lithium has been associated with cardiac (Ebstein's) anomalies; warfarin is associated with craniofacial and central nervous system anomalies; fluoroquinolones may cause fetal cartilage abnormalities; and diphenylhydantoin is associated with multiple deformities, including craniofacial, limb, central nervous system, and cardiovascular defects. Heparin does not cross the placenta and is the anticoagulant of choice in pregnancy. Some drugs, such as diphenylhydantoin (Dilantin) and lithium, may need to be given to the mother if the risk of maternal harm without the medication outweighs the risk of potential fetal harm. These are difficult decisions and are handled on a case-by-case basis. All women taking potentially teratogenic agents should be counseled about the risks should they become pregnant.

459. The answer is B. *(Obstetrics)*

If the alpha fetoprotein level is abnormal at 16 to 20 weeks, the woman often is advised to undergo ultrasound to check for accurate dates, multiple gestation, or fetal demise (all of which can cause abnormal elevation of maternal alpha fetoprotein). If the ultrasound is normal and shows a healthy, single fetus with correct estimated dates, amniocentesis (ideally done at 16 to 20 weeks) is advised for a definitive diagnosis of chromosomal disorders (cell culture) or neural tube defects (amniotic fluid alpha fetoprotein). Chorionic villus sampling is not used in this setting because of an increased rate of miscarriage and inability to detect neural tube defects. Intrauterine fetal transfusion is not relevant to this scenario.

460. The answer is D. *(Medicine—Infectious Disease)*

The patient probably has tuberculosis. The next step is respiratory isolation, followed by acquiring sputum samples for acid-fast bacilli (i.e., AFB) smears and culture. A skin test should also be placed; make sure to ask if the patient has been vaccinated to help interpret the results accurately. Those who have been vaccinated normally get a larger area of palpable induration from the vaccine exposure (the vaccine is not used in the United States, given its effect on an important diagnostic test in the setting of limited vaccine efficacy and a relatively low disease prevalence). Open surgical biopsy is not needed to confirm the diagnosis in this setting. Chemotherapy in the form of antituberculosis therapy should begin once the diagnosis can be confirmed. Granulomatous disease is one of the causes of a false positive PET scan, since metabolic activity can occur in granulomas. A PET scan would not be indicated in this setting (though a CT scan might be of some benefit to better define the cavitary lesion and detect endobronchial spread or mediastinal lymphadenopathy).

461. The answer is A. *(Psychiatry—General)*

In terms of age, the established risk factor is age greater than 45. Although suicide is the third leading cause of death in adolescents in the United States, individuals older than age 45 are more likely to commit suicide. Individuals older than age 75 commit suicide three times as often as individuals who are young. This fact often is overlooked because teen suicide receives the most attention in the media. In terms of sex, women are much more likely to attempt suicide than men, but men are much more likely to succeed owing to using more violent methods.

462. The answer is D. *(Psychiatry—General)*

It can be difficult to keep straight all of the psychotic disorders that contain "schiz-." Time course is important for a few of them. The same symptoms and signs are called *schizophrenia* if they last more than 6 months, *schizophreniform* if they last 1 to 6 months, and *acute psychotic disorder* if they last less than 1 month, as in this patient. *Schizoaffective disorder* is best thought of as coexisting schizophrenia and mood disorder—one does not cause the other. *Schizoid* is a personality disorder (long pattern of maladaptive traits) that describes the classic loner (no friends and no desire for friends). *Schizotypal* personality disorder describes a "weird," schizophrenialike person without full-blown psychosis or schizophrenia (e.g., into cults or extrasensory perception, has frequent illusions or strange speech).

463. The answer is A. *(Biostatistics)*

Power is the probability of rejecting the null hypothesis when it is false (a good thing). The best way to increase power in most circumstances is to increase the sample size.

464. The answer is B. *(Biostatistics)*

A type II error is to accept the null hypothesis when it is false. In a drug trial, the null hypothesis is usually the hypothesis that there is no effect (i.e., the drug does not work). In this setting, the experimenter has designed a study with low power because of the small sample size. This is unlikely to be a calculation error, but rather a design flaw. Two groups of 10 people are not enough to measure the effect of a drug on a variable such as blood pressure with a wide amount of intrapersonal and interpersonal fluctuation. A type I error is to reject the null hypothesis when it is true (e.g., say the drug works when it does not). The standard *p* value used in medical clinical trials is set at .05 ($p < 0.05$), which means that there is less than a 5% chance that a difference seen was due to chance. Experimenter bias generally is eliminated by double-blinding a trial.

465. The answer is C. *(Medicine—Neurology)*

This woman probably has multiple sclerosis, by far the most commonly seen clinical demyelinating disorder. The figure reveals area that fail to take up myelin stain because of demyelination. MRI has shown to be one of the most sensitive and specific tests to confirm a suspected clinical diagnosis of multiple sclerosis and is likely to be positive given the several neurologic symptoms and clinical findings. Cerebrospinal fluid usually reveals increased IgG with oligoclonal banding and increased myelin basic protein during disease flareups. The papillitis, or inflammation of the optic disk, represents optic neuritis, a fairly common site of involvement in multiple sclerosis. Dysarthric or scanning speech also is classic. A waxing and waning course with exacerbations and remissions is the norm, and a fulminant course is much less common. Persons who are born and raised in colder climates have a higher incidence of the disease.

466. The answer is B. *(Dermatology)*

This patient, with a lack of drug or environmental exposure and a positive Nikolsky's sign (epidermis easily detached from the underlying skin), most likely has pemphigus vulgaris. It is an autoimmune disorder usually seen in middle-aged or elderly individuals with antibodies directed against the skin that reveal a "lace-like" or "fish net" immunofluorescence pattern on a biopsy specimen. Treatment involves corticosteroids and other immune suppressants to prevent further skin lesions. Widespread disease is potentially fatal, and secondary infection of lesions is a concern.

467. The answer is E. *(Medicine—Infectious Disease)*

Chronic sinusitis generally is due to a bacterial or fungal infection. Any of the other choices listed as well as additional organisms are possible, including gram-negative and anaerobic bacteria, but viral causes are highly unlikely. The initial insult before a bout of acute sinusitis often is a viral infection that allows bacteria to move in, but the bacteria (or fungi) usually cause the chronic sinusitis.

468. The answer is D. *(Medicine—Infectious Disease)*

Tetracyclines (usually doxycycline) are a good empiric antibiotic for *Borrelia burgdorferi*, the cause of Lyme disease. Macrolide antibiotics have good coverage against the atypical pneumonias, including *Mycoplasma*, and are a good empirical choice. Penicillins have no significant effect against *Mycoplasma*, as it has no cell wall. Aztreonam is not effective against gram positive (e.g., streptococcal) or anaerobic bacteria. *Haemophilus* is resistant to penicillin, but may respond to broader spectrum penicillins (e.g., ampicillin). Gonococcal infections are typically treated with a third-generation cephalosporin (e.g., ceftriaxone), azithromycin or a broad-spectrum fluoroquinolone; the organism has a variable response to treatment with trimethoprim-sulfamethoxazole.

469. The answer is C. *(Medicine—Gastroenterology)*

Hemangiomas are very common, benign vascular tumors that generally are left alone unless they cause symptoms (pain, bleeding). Hepatocellular carcinoma, previously called a *hepatoma*, is the most common primary malignant tumor of the liver. Hepatoblastoma is the most common primary malignant tumor in the pediatric age group.

470. The answer is D. *(Gynecology)*

Oral contraceptive pills increase the risk of benign hepatic adenomas. The other common benign tumor in the differential diagnosis with this type of lesion (but not due to birth control pills) would be a hemangioma, a common lesion (rarely causes pain). Hepatic adenomas often regress when the pills are stopped. Repeating the ultrasound in a few months after stopping the pills would be a good idea, but first the pills should first be stopped.

471. The answer is C. *(Medicine—Hematology)*

The complete blood count and peripheral smear are inexpensive, valuable tools in initial assessment of an anemia and should be the first tests ordered. Often anemia is discovered on a routine complete blood count. The other initial test to order is a reticulocyte count. Armed with these three simple laboratory studies, you can narrow the diagnosis down to two or three possibilities and order any more specific tests you may need. The other choices are premature at this point, and you need more information before trying to ascertain a diagnosis (e.g., if the mean corpuscular volume was significantly elevated, you wouldn't want iron studies or examination of the gastrointestinal tract).

472. The answer is B. *(Medicine—Nephrology)*

Uremic pericarditis may cause a friction rub on physical examination. Patients with renal failure tend to have hyperkalemia, acidosis, and an increased risk of bleeding because of platelet malfunction. The immune system is likely to be suppressed, causing an increased risk of infection and no increase in the risk of autoimmune disease. Theoretically, one might even expect an improvement in autoimmune symptoms or disease resulting from immune suppression.

473. The answer is A. *(Medicine—Endocrinology)*

Hashimoto's thyroiditis is the most common cause of hypothyroidism in the United States, followed by iatrogenic hypothyroidism caused by treatment for Graves' disease. Subacute thyroiditis usually is due to a viral infection and causes a tender thyroid gland. Euthyroid sick syndrome describes thyroid laboratory abnormalities in the absence of true hypothyroidism and would not produce such striking symptoms of hypothyroidism. Thyroxine ingestion would cause symptoms of hyperthyroidism.

474. The answer is B. *(Medicine—Gastroenterology)*

The liver stores glycogen and is the main center for gluconeogenesis. Because of this, one would expect hypoglycemia with severe liver failure. The liver clears activated clotting factors so that disseminated intravascular coagulation may be seen with severe liver damage. Hypoalbuminemia, jaundice, and encephalopathy are classic findings of severe liver dysfunction.

475. The answer is A. *(Medicine—Infectious Disease)*

In the acute setting, all forms of viral hepatitis can present similarly and can be distinguished only by serology, although the history may suggest more likely causes. Hepatitis A, similar to all forms of hepatitis, can rarely can lead to fulminant hepatic failure and death. Chronic infection is not seen with hepatitis A, and it does not generally lead to cirrhosis. It is obtained through the fecal-oral route, with food-borne outbreaks being common.

476. The answer is E. *(Medicine—Pulmonology)*

The FEV_1 is the maximum volume that can be exhaled in 1 second—usually the first second of expiratory effort. This value can be compared with the total FEV, or the total volume of air that can be exhaled after taking in a deep breath. By definition, obstructive disease has a decreased FEV_1 to FEV ratio, whereas the ratio is often close to normal or slightly increased with restrictive disease. The FEV_1 may be the same in these conditions, but the ratio is different. Prognosis and exercise tolerance depend on the underlying cause and the severity of the disease. Obstructive disease, the pattern seen with smoking, is more common than restrictive disease.

477. The answer is B. *(Pediatrics—Cardiology)*

This child has the murmur of a patent ductus arteriosus, which can result in dyspnea and congestive heart failure. Indomethacin is used first in an attempt to induce closure of the ductus when it results in significant hemodynamic consequences (otherwise it is left alone to close on its own). If that fails, surgical correction usually is indicated.

478. The answer is D. *(Medicine—Cardiology)*

This is a classic description of a secundum atrial septal defect, which often causes no problems until adulthood. Patients may complain of palpitations resulting from sinus or atrial arrhythmias that commonly develop. A fixed, split S_2 heart sound is the most important buzz phrase for an atrial septal defect. Surgical treatment is advised in larger and/or symptomatic lesions to avoid severe right-to-left shunt and/or pulmonary hypertension.

479. The answer is C. *(Dermatology)*

The picture shows herpes zoster in a typical dermatomal pattern (in this case, the V1 distribution of the trigeminal nerve). This condition occurs as a result of reactivation of the varicella-zoster virus, which usually is acquired during childhood (not from sexual contract, which is the primary mode of spread of herpes simplex type II) and causes chickenpox. If you see zoster in a young person, consider the possibility of immune deficiency (e.g., HIV), although not always present. It will be interesting to see what happens to the incidence of zoster now that the chickenpox vaccine is in widespread use. Antiherpes agents (e.g., valacyclovir) can reduce the duration and severity of symptoms.

480. The answer is A. *(Orthopedic Surgery)*

The three classic pediatric hip disorders all can cause osteoarthritis when the patient reaches adulthood. They can be differentiated by age of onset, epidemiology, and radiographic findings.

Name	Age	Epidemiology	Symptoms/Signs	Treatment
Congenital hip dysplasia	At birth	Female, first-borns, breech delivery	Barlow's and Ortolani's signs	Harness
Legg-Calvé-Perthes disease	4–10 yr	Short male with delayed bone age	Knee, thigh, groin pain, limp	Orthoses
Slipped capital femoral epiphysis	9–13 yr	Overweight male adolescent	Knee, thigh, groin pain, limp	Surgical pinning

Osgood-Schlatter disease tends to affect boys 10 to 15 years of age. In this condition, which is essentially osteochondritis of the tibial tubercle, the knee (tibial tubercle) is tender to palpation, which does not occur with the above pediatric hip disorders. Septic arthritis would be likely to cause a fever and elevated white blood cell count. If avascular necrosis occurs in a black child, consider sickle cell disease.

481. The answer is B. *(Pediatrics—Neonates)*

The woman, given her history of hepatitis and current serology, has chronic hepatitis B. The infant should receive hepatitis B immune globulin and a first hepatitis B vaccine shot at birth to decrease the risk of contracting hepatitis. Maternal hepatitis B immune globulin is not thought to be helpful in this setting. Immunization would cause the surface antibody to be positive and all other serology to be within normal limits. Whenever the surface antigen is present, the hepatitis B infection is still active, whether acute or chronic, as this is a viral particle.

482. The answer is A. *(Pediatrics—Infectious Disease)*

Many children appear normal at birth, and only later in childhood are they noted to have a learning disability or cognitive delay or deficit. Rubella is worst when the mother becomes infected in the first trimester. *Toxoplasma* is the TORCH infection associated with maternal exposure to cats, and cytomegalovirus is probably the most common TORCH infection. TORCH infections include *T*oxoplasma, **o**ther (such as varicella-zoster and syphilis), **r**ubella, **c**ytomegalovirus and **h**erpes. They tend to cause microsomia or intrauterine growth retardation (not macrosomia), mental retardation, microcephaly, hydrocephalus, hepatosplenomegaly, jaundice, anemia, low birth weight, cataracts (especially rubella), cardiovascular defects (especially rubella), deafness (rubella and cytomegalovirus), cerebral calcifications (*Toxoplasma* and cytomegalovirus), and skin lesions (especially herpes).

483. The answer is D. *(Gynecology)*

This is a classic description of a fibroadenoma, the most common tumor of the breast. Breast cancer is extremely unlikely in this age group. Fibrocystic disease tends to be bilateral, is often painful or tender, and is cystic and less well circumscribed. A breast abscess usually causes a hot, fluctuant, erythematous breast and normally is seen in the setting of breast-feeding. Women with fat necrosis of the breast, which is uncommon, often have a history of trauma and usually have a less well-circumscribed and harder mass (can mimic cancer without appropriate history) owing to calcification.

484. The answer is A. *(Psychiatry—Addiction Psychiatry)*

This patient is most likely abusing phencyclidine (PCP). The giveaway is horizontal and vertical nystagmus, or rotary nystagmus, in the presence of schizophrenia-like symptoms. The patient may need short-term antipsychotics or sedatives (or both), but once the drug wears off, these most likely will not be needed. Acidification of the urine and gastric lavage can help eliminate PCP and can be useful adjuncts in PCP overdose, which may be fatal (coma, convulsions, respiratory arrest). A withdrawal syndrome has not been recognized with PCP. Most users take the drug as a pill or smoke it.

485. The answer is C. *(General Knowledge and Principles)*

An organic cause is most likely to be found in severe or profound mental retardation, which comprises a minority of cases. Approximately 85% of cases of mental retardation are mild, and these patients normally can achieve a reasonable level of independence, with assistance or guidance during times of stress. Fetal alcohol syndrome is the number one known preventable cause of mental retardation; the contribution of neglect to ultimate intelligence as measured by currently available tests is much harder to quantify (although the contribution may be significant). The most common known cause of mental retardation in both sexes is either Down syndrome or fetal alcohol syndrome. Down syndrome is much easier to diagnose definitively, so it is usually listed as the number one cause. Fragile X syndrome is the second or third most common cause of mental retardation in males.

486. The answer is D. *(Psychiatry—General)*

Serotonin-specific reuptake inhibitors (particularly fluvoxamine) are first-line agents in obsessive-compulsive disorder, which this patient most likely has. This disorder is not to be confused with obsessive-compulsive personality disorder, which describes an anal-retentive, stubborn personality. Obsessive-compulsive disorder is characterized by recurrent thoughts (obsessions) or actions (compulsions) that interfere with functioning. The most common activities include washing or checking rituals (e.g., a person checks to see if the door is locked 30 times a day), and fear of dirt or bacteria is common. Behavioral therapy, such as flooding or systematic desensitization, may be effective in some patients and is probably similar in efficacy to drug therapy. This patient can be managed as an outpatient.

487. The answer is D. *(Medicine—Infectious Disease)*

Klebsiella is a classic cause of pneumonia in homeless alcoholics and often causes *currant jelly* sputum. Bacterial colonies appear as described in the question.

488. The answer is A. *(Medicine—Gastroenterology)*

Patients with hemochromatosis have a markedly increased incidence of hepatocellular carcinoma that can be significantly reduced by catching the disease early and instituting therapy (phlebotomy). Patients exposed to vinyl chloride have an increased risk of angiosarcoma. Hepatitis A does not result in chronic infection, although it rarely may cause fulminant hepatic failure. Down syndrome is associated with a markedly increased risk of leukemia. Cystic fibrosis patients die at an early age (survival only into the twenties and thirties is typical) and are not particularly prone to develop hepatocellular carcinoma.

489. The answer is C. *(Medicine—Oncology)*

Nasopharyngeal carcinoma, seen most commonly in Asians, and Burkitt's lymphoma in Africa have been linked to Epstein-Barr virus, and Epstein-Barr virus also plays a role in other lymphoproliferative malignancies.

490. The answer is C. *(Medicine—Pulmonology)*

Alpha$_1$-antitrypsin deficiency can present in the neonatal period but often does not present until early adulthood. Emphysema is usually caused by smoking, and antitrypsin deficiency is quite rare. This deficiency also results in liver disease and possibly cirrhosis in many affected individuals and is probably the reason for the elevated liver enzymes. The given smoking history is not enough to cause emphysema at such a young age. The other choices generally do not cause emphysema.

491. The answer is D. *(Pediatrics—Cardiology)*

Tetralogy of Fallot is the most common congenital cyanotic heart defect after the neonatal period; as a whole, cyanotic heart defects are less common than noncyanotic heart defects. Cyanotic defects cause a right-to-left circulatory shunt (i.e., blood goes from the right side of the heart to the left side of the heart without going through the lungs), whereas noncyanotic lesions have a left-to-right shunt or no shunt. Patent ductus arteriosus causes a left-to-right shunt and is a noncyanotic defect. The five "Ts" describe the cyanotic heart diseases: **t**etralogy of Fallot, **t**ransposition of the great arteries, **t**ricuspid atresia, **t**runcus arteriosus, and **t**otal anomalous pulmonary venous return.

492. The answer is E. *(Surgery—Trauma)*

The ABCDEs are the key to initial management of trauma patients when you first see them. Always do them in order (e.g., if the person is bleeding to death and has a blocked airway, and you have to choose which issue to address first, the answer is airway management).

Airway reminds you to provide, protect, and maintain an adequate airway at all times. If the patient can answer questions, the airway is fine. You can use an oropharyngeal airway in uncomplicated cases and give supplemental oxygen. When in doubt or the patient's airway is blocked, intubate. If intubation fails, do a cricothyroidotomy.

Breathing is similar to airway, but even when the patient's airway is patent, he or she may not be breathing spontaneously. The end result is the same—when in doubt or the patient is not breathing, intubate. If intubation fails, do a cricothyroidotomy.

Circulation basically means that if the patient seems hypovolemic (tachycardic, bleeding, weak pulse, pale, diaphoretic, capillary refill > 2 seconds), give intravenous fluids, blood products, or both. The initial procedure is to start 2 large-bore intravenous catheters and give a bolus of 10 to 20 mL/kg (roughly 1 L) of lactated Ringer's solution (the intravenous fluid of choice in trauma). Then reassess the patient after bolus for improvement. Rebolus if needed.

Disability reminds you to check neurologic function (i.e., perform the Glasgow Coma Scale).

Exposure reminds you to strip the person naked and "put a finger in every orifice" so that you do not miss any occult injuries.

493. The answer is B. *(Neurosurgery)*

Although ruptured berry aneurysms (classically caused by polycystic kidney disease) are classically described, trauma is another frequent cause of subarachnoid hemorrhage (trauma is probably more common overall). The other choices are possible but less likely.

494. The answer is B. *(Obstetrics)*

Postpartum hemorrhage is defined as an estimated blood loss greater than 500 mL during a vaginal delivery (> 1000 mL during a cesarean section). The most common cause is uterine atony, responsible for roughly 75% to 80% of cases. Hemorrhage may also be caused by lacerations, retained placental tissue (placenta accreta, increta, percreta), coagulation disorders (e.g., disseminated intravascular coagulation, von Willebrand's disease), low placental implantation, and uterine inversion.

495. The answer is C. *(Obstetrics)*

The Betke-Kleihauer test is used to check for the presence of and quantify the amount of fetal blood in a maternal blood sample with suspected fetomaternal hemorrhage, sometimes used when trying to decide how much RhoGAM to give an Rh-negative mother. The others are all evidence of rupture of the amniotic sac. The nitrazine test involves placing a drop of the fluid from a speculum examination onto a piece of nitrazine paper, which turns blue in the presence of amniotic fluid.

496–500. *(Medicine—Nutrition)*

The answers are the following: 496. A, G, H, I   497. G, K   498. M   499. D   500. B.

Fat-soluble vitamin supplements may be needed in cystic fibrosis and other conditions because of fat malabsorption. Osteoporosis is common in postmenopausal women, especially thin white or Asian women who smoke. Calcium and vitamin D supplements can help reduce the risk. Folate can help reduce the risk of neural tube defects in offspring and should be considered in childbearing-age women who are sexually active. Three glasses of milk per day would give this patient adequate calcium. Isoniazid can cause pyridoxine (vitamin B_6) deficiency and supplements should be considered, especially in younger patients on prolonged therapy. Confusion and ataxia in alcoholics should make you consider Wernicke's encephalopathy, which is due to thiamine (vitamin B_1) deficiency.

ANSWERS AND EXPLANATIONS

501. The answer is C. *(Radiology)*

The description of the calculi is consistent with bilateral large staghorn calculi, which are often described as forming a "cast" of the renal collecting system (i.e., calices, infundibuli and pelvis), much like what would be seen when IV contrast is given for an intravenous pyelogram. Staghorn calculi are associated with recurrent urinary tract infections with urease-producing bacteria, such as *Proteus* and *Pseudomonas*, and would not be expected from hypercalcemia or hyperuricemia. The stones usually are of struvite (i.e., magnesium-ammonium-phosphate) composition in this setting. Stones of the size described (and staghorn calculi in general) are not going to pass spontaneously, and the patient will need surgical intervention to remove these stones.

502. The answer is B. *(Vascular Surgery)*

This lesion has a typical appearance and location (usually over or adjacent to the lateral or medial malleolus) of a venous stasis/insufficiency ulcer. The increased skin pigmentation around the ulcer and lack of pain are important signs of venous insufficiency, though some lesions are painful. Arterial insufficiency ulcers tend to occur on the underside of the distal foot (in the area of the metatarsal heads) or toes and are exquisitely painful. Neuropathic ulcers also occur on the underside of the foot at pressure points (e.g., metatarsal heads, heels) but are painless and associated with peripheral neuropathy. Embolic phenomenon would not be expected to cause the appearance of the lesion, rather causing sudden pain (almost always present acutely) and an area of swelling without pigmentary skin changes. Fungal infections do not tend to progress beyond the skin surface and would be more common between the toes (i.e. athlete's foot) or around the nails (i.e., onychomycosis). Treatment for venous stasis ulcers is conservative, with compression stockings, wet-to-dry dressings, and leg elevation. Superimposed bacterial cellulitis is not uncommon, tends to cause symptoms, and requires antibiotic treatment.

503. The answer is A. *(Dermatology)*

The appearance of this lesion and the clinical history are highly suspicious for malignant melanoma. Any mole that develops the **ABCD** changes (**a**symmetry, irregular **b**orders, **c**olor variation, and large **d**iameter) or begins to itch, bleed, or hurt should be looked on with suspicion. Excisional biopsy is advised and may be curative if metastases have not already occurred. The lesion is an acral lentiginous melanoma, the rarest melanoma subtype, which usually occurs in dark-skinned individuals on the soles or palms or sometimes under the fingernails.

504. The answer is D. *(Pharmacology)*

Beta blockers block the beta$_2$ receptors in the lungs, which stimulate bronchodilation. Beta blockers may precipitate acute asthma exacerbation in these patients.

505. The answer is B. *(Medicine—Pulmonology)*

This patient has findings of emphysema, which almost always is due to smoking. The classic *barrel chest* is described, and pursed-lip breathing is classic for emphysema. Hyperinflation of the lungs with bullous changes often is present on radiographs. Alpha-one antitrypsin deficiency and cystic fibrosis can also cause obstructive lung physiology, but are much less common. Additionally, it would be exceptionally rare for a patient with cystic fibrosis to live to the age of 56.

506. The answer is D. *(Medicine—Cardiology)*

Coarctation of the aorta is associated with Turner's syndrome and is associated with a radiofemoral delay when checking the peripheral pulses and rib notching on chest radiograph. A systolic murmur sometimes may be heard over the back as the blood flows through the stenotic portion of the aorta.

507. The answer is D. *(Medicine—Cardiology)*

Beta blockers and centrally acting calcium channel blockers (e.g., verapamil) would be expected to worsen bradycardia and should be avoided in this setting. Lidocaine is not generally effective for bradycardia, but is useful for ventricular tachycardias. Procainamide sometimes is used in the setting of certain atrial tachycardias, such as atrial fibrillation. Amiodarone is useful for a various atrial and ventricular arrhythmias, but not sinus bradycardia. Atropine, by blocking vagal tone to the heart, often increases the heart rate.

508. The answer is A. *(Medicine—Endocrinology)*

This patient has classic findings of hyperthyroidism, usually resulting from Graves' disease, a type II or antibody-mediated hypersensitivity reaction. Because the gland is overfunctioning (due to antibody-mediated stimulation), thyroid-stimulating hormone (TSH) is suppressed and should be low. In secondary hyperthyroidism (choice **B**), the TSH is high, typically due to a TSH-secreting pituitary adenoma, which is quite rare and much less common than Graves' disease. Patients tend to have weight loss in the setting of hyperthyroidism, whereas weight gain can be seen in hypothyroidism. Panic attacks should not cause atrial fibrillation but do cause severe anxiety.

509. The answer is B. *(Medicine—Gastroenterology)*

A positive antibody to hepatitis C does not mean that the patient has cleared the infection. Chronic infections are thought to be quite frequent with hepatitis C, and a polymerase chain reaction for viral RNA should eventually be done in an attempt to detect the virus. The patient has been exposed to hepatitis B but most likely has cleared the infection (because the surface antigen is negative) and is immune. The core antibody does not become positive with vaccination. Laboratory error resulting from dehydration would not cause such a significant elevation in hepatic transaminases. Alcoholic hepatitis characteristically causes an elevation of AST that is at least twice the value of the ALT.

510. The answer is D. *(Medicine—Gastroenterology)*

The classic differentiating features are presented in the table below. Although there may be overlap of these features in individual cases, these are unlikely to be asked about on USMLE exams.

	Crohn Disease	Ulcerative Colitis
Place it starts	Distal ileum, proximal colon	Rectum
Thickness of pathology	Transmural	Mucosa/submucosa only
Progression	Irregular (skip lesions)	Proximal, continuous from rectum; no skipped areas
Location	From mouth to anus	Involves colon only, rarely extends to ileum
Bowel habits change to	Obstruction, abdominal pain	Bloody diarrhea
Classic lesions	Fistulas/abscesses, cobblestoning, string sign on barium radiograph	Pseudopolyps, lead-pipe colon on barium radiographs, toxic megacolon
Colon cancer risk	Slightly increased	Markedly increased
Surgery cures bowel disease?	No (may make worse)	Yes (proctocolectomy with ileoanal anastomosis)

511. The answer is E. *(Medicine—Hematology)*

This woman has beta thalassemia minor and requires no treatment. She should not be given iron because this may cause iron overload with its resultant consequences. Affected individuals usually are asymptomatic because they have lived at a lower level of hemoglobin for their entire lives. The hallmark of β-thalassemia is elevated hemoglobin A_2 and sometimes fetal hemoglobin (hemoglobin F). Especially in a person of Mediterranean descent, no further workup is required, and a presumptive diagnosis can be made. β-thalassemia symptoms start at 6 months of life, whereas α-thalassemia symptoms start in utero or at birth.

512. The answer is C. *(Medicine—General)*

The patient most likely has a vitamin B_{12} deficiency as the cause for her neurologic symptoms. The Schilling test is used to determine the cause of a vitamin B_{12} deficiency, which most commonly is pernicious anemia but also can be bacterial overgrowth or other intestinal malabsorption syndromes. Folate deficiency can also cause megaloblastic anemia but does not cause neurologic symptoms.

513. The answer is C. *(Medicine—Nephrology)*

Proteinuria may be seen in nephritic syndromes, but it is usually not in the nephrotic range (i.e., usually < 3.5 gm/day). The others commonly are seen in the nephritic syndrome.

514. The answer is A. *(Medicine—Nephrology)*

Hyperlipidemia and lipiduria are two of the classic signs of a nephrotic syndrome, which by definition includes proteinuria of more than 3.5 gm/day. Patients also may have edema and hypoalbuminemia but do not often develop complete renal failure initially; azotemia, uremia and hypertension would be unusual. Red blood cell casts usually point to a glomerulonephritis or nephritic syndrome.

515. The answer is B. *(Obstetrics)*

Epidural anesthesia is safe and effective and is preferred in most obstetric settings if the patient is comfortable with it. If the woman started out as an attempt at vaginal delivery and ends up requiring a cesarean section, the epidural can continue to be used for this procedure without undue delay. General anesthesia introduces not only the general maternal and fetal risks associated with it, but also an increased risk of aspiration and pneumonia secondary to relaxation of the lower esophageal sphincter in pregnant women and the fact that many women have not avoided oral intake in the 8 hours before going into active labor. Spinal anesthesia carries a higher risk of hypotension and uterine muscle relaxation. Caudal anesthesia has technical difficulties associated with it and requires higher doses of local anesthetic than other techniques, which increases the risk of systemic toxicity. Paracervical block provides only relief from the pain associated with uterine contraction and the early stages of labor, not pain in the vaginal canal and perineum.

516. The answer is B. *(Obstetrics)*

Visualization of the uterus at the introitus indicates likely uterine inversion, which may occur when overaggressive pulling on the cord is used in an attempt to hasten the process of placental separation. The other four choices are the classic signs of placental separation.

517. The answer is C. *(Obstetrics)*

Tetracyclines should not be used during pregnancy, although they are an appropriate first-line agent in nonpregnant women (doxycycline typically used). Erythromycin (or azithromycin) can be used safely during pregnancy and is effective against *Chlamydia*. Cotreatment for *Chlamydia* often is done when gonorrhea is present, but the reverse is not true because gonorrhea infections tend to be more noticeable. False-positive culture results are not more likely in pregnancy, and treatment should be instituted promptly because of possible complications with the pregnancy and fetus, including prematurity, premature rupture of the membranes, endometritis, and passage of *Chlamydia* to the fetus at the time of delivery.

518. The answer is A. *(Gynecology)*

This woman has fibrocystic disease of the breast, which is estimated to affect as many as half of all premenopausal women. The lesions characteristically become more tender in the premenstrual phase and usually are bilateral. A classic description is "*lumpy-bumpy*" breasts. In a woman of this age with the given case description, no further workup is required, although follow-up is a good idea. If symptoms persist or a dominant lesion is palpable, ultrasound (not MRI, which is not a first-line diagnostic test for breast disease at this time) of the breast could be obtained. Nonsteroidal anti-inflammatory drugs, progesterone, birth control pills, and danazol all may be effective in relieving symptoms if needed. If fibrocystic disease is suspected in a woman older than 35 (or possibly younger if she has multiple strong breast cancer risk factors), further workup and baseline mammography often are recommended because the incidence of malignancy is increased in these patients.

519. The answer is C. *(Psychiatry—General)*

Dopamine inhibits prolactin secretion in the hypothalamus. Giving an antipsychotic, which works partially through dopamine blockade, may increase prolactin secretion and result in decreased libido, nonbloody nipple discharge (usually bilateral), amenorrhea and decreased libido. Although a delusion is possible in a schizophrenic, most would not have the ability to describe their symptoms so exactly, and the patient is described as coherent and appropriate, suggesting control of positive symptoms. Malingering is rare in schizophrenics because they lack the capacity to muster the necessary acting skills. Breast cancer would be exceedingly rare as a cause of a bilateral, clear nipple discharge in a patient this age. Polycystic ovary syndrome is a common cause for hypo- or amenorrhea, but tends to occur in overweight women and does not normally cause nipple discharge or decreased libido.

520. The answer is C. *(Medicine—Infectious Disease)*

In the absence of other risk factors, a man with hypertension would not be expected to develop a gram-negative pneumonia. Cystic fibrosis patients commonly develop *Pseudomonas* pneumonia; alcoholics and others with a risk of aspiration commonly develop gram-negative pneumonias with enteric organisms; and hospitalized patients develop nosocomial pneumonias, which are commonly gram-negative.

521. The answer is E. *(Preventive Medicine)*

The pneumococcal vaccine is now universally recommended for newborns, as well as all adults older than age 65. Other indications include all patients with splenectomy or functional asplenia (e.g., sickle cell disease), patients with immunodeficiency, and patients with chronic diseases such as diabetes and renal disease that place them at higher risk for contracting pneumococcal pneumonia.

522. The answer is C. *(Urology)*

A history of cryptorchidism is the most potent known risk factor for testicular cancer, increasing the risk by up to 50 times above that of the general population. Surgical correction of cryptorchidism does not lower the incidence of (or only mildly decreases the risk of) cancer but is done in an attempt to preserve fertility and facilitate testicular examinations. Although prior chemotherapy and family history can increase the risk of neoplasm, the other two choices are not associated with an increased risk of cancer of any kind.

523. The answer is C. *(Medicine—Gastroenterology)*

Chronic alcohol abuse and tobacco abuse are the primary modifiable risk factors for squamous cell esophageal cancer, and a history of one or both can be found in 85% of affected patients. This type of weight loss should always make you think about a possible malignancy in an adult, and food sticking in the throat or chest is the classic esophageal carcinoma complaint. Most esophageal cancers are adenocarcinomas, but these are related primarily to chronic gastroesophageal reflux, esophagitis and subsequent development of metaplasia (Barrett esophagus), not alcohol and tobacco abuse.

524. The answer is D. *(Pediatrics—Oncology)*

The posterior fossa includes the cerebellum, medulla oblongata, and pons. The two most common primary brain tumors in children are cerebellar astrocytomas and medulloblastomas, which both commonly arise from the posterior fossa. The third most common neoplasm is probably ependymoma, which tends to arise from the fourth ventricle. Because of this, children with brain tumors primarily present with cerebellar signs and signs of increased intracranial pressure. MRI is far superior to CT in imaging the posterior fossa because of artifacts in this area with CT scanning. It is often said that two thirds of adult primary brain tumors are supratentorial, whereas two thirds of childhood primary brain tumors are infratentorial. The other choices are much less common sites of tumors in children but do occur.

525. The answer is D. *(Medicine—Neurology)*

The hallmark of demyelinating disorders and peripheral neuropathies is that they slow nerve conduction velocity. The amplitude of muscle contraction decreases with repetitive stimulation in myasthenia gravis but increases with repetitive stimulation with the paraneoplastic Eaton-Lambert syndrome. Lower motor neuron lesions produce increased fasciculations and fibrillations at rest. Intrinsic muscle disease gives decreased muscle contraction amplitude. There is normally little electric activity at rest in a normal muscle other than occasional random discharges.

526. The answer is B. *(Medicine—Neurology)*

This patient most likely has Guillain-Barré syndrome, which normally starts roughly 1 week after mild (commonly upper respiratory) infection or immunization. Ascending paralysis with usually intact sensation and decreased reflexes in the affected areas is due to a peripheral neuropathy (which would cause the nerve conduction velocity to be slowed). Corticosteroids generally are not effective and occasionally worsen symptoms. Plasmapheresis may shorten the severity or duration of symptoms, but treatment is otherwise supportive. Head CT scan or MRI is normal because this is a condition affecting the peripheral nervous system. Lumbar puncture usually reveals mildly elevated protein but not an increased opening pressure.

527. The answer is A. *(Dermatology)*

This question describes pityriasis rosea. It usually starts out with the classic "herald" patch 1 week before the generalized eruption that tends to affect the trunk. The scaly, erythematous patches are classically in a *Christmas tree* pattern on the back, following the skin lines of Langerhans. The lesions usually remit spontaneously in about 1 month, and supportive treatment (e.g., antihistamine for itching) is all that usually is required.

528. The answer is E. *(Biostatistics)*

Incidence is defined as the number of new cases of a disease in the population of interest over a given length of time. The length of time is often 1 year, but any time frame can be used. In this case, no information is given about when the people with *Chlamydia* acquired their infection, so the incidence cannot be calculated. The prevalence can be calculated, however, and would be 50 in 1000.

529. The answer is E. *(Biostatistics)*

This is a retrospective study (case-control), and a relative risk cannot be calculated. Relative risk can be calculated only when a prospective study is done. For a retrospective study, an odds ratio can be used to estimate relative risk. The formula for relative risk, if this was a prospective study, is the following:

[(number of cases of disease in people exposed) / (total number of people exposed)] /
[(number of cases of disease in people not exposed) / (total number of people not exposed)]

530. The answer is E. *(Psychiatry—Addiction Psychiatry)*

Inhalant abuse (e.g., gasoline, glue, varnish remover) classically causes euphoria, dizziness, ataxia, slurred speech, and a heightened sense of power. The effects often wear off in a matter of minutes to an hour. Abuse of this agent is most common in the 11- to 15-year-old age group and can be fatal in overdose and cause severe permanent sequelae (central and peripheral nervous system, liver, and kidney toxicity). There is no recognized withdrawal syndrome, which is seen commonly with cocaine and heroin, substances rarely abused at this age. LSD usually lasts 6 to 18 hours, so is unlikely in the scenario described. Marijuana does not cause slurred speech and does not usually cause a heightened sense of power or loss of balance, although it may cause euphoria and should be considered as a possibility because of its frequency of use and widespread availability.

531. The answer is E. *(Psychiatry—General)*

There is a wide range of individual behavior, and you must be careful on the boards not to label every variant as pathologic. Transsexuals believe that they are the opposite sex and usually desire a sex change operation. Transvestites engage in cross-dressing (not just the underwear) so that they look like the opposite sex or have recurrent fantasies about cross-dressing. Fetishism is arousal from nonliving objects that become more important than the person with whom the individuals are supposed to be having sex. All three of these disorders, similar to most psychiatric diagnoses, require coexisting distress or occupational, social, or other functioning impairment, which this man lacks. There is no indication of homosexuality, or being sexually attracted to the same sex, and this is not a diagnosis any more than heterosexuality is a diagnosis. Homosexuality and occasionally kinky thoughts, activities, or fetishes are considered within the normal limits of sexual behavior.

532. The answer is B. *(General Knowledge and Principles)*

For the boards (where the chronic lack of time available to spend with patients is not an issue), it is preferable to ask open-ended questions. Especially at the beginning of the interview, this allows patients the chance to explain fully what they are experiencing. The other questions may be asked later on, after the woman has had adequate opportunity to express her symptoms.

533. The answer is D. *(Obstetrics)*

LSD and marijuana have not been well-established as teratogens. The others are all highly teratogenic. Alcohol is the number one cause of preventable mental retardation in the United States, and the fetal alcohol syndrome includes a well-characterized list of fetal malformations. Cocaine can cause gastrointestinal, genitourinary, and limb defects in the fetus. Almost all antiepileptic agents are teratogenic, and trimethadione is one of the worst offenders. Isotretinoin, a vitamin A derivative used to treat acne, is highly teratogenic.

534. The answer is E. *(Obstetrics)*

Group B streptococcus is a gram-positive cocci that is part of the normal vaginal flora in a significant minority of women, and its presence does not indicate an infection. Women with this organism are treated during labor, however, to reduce the incidence of neonatal sepsis (from vertical transmission of the organism) and endometritis. Amoxicillin or a similar penicillin agent is the treatment of choice to eliminate this organism.

535. The answer is D. *(Obstetrics)*

Other sexually transmitted diseases are common in HIV-infected women, and screening is indicated, even in the absence of symptoms, to reduce complications of the pregnancy via treatment of any infections present. HIV transmission occurs in approximately 25% of cases in the absence of treatment, and this can be reduced to approximately 8% by administering antiretroviral therapy to the mother during pregnancy and to the infant for the first 6 weeks after delivery. Breast-feeding should not be done by HIV-positive mothers because transmission of HIV to the baby can occur. A false-positive HIV enzyme-linked immunosorbent assay (i.e. ELISA) test may occur in the neonate because of transplacental passage of maternal antibodies. These antibodies generally disappear by 6 to 8 months after delivery.

536. The answer is C. *(Gynecology)*

This woman is most likely going through menopause, and her irregular periods are considered physiologic. Major depression does not have mood swings (patients are always depressed) or hot flashes. Cancer also should not cause moods swings or hot flashes, although abnormal uterine bleeding should always make you consider the possibility in a woman of this age. An elevated follicle-stimulating hormone level tentatively confirms the diagnosis of menopause.

537. The answer is A. *(Gynecology)*

The first step in evaluating a complaint of amenorrhea, whether primary or secondary, is to order a pregnancy test. beta human chorionic gonadotropin is a quick, easy way to determine pregnancy and can be done on urine (cheaper, less sensitive) or serum. The other choices are used later in the amenorrhea algorithm, after pregnancy has been ruled out.

538. The answer is A. *(Ophthalmology)*

Choice A describes panretinal photocoagulation, a treatment that often causes regression of the retinal neovascularization (the hallmark of proliferative retinopathy) and helps to prevent other new vessels from forming. This treatment is thought to work by destroying the portions of the retina that are releasing the intercellular signals (owing to ischemia) thought to be responsible for the formation of new retinal vessels. Focal laser photocoagulation, described in choice **B**, is used for nonproliferative diabetic retinopathy (background retinopathy, including dot-blot hemorrhages, microaneurysms, exudates, and edema) when it affects the macula (area of highest visual acuity) to preserve as much vision as possible. The other choices have not been shown to be effective in treating proliferative retinopathy, although vitrectomy (removal of the vitreous jelly and replacement with an artificial solution) may be an adjunctive treatment for vision-reducing hemorrhage into the vitreous resulting from neovascularization. Vitrectomy does not treat the neovascularization itself, however.

539. The answer is A. *(Ophthalmology)*

Glaucoma is more common in blacks than whites and is the number one cause of acquired blindness in black adults. Annual screening for glaucoma (by tonometric measurement of intraocular pressure) is recommended in all adults older than age 40, especially if the person is black, is diabetic, or has a family history. Glaucoma is the number three overall cause of blindness in the United States. Diabetes is a common cause of acquired vision loss, but is most often due to type II diabetes. Diabetes is probably the number one cause of acquired blindness in whites younger than age 55, and macular degeneration is the probably most common cause of acquired blindness in whites older than age 55. Both wet (exudative, 10% of cases) and dry (nonexudative, 90% of cases) types of macular degeneration can cause blindness. Trauma is unlikely to make someone legally blind, because it most commonly causes unilateral vision loss.

540. The answer is B. *(Surgery—Trauma)*

A simple pneumothorax usually can be compensated for by the other lung. A tension pneumothorax or open pneumothorax can be rapidly fatal, however, and is much more concerning because of the effect on both lungs and possibly the heart. A simple pneumothorax is much more common and is implied when no descriptive adjective is used (as in the question). The other choices are all rapidly fatal, and immediate heroic measures usually are typically required if the patient is to survive.

541. The answer is D. *(Surgery—Trauma)*

With blunt abdominal trauma, stable patients with benign abdominal examination may be observed with serial abdominal examinations. If patients are unstable, they should go immediately to laparotomy. If patients are stable with abdominal pain/tenderness or have an unreliable abdominal examination because of altered mental status or blood loss elsewhere, abdominal and pelvic CT scan *with contrast* should be performed to determine the need for laparotomy. With penetrating gunshot wounds to the abdomen, many surgeons proceed directly to laparotomy. With stab wounds or other penetrating abdominal trauma besides gunshots, laparotomy or CT scan of the abdomen and pelvis *with contrast* are used, depending on whether or not the patient is stable (unstable patients go directly to laparotomy). Abdominal angiography is not performed normally in the setting of acute abdominal trauma, unless vascular injury or active bleeding are supected (embolization of the bleeding vessels may then be performed).

542. The answer is A. *(Pediatrics—Gastroenterology)*

An omphalocele is in the midline, the umbilical ring is absent, and other physical anomalies are common. Affected fetuses may have herniation of bowel and/or liver into the defect. Aneuploidy, or an abnormal number of chromosomes, is present in up to 1/3 of fetuses with an omphalocele (e.g., trisomy 13, 18, 21; Turner syndrome). Gastroschisis is to the right of the midline, typically only bowel is exposed (there is no true hernia sac), the umbilical ring is present, and other anomalies and aneuploidy are rare.

543. The answer is A. *(Pediatrics—General)*

This newborn most likely has a congenital diaphragmatic hernia, which is due to Bochdalek-type hernias in roughly 90% of cases. These almost always occur on the left side (posterolateral location) and result in bowel herniation into the left hemithorax. The main complication of this condition is pulmonary hypoplasia that develops on the side of the lesion and sometimes both sides because of bowel compressing the developing lungs. Preferred treatment is surgical correction of the defect because the defect will not resolve on its own. Prognosis is most closely related to pulmonary function.

Morgagni hernias are the other commonly encountered congenital diaphragmatic hernia (roughly 10% of cases) and are more common on the right side (anteromedial location). Omentum, bowel and/or liver may herniate through the defect and result in a right cardiophrenic angle mass on x-ray. Many cases are asymptomatic as the defect is often too small to significantly affect pulmonary function. The other two hernia choices are hernias through the esophageal hiatus of the diaphragm and are typically seen in adults. Sliding-type hernias (gastroesophageal junction slides above the diaphragm) are associated with gastroesophageal reflux, but otherwise have little significance. Paraesophageal hernias (gastroesophageal junction stays below the diaphragm) are at fairly high risk for entrapment and strangulation of the herniated stomach and are typically repaired surgically when found.

544. The answer is A. *(Pediatrics—Gastroenterology)*

The other conditions generally present in the first month of life. Bilious vomiting, currant-jelly stools, and a palpable sausage-shaped mass in the abdomen are classic for intussusception, which usually occurs between 4 months and 2 years of age. An air or barium enema often reduces the deficit and prevents the need for surgery.

545. The answer is C. *(Orthopedic Surgery)*

This is the classic history for a scaphoid bone (also known as the navicular bone of the hand) fracture.

546–550. *(Medicine—Nutrition)*

The answers are the following: 546. A   547. O   548. J   549. A   550. L.

Vitamin A can be teratogenic in high doses, which is the reason vitamin A analogues such as isotretinoin should not be given to women of childbearing age before a negative pregnancy test is obtained. Deficiency of this vitamin can cause night blindness as well as dry eyes and skin. *Pellagra* is the term used to describe niacin (vitamin B_3) deficiency and is associated classically with the *three Ds*—diarrhea, dementia, and dermatitis. Stomatitis also may be seen, as in other B vitamin deficiencies. Hemochromatosis is a condition caused by iron overload and is classically referred to as bronze diabetes because patients may develop skin colored bronze (or greyish), diabetes, cardiomegaly and heart failure, and cirrhosis from iron deposits into the tissues. Impotence is a common complaint in affected male patients. Hypermagnesemia can occur in pregnant women when they are given too much magnesium for tocolysis. Hyporeflexia, weakness, respiratory depression, and respiratory arrest can be seen with increasing serum magnesium levels.

BLOCK 12

ANSWERS AND EXPLANATIONS

551. The answer is C. *(Ethics)*

You must respect the patient's wishes in this circumstance. No one else should be contacted because the patient is the one who should make the decision, and she was warned before the surgery of the risks and agreed to proceed with her stipulations. Never conceal a treatment from the patient. If you give a transfusion in this case, you may be charged with a crime.

552. The answer is A. *(Pediatrics—General)*

Lead screening is generally done at 12 and 24 months for low-risk children (though somewhat controversial due to its low yield) and started at 6 months of age for high-risk children (live in old building [lead paint was still in use], eat paint chips, live near or parents work at battery recycling plant). Fluoride supplementation, vitamin D supplementation, and tuberculosis screening are reserved for high-risk children. Sickle cell disease screening generally is done at birth and would have caused problems by now if the child had it.

553. The answer is D. *(Pediatrics—General)*

Most children who are obese have no organic disease. Most take in an excessive number of calories relative to their need, which often is in part due to a sedentary lifestyle. The trend of childhood obesity is alarming. Adolescents are among the fastest growing group of persons that are at risk for developing type II diabetes. There is no reason to suspect an organic cause in this child because the examination and laboratory values are within normal limits.

554. The answer is D. *(Pediatrics—General)*

The infant has normal development for his age. Infants at this age, on average, are just becoming able to sit without support, generally have a voluntary grasp without good voluntary release of the grasp, babble incoherently, and can transfer objects from one hand to the other. At this age, infants are not expected to be able to say any words (first word around 9 to 12 months), play pat-a-cake (9 to 10 months), or understand one-step commands (15 months). Rolling front to back generally can be performed starting at 4 to 5 months, and infants usually can lift the head up 90° while prone at the age of 3 to 4 months. The mother has no reason for concern—her infant is progressing normally.

555. The answer is D. *(Orthopedic Surgery)*

Pulses usually are palpable in compartment syndrome because muscle compartment pressures rarely rise above 80 mmHg, and pressures of only 30 to 40 mmHg can cause permanent neurologic injury and muscle necrosis. Lack of pulses is a late, ominous finding. The microvascular circulation is affected by the increased compartment pressure and contributes to a vicious cycle of increasing edema and pressure in this syndrome. Pain out of proportion to the injury and with passive motion are important clues in the correct setting. Compartment syndrome commonly occurs after trauma (classic are tibial and supracondylar elbow fractures), revascularization procedures, electric burns, and arterial or venous disruption. Paralysis is a late, ominous finding, but hypoesthesia or worsened two-point discrimination and a firm or tight-feeling muscle compartment may be present relatively early. Treatment usually involves a fasciotomy to relieve the elevated pressure within the muscle compartment.

556. The answer is A. *(Ophthalmology)*

Microvascular complications of hypertension and diabetes not uncommonly cause cranial nerve palsies. When the oculomotor nerve is involved, the hallmark of microvascular disease is that it spares the pupil, whereas an aneurysm or tumor normally affects the pupil (causing it to be dilated and poorly reactive or *"blown"*). A stroke involving the oculomotor nerve usually causes other neurologic findings or complaints and often does not spare the pupil. Exotropia describes an eye that deviates outward, which would occur in an oculomotor palsy but does not explain cause (physical finding, not a diagnosis or etiology). Cranial nerve palsies caused by microvascular disease normally resolve spontaneously within 1–2 months and require no treatment. If the pupil is involved, the palsy does not resolve, other neurologic symptoms or signs are present, or the history does not fit, CT or MRI of the brain should be ordered to rule out a more serious cause.

557. The answer is C. *(Ophthalmology)*

The question is describing bitemporal hemianopia, which is caused by a lesion at the optic chiasm, classically a pituitary tumor. Bilateral optic neuritis may cause globally decreased visual acuity bilaterally but generally would not produce specific, well-demarcated visual field loss. Parietal, temporal, and occipital lobe lesions generally cause a homonymous hemianopia or quadrantanopia, not bitemporal hemianopia).

558. The answer is C. *(Surgery—Trauma)*

This patient has had a massive hemothorax (> 1 L of blood) and requires thoracotomy to identify and control the source of the bleeding. Observation and repeat chest radiographs are reserved for hemodynamically stable patients whose bleeding stops after the initial chest tube output. With continued bleeding more than 1 hour later (or sooner with brisker bleeds), the patient needs a thoracotomy. Pleurodesis and abdominal CT scan are not indicated for the hemothorax. Additional blood transfusion may be required, but this is a supportive measure to gain time until thoracotomy is performed, and the question does not mention clues that a further transfusion currently is needed. A chest CT or thoracic angiography may help better define the injury prior to exploratory surgery in stable patients.

559. The answer is B. *(Obstetrics)*

The risk of uterine atony, the most common cause of significant postpartum hemorrhage, is increased by situations that overdistend or exhaust the uterus. Examples include multiple gestation, polyhydramnios, macrosomia, prolonged labor, oxytocin usage, grandmultiparity (history of ≥ 5 deliveries), and precipitous labor (< 3 hours). Treatment often involves a dilute oxytocin infusion and bimanual compression with massage of the uterus. If this fails, second-line drugs, such as ergonovine, may be tried, but a hysterectomy may be required if medical management fails to stop the bleeding.

560. The answer is B. *(Obstetrics)*

Rh immune globulin (RhoGAM) is given only to women who are Rhesus factor (Rh) negative and the father of the infant is blood type unknown or positive. During routine prenatal care, check for Rh antibodies at the first visit. If they are positive, RhoGAM is not given because it is too late—sensitization already has occurred. If the Rh antibody titer is negative, RhoGAM can help prevent sensitization and generally should be given routinely at 28 weeks and immediately postpartum. Also give RhoGAM after an abortion, stillbirth, ectopic pregnancy, amniocentesis, chorionic villus sampling, and any other invasive procedure done during pregnancy that may cause transplacental bleeding.

561. The answer is C. *(Obstetrics)*

This is one of those straight memorize and regurgitate questions. Expulsion occurs after the five positions are completed.

562. The answer is D. *(Gynecology)*

Anorexia is common in this age group, and female teenage ballerinas are classic. Anorexic patients have a distorted body image and may feel fat or "bloated" even when markedly cachectic. Amenorrhea is required for a diagnosis of anorexia nervosa. After 6 months of pregnancy, the patient would have abdominal prominence and wouldn't appear abnormally thin (at least in her abdomen). Hypothyroidism normally causes weight gain, and patients would not be expected to be abnormally thin. Depression is a possibility and should be asked about but does not tend to cause amenorrhea.

563. The answer is A. *(Pharmacology)*

Lithium causes nephrogenic diabetes insipidus. The other associations are correct. With clozapine, blood counts must be monitored because of the potential for agranulocytosis. Any antipsychotic theoretically has the potential to cause tardive dyskinesia, although it may be less common with newer agents, such as risperidone or olanzapine.

564. The answer is D. *(Psychiatry—General)*

The patient is having acute dystonia in response to haloperidol, which is most common in young men. Antihistamines, such as diphenhydramine, or anticholinergics, such as benztropine or trihexyphenidyl, are effective in relieving this bothersome side effect of antipsychotics. The medication does not need to be stopped or reduced at this point. Although clozapine may have a reduced incidence of extrapyramidal side effects, it requires white blood cell count monitoring and usually is reserved for treatment failure with multiple other agents.

565. The answer is C. *(Biostatistics)*

The large hospital takes sicker patients, as evidenced by its cardiac catheterization laboratory and receiving the unstable patients. The small hospital most likely transfers all the sickest patients to the larger hospital. Naturally the mortality is worse in severe myocardial infarction, even with superior care.

566. The answer is A. *(Biostatistics)*

Prevalence greatly exceeds incidence in chronic diseases such as prostate cancer. Earlier detection does not change the true incidence but may temporarily artificially inflate incidence numbers because of an increased number of cases being detected and can increase prevalence. The incidence and prevalence of prostate cancer increase with age.

567. The answer is E. *(Biostatistics)*

Remember that relative risk cannot be calculated from a retrospective study. The odds ratio, an approximation of the relative risk, can be calculated from this retrospective data:

$$= \frac{[\text{Number of cases of disease in exposed persons}] \times [\text{Number of cases of nondisease in unexposed persons}]}{[\text{Number of cases of disease in unexposed persons}] \times [\text{Number of cases of nondisease in exposed persons}]}$$

$$= \frac{[100] \times [990]}{[10] \times [900]}$$

$$= 99000 / 9000$$

$$= 11$$

568. The answer is E. *(Medicine—Geriatrics)*

The basal metabolic rate is decreased in the elderly because of loss of lean body mass (muscle), on which the basal metabolic rate is based, resulting in lower calorie requirements. An increased basal metabolic rate in the elderly may indicate a malignancy or endocrine disorder. Presbyopia is normal and describes the hardening of the lens that decreases the ability to accommodate and results in the need for reading glasses. Presbyacusis is the normal hearing loss that occurs with age, usually affecting higher frequencies first. The brain also changes with age, resulting in decreased brain weight and an increased size of the sulci and ventricles. There is a slightly decreased ability to learn new material in the elderly.

569. The answer is B. *(Medicine—Neurology)*

This patient most likely has Huntington chorea, an autosomal dominant disorder characterized by onset in middle age, progressive intellectual deterioration, choreiform movements, emotional or psychiatric disturbances, and atrophy of the caudate nuclei. Treatment is supportive, and antipsychotics may be needed once mental deterioration begins.

570. The answer is A. *(Medicine—Neurology)*

This girl most likely is having petit mal seizures. This disorder almost never begins after the age of 20. The seizures are characterized by a loss of consciousness, although the eyes may remain open; little to no associated movement disorder; and lack of a postictal state. Finishing a sentence 30 seconds after stopping in the middle of it for no apparent reason, eye fluttering during the seizure episode, and a description of a child as "daydreaming" are all classic for petit mal epilepsy. Chemistry profiles are likely to be normal, although the electroencephalogram is probably abnormal, and seizure disorders are rarely autosomal in origin. Treatment often includes ethosuximide or valproic acid.

571. The answer is A. *(Medicine—Infectious Disease)*

Although thrush may be normal in young children, in an adult male it is likely to represent the presence of an underlying disorder that affects the immune system. AIDS or other primary immune disorder, uncontrolled diabetes, and a blood dyscrasia are all possibilities.

572. The answer is D. *(Pediatrics—Infectious Disease)*

This child has tinea capitis with the formation of a **kerion**, a benign inflammatory reaction to the fungal infection (the "skin tumor"). The usual cause is a *Trichophyton* species, but *Microsporum* infection is the presumptive diagnosis if the scalp fluoresces under a Wood's light. Topical therapy is ineffective for this highly contagious condition, and systemic therapy (e.g., griseofulvin, terbinafine, fluconzaole, itraconazole) is required. Topical therapy may be a useful adjunct to help reduce transmissibility but is inadequate as monotherapy.

573. The answer is E. *(Medicine—Infectious Disease)*

Immunocompromised persons should, in most cases, be given varicella-zoster immune globulin if you see them within 4 days of exposure to chickenpox. Chickenpox is contagious for a few days before the rash appears until the last skin lesion crusts over completely. The adoption of the varicella vaccine in the mid-1990s soon may make this question obsolete. Because it is a live attenuated virus, varicella vaccine should be avoided in those who are immunocompromised from AIDS or other conditions. Diagnosis of chickenpox usually is clinical, but a Tzanck smear of the base of the lesions shows multinucleated giant cells, and immunofluorescence for the virus itself or culture can be performed if needed.

574. The answer is D. *(General Knowledge and Principles)*

This patient most likely has primary syphilis with a classic painless chancre. Syphilis is a reportable disease, thus the health department should be notified. This organism cannot be cultured and is treated with penicillin. This patient technically is an *emancipated* minor because he lives on his own and works full-time, meaning his parents do not need to give consent for treatment. Patients who present requesting treatment for sexually transmitted disease also generally can be treated without parental consent. Although some states differ with these points of view, they should be followed for USMLE exams.

575. The answer is C. *(Medicine—Oncology)*

Small cell lung cancers usually contraindicate surgical intervention because of their propensity for early metastases. Squamous and small cell cancers tend to start centrally, whereas adenocarcinomas tend to start peripherally. Recurrent laryngeal nerve damage produces hoarseness; phrenic nerve damage can produce diaphragm paralysis. Smoking is the most potent risk factor for lung cancer, thought to be responsible for 85% to 90% of all lung cancers. Horner syndrome is due to invasion of the cervical sympathetic nerve fibers and usually occurs with an apical lesion (i.e., Pancoast tumor).

576. The answer is B. *(Preventive Medicine)*

Cigarette smoking is the number one cause of preventable disease, disability, and premature death in the United States. It causes roughly 1 of every 6 deaths in the United States, mostly as a result of increasing coronary artery disease deaths (roughly 20% to 40% of cases), deaths from stroke (roughly 20% of cases), cancer deaths (roughly 30% of cases), and chronic obstructive pulmonary disease deaths (roughly 80% of cases). Smoking is a more potent risk factor for atherosclerosis than hypercholesterolemia. Though illicit drugs garner considerable legal and media attention, the morbidity and mortality they cause is laughably small compared to the number of lives ended and ruined by alcohol and tobacco. Infectious diseases were the leading cause of death at the beginning of the 20th century, but are now much better controlled thanks to antibiotics and immunizations. Influenza&pneumonia (lumped together) and septicemia remain among the top ten leading causes of death, however (usually bacteria cause the deaths, not viruses).

577. The answer is E. *(Medicine—Oncology)*

Metastatic liver cancer is more common than all the primary liver malignancies put together. Hepatoma is the old term for hepatocellular carcinoma, and hemangioma is not a malignancy (benign tumor). Of the primary liver malignancies, hepatocellular carcinoma is the most common overall by far, though hepatoblastoma would be more common in young children.

578. The answer is C. *(Medicine—Hematology)*

The first step in any suspected transfusion reaction is to stop the transfusion, then institute further work-up and therapy based on signs, symptoms, and the type of transfusion reaction suspected. The most common cause of a blood transfusion reaction is laboratory error (e.g., sending the wrong unit of blood, mislabeling). This patient most likely is having what is termed a *febrile reaction* as a result of antibodies against white blood cells. Other reactions include hemolytic and allergic or anaphylactic. After you stop the transfusion, you should call the lab to see if an error may have occurred.

579. The answer is A. *(Medicine—Hematology)*

Different blood components have different indications. Whole blood is used only for rapid, massive blood loss or exchange transfusions (poisoning, thrombotic thrombocytopenic purpura). Packed red blood cells are used instead of whole blood in most cases. Washed red blood cells are free of traces of plasma, white blood cells, and platelets, making this product good for IgA deficiency and allergic or previously sensitized patients (the patient in choice **D**). Platelets are given for symptomatic thrombocytopenia (usually < 10,000/μL). Granulocytes are used rarely for neutropenia with sepsis caused by chemotherapy—more commonly, colony-stimulating factor products are used. Fresh-frozen plasma contains all clotting factors and is used for bleeding diathesis when one cannot wait for vitamin K to take effect (e.g., disseminated intravascular coagulation, severe warfarin poisoning) or Vitamin K will not work (e.g., liver failure). Cryoprecipitate contains fibrinogen and factor VIII and can be used in hemophilia, von Willebrand's disease, and disseminated intravascular coagulation. Specific factor VIII replacement is now used for hemophilia and is generally preferred over cryoprecipitate.

580. The answer is A. *(Medicine—General)*

Nursing home patients, especially those with dementia, are at risk for developing dehydration. The laboratory values point to dehydration as well, with a classic elevation of the BUN-to-creatinine ratio to greater than 20, a marker of prerenal renal failure. The urine is concentrated, and the sodium and chloride levels are elevated, supporting dehydration. Although acetaminophen is a definite cause of nephropathy, as are the other choices, they are intrarenal or postrenal causes of renal failure, so they do not tend to elevate the BUN-to-creatinine ratio or cause hypernatremia or increased specific gravity of urine. Uncontrolled diabetes should cause glucose to spill into the urine in large amounts, thus the lack of glucose in the urine argues against this choice.

581. The answer is A. *(Medicine—Endocrinology)*

Both forms of diabetes insipidus (DI) present with the same disturbance in fluid imbalance, but the mechanism is different. In central DI, there is no antidiuretic hormone (ADH) being made by the posterior pituitary gland. In nephrogenic DI, ADH is being produced normally, but the kidney does not respond to it. Giving ADH, then assessing for a response by measuring the serum and urine for changes in osmolarity, can differentiate these two conditions. In nephrogenic DI, no changes occur because the kidney does not respond to ADH. In central DI, giving ADH corrects the problem so that the urine and serum osmolarity begin to normalize.

582. The answer is B. *(Medicine—Gastroenterology)*

Gastroesophageal reflux is thought to be due to intermittent, inappropriate relaxation of the lower esophageal sphincter that allows gastric contents to reflux into the esophagus. This reflux may result in heartburn, chest pain, hoarseness, chronic cough, asthma, dysphagia, bloating, and early satiety. Strictures, Barrett esophagus, and esophageal adenocarcinoma are late complications of gastroesophageal reflux disease. Adenocarcinoma is the most common histologic type of esophageal carcinoma and tends to occur in the lower half of the esophagus (where reflux is most concentrated and common), while squamous cell carcinoma tends to occur in the middle or upper portion of the esophagus (from tobacco smoke and alcohol exposure).

583. The answer is D. *(Medicine—Gastroenterology)*

Peptic ulcers are located in the duodenum in approximately 75% of cases, usually in the first portion of the duodenum (often called the duodenal bulb). Smokers are twice as likely to develop peptic ulcer disease, and smoking delays healing of ulcers and increases the risk of ulcer complications. Multiple, atypical ulcers should raise the suspicion of a gastrinoma (not glucagonoma), which is known as the Zollinger-Ellison syndrome. The location of a gastric ulcer cannot tell you reliably whether or not the ulcer is benign or malignant. All gastric ulcers need endoscopy and biopsy or follow-up imaging studies (upper gastrointestinal barium series) to document healing and prove the ulcer is benign. People with gastric ulcers may have low, normal, or high levels of acid secretion (typically normal or low), and gastric ulcers are not thought to be caused by acid hypersecretion. Gastric acid generally must be present, however, for a gastric ulcer to occur (i.e., people with achlorhydria do not generally develop gastric ulcers).

584. The answer is B. *(General Knowledge and Principles)*

A consolidation usually produces the following findings in the area of consolidation: decreased breath sounds, increased tactile fremitus, increased whispered pectoriloquy, increased egophony, and a dull percussion note.

585. The answer is B. *(Medicine—General)*

This man has a hypertensive emergency, which usually occurs when the systolic blood pressure is greater than 200 mmHg or the diastolic pressure is greater than 110 mmHg. To be considered an emergency, a person must have end-organ effects from the blood pressure, such as heart failure, chest pain, myocardial infarction, new-onset renal insufficiency, or encephalopathy, which may cause headaches, papilledema, blurry vision, vomiting, or altered mental status. In this setting, a patient needs immediate treatment in a hospital (ICU) setting. If the blood pressure is lowered too quickly to normal, as in choice **A**, cerebral perfusion can drop precipitously, which may cause a stroke. A good rule of thumb is to drop the diastolic pressure immediately by one quarter to one third, but without going below 95 mmHg. Although checking the urine for cocaine is a good idea, steroids are not indicated.

586. The answer is A. *(Medicine—General)*

Although high blood pressure is the number one known modifiable risk factor for stroke or cerebrovascular accident, people with untreated (or treated) hypertension are most likely to die from coronary disease (as in the general population). Hypertension is also the second leading cause of chronic renal failure behind diabetes.

587. The answer is A. *(Medicine—Cardiology)*

This patient has multiple risk factors for a myocardial infarction (age, sex, diabetes, and presumed hypertension given his medication list) and diabetic patients classically present with "silent" infarctions (i.e. those that don't cause chest pain) due to autonomic neuropathy. An EKG, chest x-ray (to look for cardiac failure) and serial serum cardiac enzymes (e.g., troponins) should be ordered and the patient put on oxygen with close monitoring of vital signs.

Hyperkalemia is not a common cause for the presenting symptoms (not associated with diaphoresis in the absence of arrhythmias, which should have caused an abnormal pulse or heart rate on exam). Physical findings would be present with atrial fibrillation (irregularly irregular pulse) and third-degree heart block (bradycardia). Pericarditis is possible, but typically causes fever and a history of upper respiratory infection, and less important to rule out (and less common in this age group) than a myocardial infarction.

588. The answer is E. *(Medicine—Gastroenterology)*

This woman most likely has achalasia. Cancer and stricture could cause a similar appearance but are unlikely given the patient's age, lack of history of heartburn, and equal problem with solids and liquids. With a mechanical narrowing (i.e., cancer or stricture), dysphagia for solids often is greater than for liquids because liquids can pass a narrowed segment of esophagus more easily. In motility disorders such as achalasia, solids and liquids often are affected equally because the problem is functional. Endoscopy would be advised to ensure there is not a cancer or stricture, although the barium swallow findings and the clinical history are fairly classic.

Esophageal manometry is typically used to confirm the diagnosis of achalasia. Classic manometric abnormalities include poor or absent peristalsis in the esophagus, elevated lower esophageal sphincter pressure, and incomplete or absent relaxation of the lower esophageal sphincter (which prevents gastroesophageal reflux). Treatment usually involves pneumatic dilation during endoscopy or administration of botulinum toxin to paralyze the lower esophageal sphincter, both of which may need to be performed repeatedly over the years. Surgical myotomy is reserved for those that fail less invasive treatments.

589. The answer is C. *(Obstetrics)*

This woman has eclampsia, which most likely could have been prevented with regular prenatal care to detect the disease process at an earlier stage and allow proper treatment to prevent disease progression. A low-salt diet sometimes is prescribed to women with mild preeclampsia but has only a minor impact (at best) on prevention. Immediate hydralazine on presentation to the emergency department is unlikely to have stopped this scenario from evolving the way it did. Multivitamins do not prevent preeclampsia or eclampsia, and alcohol use has not been associated with preeclampsia.

590. The answer is D. *(Gynecology)*

This patient is a genotypic male with the rare androgen insensitivity syndrome, also known as *testicular feminization*. A lack of cellular response to testosterone creates the external appearance of a female, but pubic and axillary hair are lacking, and the uterus is absent. These patients have functional testicles, causing a testosterone level in the normal male range (i.e., above the normal female range). Psychologically, this patient is clearly a female (as she presented for primary amenorrhea), and this matter needs to be handled delicately. A karyotype should be ordered to confirm the diagnosis. True hermaphrodites, an extremely rare group, have both testicular and ovarian tissue present and usually have components of both male and female external genitalia. 21-Hydroxylase deficiency tends to present in the neonatal period, and there are usually signs or symptoms of adrenal insufficiency and some degree of ambiguous genitalia in females.

591. The answer is D. *(Gynecology)*

Patients with an ectopic pregnancy should have a positive pregnancy test, and the other choices should have uterine bleeding with a progesterone challenge except Turner's syndrome, which causes primary amenorrhea. Absence of uterine bleeding with a progesterone challenge in the setting of secondary amenorrhea with a negative pregnancy test generally indicates ovarian, hypothalamic, or pituitary failure.

592. The answer is C. *(Gynecology)*

Semen analysis is a cheap, noninvasive test that identifies the cause of infertility in roughly one third of cases. CT scan and progesterone challenge have no role in the evaluation of infertility in a normally menstruating woman, and the other tests are reserved for later in the testing algorithm or with a suggestive history. Laparoscopy is used as a last resort because of the associated morbidity and mortality.

593. The answer is A. *(Gynecology)*

Physiologic (normal) menstrual irregularities occur around the time of menarche (first menstrual period) and menopause. Oral contraceptive pills are used to treat dysmenorrhea and tend to decrease its occurrence. Hypothyroidism and cancer are much less common than polycystic ovary syndrome as a cause of dysmenorrhea at this age, although they are possibilities. Hypothyroidism often causes a goiter (usually due to Hashimoto thyroiditis) and other findings (e.g., bradycardia, coarsened hair, slow speech), though not always. It would be quite unusual for a patient with hypothyroidism not to have any complaints of fatigue or lethargy (often the most troubling symptoms) and present solely for menstrual irregularities. Polycystic ovary syndrome is classically seen in overweight women with hirsutism, but not always, and is probably the most common cause for dysfunctional uterine bleeding in younger women.

594–599. *(Preventive Medicine)*

The answers are the following: **594. A**   **595. A**   **596. A**   **597. C**   **598. D**   **599. A.**

Smoking is the most likely risk factor for renal cell, bladder, pancreatic, and cervical carcinomas of the choices listed. Although maternal diethylstilbestrol (DES) exposure is a classic board question for vaginal and cervical neoplasias, these are of the clear cell type, which is quite rare compared with squamous cell carcinoma of the cervix. Human papillomavirus infection is thought to be a more potent factor than smoking for cervical cancer but was not a choice. For bladder cancer, *Schistosoma* infection is a more potent risk factor in some places outside the United States, but is seen rarely in this country other than in recent immigrants. *Whenever a question asks about incidence, prevalence, or how common a condition is, you should assume that the question is referring to the United States unless otherwise instructed.*

Obesity increases the risk of endometrial carcinoma by increasing estrogen stimulation of the uterus. Previous radiation of the head and neck is a strong risk factor (and one of the few discovered identifiable causes) for thyroid cancer. Prior radiation and chemotherapy are well-known risk factors for the development of malignancy. With radiation, solid tumors tend to occur in the specific area irradiated and the latency period is typically 10-20 years. With chemotherapy, leukemia and lymphoma are more typical and the latent period is somewhat shorter, typically 1 to 10 years.

600. The answer is B. *(Pathology)*

The figure demonstrates an invasive colon adenocarcinoma. A normal mucosa (labeled "Muc" in figure) and muscularis mucosa (labeled "MM") are seen on the right side, while the adenocarcinoma (labeled "T"), which is forming irregular glands (labeled "G") and has nuclear hyperchromatism, has invaded into the submucosa (labeled "SM"). Initial treatment in the absence of known metastases is surgical resection (right hemicolectomy in this case) with local lymph node dissection to determine whether or not spread has occured. Pre-operative imaging can be helpful in staging (e.g., CT scan of the abdomen and pelvis with contrast). Chemotherapy is not indicated at this time, unless spread is detected at surgery or on pre-operative imaging.

ANSWERS AND EXPLANATIONS

601. The answer is D. *(Medicine—Gastroenterology)*

The hundreds or even thousands of polyps that may be seen in the Peutz-Jeghers syndrome, which often can be recognized by the oral or buccal facial pigmentation, are hamartomatous and generally do not become malignant. These patients are, however, at an increased risk for cancer of the pancreas, breast, lung, ovary, and uterus. Patients with familial adenomatous polyposis are considered to have a 100% chance of getting colon cancer if they live long enough and are advised to have a prophylactic colectomy. Prior to colectomy, colonoscopic surveillance is undertaken. Long-standing ulcerative colitis increases colon cancer incidence markedly, and it is said that after roughly 10 years of moderately severe disease, colon cancer develops in about 33% of affected individuals. The patient in choice **E** should have annual colonic examination at this point in his life, or preferably, proctocolectomy. Blood in the stool of a patient older than age 40, whether occult or visible in the form of hematochezia or melena, is colon cancer *until proved otherwise*, especially in the presence of weight loss or a change in the caliber of the stool.

602. The answer is A. *(Medicine—Oncology)*

This patient most likely has prostate cancer with osteoblastic metastases to the lumbar vertebrae, a not unusual presentation. Prostate-specific antigen (PSA) becomes positive before prostate cancer breaks through the capsule, thus is useful for early detection and follow-up during and after treatment. The PSA level can also become mildly elevated in the setting of benign prostatic hyperplasia. Standard chemotherapy agents rarely are effective against prostate cancer, and the therapy of choice is hormonal therapy, with palliative local radiation to the spine if medications fail. Orchiectomy, gonadotropin-releasing hormone agonists, androgen-receptor antagonists, estrogen, and others can be used and often are effective.

603. The answer is C. *(Medicine—Oncology)*

Syndrome of inappropriate antidiuretic hormone secretion, Eaton-Lambert syndrome, and Cushing syndrome (as paraneoplastic syndromes) all are most commonly due to small cell lung cancer. Thymomas are associated with myasthenia gravis, and polycythemia classically is associated with renal cell carcinoma. Hypercalcemia is a recognized consequence of head and neck squamous cell cancers as well as squamous cell lung cancers. It can also occur in any cancer secondary to widespread bone metastases and destruction, though this would not be considered a paraneoplastic syndrome.

604. The answer is A. *(Medicine—Hematology)*

This patient most likely has glucose-6-phosphate dehydrogenase (i.e., G6PD) deficiency, an X-linked recessive condition thought to affect 10% of all black males in the United States. It classically causes bite cells because of splenic macrophages taking a *bite* out of cells with *Heinz bodies* in them. Sulfa drugs commonly precipitate hemolysis in this condition through oxidative stress, not antibody formation. Antibody-mediated hemolysis usually requires several days to a few weeks to develop. There is no reason to suspect disseminated intravascular coagulation or occult blood loss in this patient.

605. The answer is E. *(Pediatrics—Hematology)*

This child has pancytopenia caused by bone marrow failure, also known as *aplastic anemia*. The inappropriately low reticulocyte count should alert you to the fact that the bone marrow is not responding adequately to the anemia. One of the causes of this scenario is leukemia that has overrun the normal bone marrow. The other causes do not explain the simultaneous reduction in hemoglobin, white blood cells, and platelets, with the exception of autoimmune disorders (e.g., lupus), which are quite rare at this age.

606. The answer is B. *(Medicine—Nephrology)*

This patient most likely has developed worsening benign prostatic hypertrophy, a fairly common cause of acute renal failure in older men. The other choices would tend to cause other symptoms or history.

607. The answer is A. *(Medicine—Endocrinology)*

Thiazide diuretics have a paradoxic effect of decreasing the urine output in nephrogenic diabetes insipidus. Vasopressin is ineffective in nephrogenic diabetes insipidus; demeclocycline and lithium are causes of diabetes insipidus.

608. The answer is A. *(Medicine—General)*

Metanephrines are catecholamine breakdown products that can be used as a marker for a pheochromocytoma. A carcinoid tends to elevate urinary 5-hydroxyindoleacetic acid (i.e., 5-HIAA), a serotonin breakdown product, and does not often cause hypertension. Wild swings in blood pressure are highly suspicious for pheochromocytoma.

609. The answer is D. *(Medicine—Gastroenterology)*

Although seen only in severe cases, chronic pancreatitis can destroy enough of the insulin-secreting β cells to cause glucose intolerance or frank diabetes. Frequent stooling and steatorrhea also occur in severe cases, not constipation. Fat-soluble vitamin supplements, not B-vitamin supplements, also may be required. Diffuse pancreatic calcifications are not sensitive but are fairly specific for chronic pancreatitis. The calcifications represent intraductal stones that are thought to form as a result of stasis and inflammation. The most common cause of chronic pancreatitis is alcoholism in the United States. Although gallstones are one of the most common causes of acute pancreatitis, they do not generally result in chronic pancreatitis (at least in part because cholecystectomy is advised after a bout of gallstone pancreatitis).

610. The answer is B. *(Medicine—Gastroenterology)*

Irritable bowel syndrome is extremely common and tends to present with waxing and waning symptoms over years without evidence of pathology. A normal sigmoidoscopy and temperature help exclude *C. difficile* colitis and ulcerative colitis. Crohn disease is likely to produce more serious symptoms, and a fever would be fairly common during an acute flare of the disease. Although it cannot be ruled out after this scenario, it is less likely and much less common than irritable bowel syndrome. The history of antibiotic use should always make you think of *C. difficile*, but in this case *C. difficile* was mentioned only as a distracter. Symptoms started long before the use of antibiotics.

611. The answer is B. *(Medicine—General)*

Community-acquired pneumonia usually begins as primarily a focal or diffuse area of consolidation, not pulmonary edema. Pulmonary edema from cardiac causes is usually fairly symmetric, and cardiomegaly often is present. Hypoxia secondary to pulmonary edema from heart failure or a myocardial infarction usually improves with oxygen and diuretics. Patients often have some type of cardiac history. This description is fairly typical for adult respiratory distress syndrome, and sepsis is a known cause.

612. The answer is B. *(Medicine—Infectious Disease)*

If the boards mention a trip to the desert regions of southern California or Arizona, it is significant and most likely indicates *Coccidioides* infection, which can cause pulmonary infection as well as *erythema nodosum* in about 10% of cases, as in this woman.

613. The answer is C. *(Medicine—Pulmonology)*

In a patient with such a strong smoking history and an ill-defined lesion on chest radiograph without any symptoms or sick contacts, lung cancer should be first on the list of differential diagnoses. A hamartoma would have shown up on the radiograph 1 year ago. Reactivation tuberculosis typically occurs in the upper lobes, is classically cavitary, and causes symptoms. This patient needs a CT scan of the chest (to further characterize the lesion and look for mediastinal adenopathy) and biopsy of the lesion to obtain a tissue diagnosis. Coccidiomycosis is a possibility, but the question does not mention the southwestern United States and this would be less common than cancer in a patient with such a significant smoking history.

614. The answer is D. *(Medicine—Pulmonology)*

β_2-agonists, such as albuterol, are preferred for relief from acute asthma exacerbation. Ipratropium often is effective in chronic obstructive pulmonary disease exacerbation, but its efficacy is much lower in asthma. Cromolyn and zafirlukast are used as prophylaxis, not to break an attack. Corticosteroids, such as prednisone, do not provide immediate relief but reduce inflammation several hours later and often are useful adjuncts to beta$_2$-agonist therapy.

615. The answer is D. *(Obstetrics)*

Polyhydramnios may result in an overdistended uterus that compromises maternal pulmonary function. Normal amniotic fluid volume is 500 to 2000 mL. Polyhydramnios generally is defined as an amniotic fluid volume greater than 2 L or by using ultrasound criteria. It is associated with maternal diabetes, multiple gestation, neural tube defects (anencephaly, spina bifida), gastrointestinal anomalies (omphalocele, esophageal atresia), and fetal hydrops. Polyhydramnios increases the risk for postpartum uterine atony. Renal agenesis and pulmonary hypoplasia are associated with oligohydramnios. Treatment generally is supportive and rarely includes amniocentesis because reaccumulation of fluid occurs quickly and there are risks associated with this procedure, but it can be used in extreme cases that cause significant maternal discomfort. Amniotomy is used to hasten labor, but is not a standard treatment for polyhydramnios and introduces the risk of fetal and maternal infection. Labor induction may be required in severe cases causing maternal deterioration.

616. The answer is A. *(Obstetrics)*

Pulmonary embolus is one of the leading causes of maternal mortality and may be secondary to an amniotic fluid embolus, which also can cause disseminated intravascular coagulation. This woman has several classic symptoms and signs of a pulmonary embolus. The other listed causes are much less likely with the given description and/or rarely cause death so quickly after the onset of symptoms.

617. The answer is C. *(Obstetrics)*

This woman has developed moderate-to-severe preeclampsia. She should be admitted to the hospital for observation, laboratory work, and blood pressure control. If she does well, she may be discharged with close outpatient follow-up. If not, she needs labor induction. Cesarean section is premature at this point. Follow-up in 1 week is too long and may have disastrous consequences. Angiotensin-converting enzyme inhibitors should be avoided in pregnancy because of the possibility of causing renal damage in the fetus.

618. The answer is A. *(Gynecology)*

Leiomyomas are the most common tumors in women, and approximately 20% of women have at least one leiomyoma by age 40. They are the most frequent indication for hysterectomy because they may grow to massive proportions, may cause anemia secondary to menorrhagia, and may cause disabling pelvic pain. These benign tumors are estrogen dependent, so they may enlarge markedly during pregnancy or with oral contraceptive pill use and tend to regress after menopause. They are a relatively common cause of infertility (by interfering with implantation or embryo growth), and uterine myomectomy may restore fertility in this setting. Malignant transformation is extremely rare, with less than 1% of cases progressing to leiomyosarcoma.

619. The answer is D. *(Gynecology)*

This woman has adenomyosis, a common cause of the mentioned symptoms and physical findings in women older than age 40. The slide reveals the presence of endometrial glands (labeled "G" in th slide) and stroma (labeled "S") situated within normal-appearing myometrium (labeled "M"). There is no particular reason to suspect menopause in a woman who is 41 years old without additional information. Though endometrial carcinoma should always be in the differential with unexplained gynecologic bleeding in a woman over the age of 35, a negative dilatation and curettage makes it very unlikely. Endometriosis is similar to adenomyosis in terms of pathophysiology and these conditions not uncommonly coexist, but by definition, endometrial glands must be located outside the uterus to make the diagnosis of endometriosis.

620. The answer is C. *(Medicine—Cardiology)*

Although not a first-line agent, milrinone has inotropic cardiac effects and can be used in the setting of severe heart failure. Beta blockers and centrally acting calcium channel blockers should be avoided in this setting. Corticosteroids and lidocaine would not be of use in this setting unless the heart failure was due to hypoadrenalism or ventricular arrhythmias, respectively.

621. The answer is C. *(Medicine—General)*

Although severe psychogenic polydipsia (or drinking large amounts of water because of a psychiatric disturbance) may cause hyponatremia, it has not been associated with hypertension. Both hypothyroidism and hyperthyroidism can be associated with high blood pressure. Cocaine abuse and hyperadrenalism are well-known causes of secondary hypertension.

622. The answer is B. *(Medicine—General)*

The patient has acute gouty arthritis. Allopurinol should not be used in acute attacks of gout because it can make symptoms worse (maintenance therapy, not for acute exacerbations). The other choices are true. Gout results in needle-shaped crystals (sometimes within leukocytes) with *negative birefringence* using polarized light microscopy.

623. The answer is E. *(Medicine—Oncology)*

This patient has an extensive gastric malignancy involving the distal stomach (the thin, irregular, curvilinear contrast focus in the center of the x-ray image), which is most likely to be an adenocarcinoma (accounts for ≥ 95% of primary gastric malignancies). Risk factors include Japanese race, male sex, age greater than 40, eating smoked meats and fish, family history and *Helicobacter pylori* infection. A gastric lymphoma and leiomyosarcoma would be other differential considerations given the history and x-ray findings, but are much less common than adenocarcinoma.

624. The answer is A. *(Ethics)*

Depression is a valid reason for a patient to be considered incompetent to make treatment decisions. This woman believes her situation is hopeless and is depressed enough to be unable to see the benefits of proposed treatment. Only after her depression is treated adequately should a living will be honored. You cannot force treatment on the woman, but treatment decisions should be delayed until the woman has better (i.e., depression-free) judgment. It is inappropriate to contact anyone about this patient's condition because of physician-patient confidentiality (unless she asks you to do so), and you should not lie to the woman about a treatment that you are giving her. She is not causing a current and immediate danger to herself or others; therefore, involuntary hospitalization is not a valid option.

625. The answer is A. *(Ethics)*

This patient has a history of violence and is expressing acute homicidal ideation and paranoid delusions. He needs hospital admission, and the authorities should be alerted so that they can warn the woman. Physician-patient confidentiality should be broken in certain circumstances, including child abuse and the duty to protect and warn in situations such as this. When patients are a danger to others, the physician has a duty to warn the local authorities. Outpatient medication and follow-up eventually will be needed but not until stabilization has been confirmed on an inpatient basis. This patient may be a good candidate for long-acting depot injections in the future given his history but needs inpatient stabilization first.

626. The answer is A. *(Pediatrics—General)*

Shoelace tying is generally not mastered until around the age of 5. Good use of a cup and spoon (15 to 18 months), running well (2 years), understanding one-step commands (15 months), and building a tower of six blocks (2 years) would all be expected in a 3-year-old child.

627. The answer is A. *(Pediatrics—Infectious Disease)*

This child most likely has epiglottitis and may need intubation. Affected patients usually are between the ages of 2 and 5. Further history, physical examination, imaging tests, and/or blood draws may irritate the child and precipitate acute airway obstruction. These can be done later, once the child is stabilized. Never forget the ABCs. Drooling often is an ominous sign in a child with labored respirations. Broad-spectrum antibiotics are indicated to treat the likely bacteria, which often is either *Haemophilus influenzae* or *Staphyloccus aureus*. Disease confirmation can be done via direct visualization (often endoscopically) in the operating room once appropriate equipment is available for intubation with experienced personnel ready to secure the airway. Lateral neck radiographs are used in milder cases (not CT) to confirm the diagnosis and reveal a "thumb" sign, which describes the appearance of a swollen, edematous epiglottis.

628. The answer is A. *(Pediatrics—Infectious Disease)*

Corynebacterium diphtheriae is a gram-positive rod that causes diphtheria, an infection that rarely is seen in the United States because of mandatory vaccination. The grayish pseudomembranes and rapidity of onset are the hallmarks of the disease. Always keep diphtheria in the differential diagnosis in a child who may not have been immunized (very rarely occurs in immunized persons). The complications of diphtheria are due to the production of toxins by the bacteria, which may result in myocarditis and peripheral neuritis. Antitoxin is the most important aspects of initial treatment. Patients should be admitted to a hospital and watched for respiratory decompensation because they may need airway management. Eradication of the bacteria is an important adjunctive/secondary measure; penicillin or erythromycin are the preferred agents.

629. The answer is C. *(Orthopedic Surgery)*

The radial nerve is involved in wrist extension, and lesions may produce wristdrop. The ulnar nerve is involved in finger abduction, and lesions may produce a *claw* hand with hypothenar wasting. The median nerve is involved in wrist pronation and thumb opposition, and thenar eminence wasting is classic. The musculocutaneous nerve is involved in elbow flexion, and the axillary nerve supplies muscles in the shoulder and is involved in abduction and lateral rotation of the arm.

630. The answer is C. *(Orthopedic Surgery)*

The other choices are valid indications for open reduction, in addition to the presence of an intra-articular fracture and nonunion or failed closed reduction. Fractures in children tend to do well (often better than adults), and there is no special reason to do an open reduction in an uncomplicated closed fracture.

631. The answer is C. *(Ophthalmology)*

The red reflex usually becomes abnormal because cataracts interrupt the beam of light on its way to the retina and cause the red reflex to become black or white in the areas where the lens has cataract formation. Gradual onset is the rule and bilateral involvement is common (although often asymmetric). Corticosteroid use is associated with an increased incidence of cataracts. Cataracts are a common cause of gradually progressive loss of vision and surgery is often postponed until the visual changes interfere with patient's daily activities.

632. The answer is A. *(Ophthalmology)*

Retinal detachment usually is painless. The other choices accurately describe retinal detachment. Another classic history is a patient who complains of a curtain or veil coming down in front of the eye. Immediate ophthalmologic referral is needed with suspicion of retinal detachment because surgery may save vision in the affected eye.

633. The answer is A. *(Obstetrics)*

This woman is unstable most likely because of a ruptured ectopic pregnancy. She needs an urgent laparotomy to confirm the diagnosis and to institute treatment. Although intravenous fluids and other supportive measures are appropriate, waiting 1 hour to repeat the physical examination is not (the woman may be dead by that time). Culdocentesis, CT scan, and ordering a quantitative human chorionic gonadotropin may help confirm the diagnosis but only would delay the needed therapy in this setting. Regardless of what these tests showed, the woman still would need a laparotomy.

634. The answer is D. *(Obstetrics)*

Nulliparity is not thought to be associated with ectopic pregnancy, unless there is a specific underlying pathologic tubal cause that has resulted in involuntary nulliparity (rare). The most potent risk factors for ectopic pregnancy are pelvic inflammatory disease and prior ectopic pregnancy. The other choices also are common risk factors for ectopic pregnancy development. Any history of tubal surgery (including tubal ligation, which is not 100% effective), prolonged infertility (may indicate tubal abnormality), or in utero diethylstilbestrol exposure increases the risk of developing an ectopic pregnancy. An intrauterine device is an effective method of contraception that prevents implantation into the endometrium, thus if a pregnancy does occur, it is often an ectopic gestation (can't be reached by the device).

635. The answer is D. *(Obstetrics)*

Abortion, by convention, implies less than 20 weeks' gestation. Threatened abortion is uterine bleeding without cervical dilation or expulsion of products of conception. Inevitable abortion is uterine bleeding with cervical dilation and crampy abdominal pain and no tissue expulsion. Incomplete abortion is passage of some products of conception through the cervix. Complete abortion is expulsion of all products of conception from the uterus. Missed abortion is fetal death with no expulsion of tissue (often for several weeks). An elective induced abortion is one that is requested by the mother, whereas a therapeutic induced abortion is done for maternal health reasons.

636. The answer is A. *(Obstetrics)*

The classic or vertical uterine incision causes an increased rate of uterine rupture when vaginal delivery is attempted with future pregnancies. The modern or horizontal uterine incision should not prevent a woman from attempting a vaginal delivery or receiving labor-inducing agents. Nulliparity is not a consideration, and a term gestation is not a consideration if there is an indication for delivery. Preeclampsia often is a reason to induce labor because delivery is the only known definitive treatment. A history of genital herpes does not prevent vaginal delivery or labor induction, but the presence of active genital herpes would be considered a contraindication to vaginal delivery and labor induction.

637. The answer is E. *(Psychiatry—Addiction Psychiatry)*

Barbiturate, benzodiazepine, and alcohol withdrawal all can be fatal. Seizures and cardiovascular collapse may occur with abrupt cessation of benzodiazepines or barbiturates. Patients who have been on either of these drugs need to have the dose tapered gradually. Patients who are addicted and cease using abruptly need to be admitted to the hospital (they may appear in the emergency department with seizures). Gradually decreasing doses of a member of the class to which the patient is addicted (usually a long-acting preparation and sometimes a similar agent from another class, such as benzodiazepines used in alcohol withdrawal) are used to prevent seizures and other withdrawal effects.

638. The answer is A. *(Psychiatry—General)*

This patient had a panic attack, which is associated with agoraphobia (fear of leaving the house) in roughly half of cases. The workup is negative, and the patient returned to baseline with each attack. The primary respiratory alkalosis is due to anxiety-induced hyperventilation. Hyperthyroidism and pulmonary emboli would not wax and wane so dramatically. Treatment often involves serotonin-specific reuptake inhibitors. Generalized anxiety disorder presents in a much less dramatic fashion, with constant worrying and anxiety about multiple aspects of one's life.

639. The answer is C. *(Psychiatry—General)*

Normal versus pathologic grief, mourning, or bereavement is a popular board question. Initial grief after a loss (e.g., death of a loved one) may include a state of shock, feeling of numbness or bewilderment, distress, crying, sleep disturbances, decreased appetite, difficulty concentrating, weight loss, and guilt (survivor guilt) *for as long as 1 year*. These are some of the same symptoms as depression. It is normal to have an illusion or hallucination about the deceased (but a normal grieving person knows it was an illusion or hallucination, whereas a depressed person believes the illusion or hallucination is real). Intense yearning (even years after the death) and searching for the deceased are normal. Feelings of worthlessness, psychomotor retardation, and suicidal ideation are *not* normal grief; they are signs of depression. With the brief amount of information given, normal grief is the best answer.

640. The answer is D. *(Pharmacology)*

Priapism, or a painful prolonged erection not associated with sexual arousal, may result in permanent impotence if not treated promptly. Trazodone is the classic offender (other antidepressants have also been implicated but cause it much less often); cocaine and anti-impotence drugs are other common drug-related causes. Sickle cell disease and leukemia are common non-drug related causes. Needle decompression is the usual treatment; if this fails, open surgical decompression is needed.

641. The answer is C. *(Pharmacology)*

Tranylcypromine is a monoamine oxidase inhibitor, a class of antidepressants that has fallen out of favor because of restrictions placed on individuals who take it. Persons on a monoamine oxidase inhibitor must avoid tyramine-containing foods (long list, but classic *no-no's* are wine and cheese), meperidine, sympathomimetic drugs and serotonin-specific reuptake inhibitors. Tyramine and sympathomimetic drugs can precipitate a hypertensive crisis, for which nifedipine sometimes is used to control the blood pressure. Giving meperidine or a serotonin-specific reuptake inhibitor to someone on a monoamine oxidase inhibitor may result in death.

642. The answer is C. *(Biostatistics)*

The negative predictive value tells you how likely it is that a negative test represents true absence of the condition you are testing for (a *true* negative). It is calculated by dividing the number of true negatives by the total number of persons with a negative test. This value is affected by the prevalence and decreases with increasing prevalence. An overly sensitive test with a large number of false-positive results makes it more likely that a negative test is truly negative, increasing the negative predictive value.

643. The answer is A. *(Biostatistics)*

A variation of this question frequently has appeared on the boards. Changing the cutoff value of the fasting glucose test to diagnose diabetes (which was done in the 1990s) has some important ramifications. The absolute risk of true diabetes does not change by changing a test because diabetes is a disease and will continue to be regardless of how it is defined by the medical community. Changing the cutoff value of the test causes physicians to label an increasing number of people diabetic, however, resulting in more false-positives, fewer false-negatives, increased sensitivity, decreased specificity, a decreased positive predictive value, and an increased negative predictive value. The thought in changing the cut-off value was that identifying more people with borderline diabetes may result in earlier intervention and treatment to prevent the development of the complications of true diabetes. This change is at the expense, however, of labeling some people diabetic who may be normal.

644. The answer is E. *(Biostatistics)*

Specificity is defined as the number of true negatives divided by the number of people who are disease-free. In this example, 96,000 people tested negative, but 2000 of those actually had the disease, giving a true-negative value of 94,000. The number of people without the disease is 95,000 because the gold standard detected 5000 cases in a city of 100,000. 94,000/95,000 = 0.99 = > 95%.

645. The answer is B. *(Biostatistics)*

The attributable risk is the additional incidence of a disease that can be linked directly to the risk factor being examined. In this case, attributable risk would represent the number of cases that are entirely due to smoking. The way to calculate attributable risk is the following:

[(Number of disease cases in those exposed) / (total number of people exposed)] –
[(Number of disease cases in those not exposed) / (total number of people not exposed)].

As opposed to relative risk, the two division products are subtracted (as opposed to divided in relative risk). In this example, the calculation would be the following:

$$[(300)/(10,000)] - [(200)/(20,000)] = 0.03 - 0.01 = 0.02 = 2/100 = 20/1000$$

646–649. *(Medicine—Neurology)*

The answers are the following: **646. C**   **647. A**   **648. I**   **649. B.**

See the table. Chronic alcoholics commonly develop cerebellar atrophy that may cause symptoms.

Symptom/Sign	Think of This Area
Apathy, inattention, uninhibited, labile affect	Frontal lobes
Broca's (motor) aphasia	Dominant frontal lobe*
Wernicke's (sensory) aphasia	Dominant temporal lobe*
Memory impairment, aggressive, sexual	Temporal lobes
Cannot read, write, name, do math	Dominant parietal lobe*
Ignore one side of body, trouble dressing	Nondominant parietal lobe*
Visual hallucinations, illusions	Occipital lobes
Ataxia, dysarthria, nystagmus, intention tremor, dysmetria, scanning speech	Cerebellum

* Left side is dominant in > 95% of population (99% of right-handed people and 60% to 70% of left-handed people).

650. The answer is E. *(Medicine—Pulmonology)*

The patient has clubbing of the fingers, which is classically due to respiratory disorders, such as emphysema, bronchiectasis, tuberculosis, lung abscess, cystic fibrosis or bronchogenic carcinoma. Given the patient's smoking history, it is likely that his clubbing is related to a respiratory complication of smoking, and an investigation to rule out lung cancer would be appropriate. However, clubbing has been associated with multiple other conditions, including cyanotic congenital heart disease, cardiac tumors, inflammatory bowel disease, celiac disease, cirrhosis, chronic active hepatitis, and lymphoma. Clubbing is easier recognized than described, but involves a broadening and thickening of the distal phalanges with increased lengthwise curvature and flattening of the angle between the cuticle and nail.

ANSWERS AND EXPLANATIONS

651. The answer is C. *(Pediatrics—Infectious Disease)*

This infant most likely has roseola infantum, usually caused by human herpesvirus type 6. The hallmark of the condition is extremely high fevers for 3 to 5 days without localizing signs that may result in febrile seizures. The child is classically alert and active. The fever stops abruptly (as it usually begins), then a mild maculopapular rash classically appears on the chest and abdomen. Acetaminophen to reduce fever can help prevent further febrile seizures, but given the classic history and a neighbor child that completed the classic infectious course on the boards, further aggressive workup is not required, although close follow-up is.

652. The answer is A. *(Pediatrics—Neonates)*

This infant likely has herpes encephalitis. Though this disorder is classically described as causing temporal lobe enhancement or inflammation on MRI or CT scan, this is the type I herpes simplex (i.e., HSV-1) that typically presents in children after the neonatal period. Neonatal herpes encephalitis is typically due to herpes simplex type two virus (i.e., HSV-2) and often causes inflammatory changes in a more diffuse manner, classically with an associated vesicular rash and seizures when when maternally transmitted to neonates. A lumbar puncture would most likely show mild pleocytosis with a predominance of lymphocytes and red blood cells. Treatment is with intravenous acyclovir, and neurologic morbidity is high if the child survives. If the child had been born at the hospital, the lesions should have been identified and a cesarean section performed in an attempt to reduce maternal transmission. Maternal chickenpox (i.e., varicella-zoster virus infection) could also cause such a scenario if the rash was different; affected neonates classically develop pneumonia with systemic infection.

653. The answer is C. *(Pediatrics—Infectious Disease)*

Kawasaki disease (also called syndrome) is currently an idiopathic febrile disorder that can cause coronary aneurysms and arteritis, which have resulted in myocardial infarction (MI) in young children. The other conditions have not been significantly associated with myocardial infarction. Homozygous familial *hypercholesterolemia* can cause myocardial infarcts in teenagers, but rarely before the age of 10. Those with familial hypertriglyceridemia are more at risk for pancreatitis than coronary artery disease and MI. Duchenne muscular dystrophy patients can experience congestive failure or arrhythmias from cardiac muscle involvement, a common causes of death. Affected patients often die in their teens. Cardiac involvement is only rarely described in neurofibromatosis (e.g., tumors, arrhythmias).

654. The answer is D. *(Orthopedic Surgery)*

A Charcot joint, also known as a *neuropathic joint*, is a joint that becomes severely deformed secondary to loss of proprioception and/or pain sensation. This causes the joint to be overused or used inappropriately. Patients may break bones and disrupt joints and lack any sensation of pain or discomfort (may present with swelling or infection). Patients with decreased sensation should have radiographs done for minor trauma to prevent complications. Clinically, Charcot joints are seen most commonly in diabetics but may occur in other conditions affecting peripheral sensation, such as syringomyelia, syphilis and vitamin B_{12} deficiency.

655. The answer is D. *(Orthopedic Surgery)*

Urinary retention usually is not seen with typical L5–S1 posterolateral disk herniation, which affects the ipsilateral S1 nerve root and causes the other choices to occur. In rare cases, disks can compress the cauda equina, causing *cauda equina syndrome*, with resultant urinary retention that is associated with incontinence, perineal anesthesia and poor anal sphincter tone.

656. The answer is D. *(Ophthalmology)*

This is one of the few instances in which obtaining more history or performing a full physical examination should be avoided because of the need for immediate treatment. Immediate copious irrigation of the eye with the nearest source of water, with or without salt and whether sterile or not, should be performed. The sooner this is performed, the less damage will be done to the eye. Alkaline burns generally are worse than acidic burns because they tend to penetrate deeper into the eye. Dilution, not neutralization, is the preferred treatment for acidic or alkaline burn because the chemical reaction of neutralization may increase tissue damage.

657. The answer is A. *(Ophthalmology)*

Proptosis, or *exophthalmos*, is protrusion of the eye and does not occur with preseptal cellulitis. Fever, lid swelling, history of trauma (or sinusitis), and chemosis (edema of the bulbar conjunctiva) can be present in both conditions. Orbital cellulitis also may cause ophthalmoplegia, decreased visual acuity, and severe eye pain, none of which generally occur with preorbital cellulitis. The distinction is important because preseptal cellulitis has a better prognosis than orbital cellulitis, an ophthalmologic emergency (i.e. warning, may cause blindness) requiring inpatient management with intravenous antibiotics. A CT scan can help detect intraorbital abscess (often needs surgical drainage) and the feared but rare intracranial extension. The bacterial causes of the two conditions are similar, most commonly *Streptococcus pneumoniae* or *Haemophilus influenzae* in cases resulting from sinusitis and *Streptococcus* or *Staphylococcus* species with a history of facial trauma.

658. The answer is A. *(Surgery—Trauma)*

CT is preferred over MRI in the setting of acute trauma, and contrast material is not used. This reduces any confusion about the presence of an intracranial bleed (contrast material and blood both appear white on a standard CT scan). Plain skull films are nearly obsolete for acute trauma because they cannot detect most life-threatening intracranial injuries. Positron emission tomography (i.e., PET) scanning and MRI generally are not used in the setting of acute trauma, but have both played a role in improving our understanding of pathophysiology and prognosis in closed-head injury.

659. The answer is D. *(Surgery—Trauma)*

Flail chest describes a situation in which a portion of the chest wall moves paradoxically during respiration (in during inspiration, out during expiration). It is seen most commonly in patients with multiple, multifocal rib fractures. These patients may need to be intubated secondary to the ineffective respirations and frequently associated pulmonary contusions.

660. The answer is C. *(Obstetrics)*

An ultrasound must be done first before a pelvic examination because placenta previa may change from a semiurgent situation to an emergency if the placenta is disturbed on physical examination. Urine drug screen may be appropriate because cocaine increases markedly the risk of placental abruption. A complete blood count is useful to help determine the presence of anemia or infection, although this test is sometimes inaccurate in the setting of hyperacute hemorrhage. Intravenous fluids and maternal and fetal monitoring are basic aspects of care in third-trimester bleeding, as are oxygen and other supportive measures.

661. The answer is A. *(Obstetrics)*

The risks of tocolysis with ritodrine generally outweigh the benefits (i.e., avoid) if the mother has heart disease, hypertension, diabetes, severe hemorrhage, chorioamnionitis, ruptured membranes, or a cervix dilated more than 4 cm. Tocolysis should not be attempted if the fetus has severe intrauterine growth retardation, if the fetus has anomalies incompatible with life, or in the setting of fetal demise. Corticosteroids sometimes are given in the clinical setting described in the question to hasten fetal lung maturity (usually only between 24 and 34 weeks). Amniotic fluid testing to determine whether or not the lungs are mature is preferred before giving the steroids, but in some circumstances they are given empirically. Hydralazine is known to be safe in pregnancy and would be an appropriate choice for blood pressure control. The other choices are fairly routine and though they may not make a big difference, they wouldn't hurt either.

662. The answer is C. *(Obstetrics)*

A vertex presentation is the normal presentation and its absence is a cause for performing caesarian section. Early decelerations indicate fetal head compression from uterine contractions and are a normal part of the labor process. The other choices are all indications for cesarean section.

663. The answer is E. *(Pharmacology)*

Tricyclic antidepressants have anticholinergic and adrenergic alpha$_1$ receptor antagonism properties and typically cause tachycardia when they affect the heart rate. Blurry vision (paralysis of accommodation), dry mouth, urinary hesitancy, tachycardia, and constipation all may result from the anticholinergic effects. Orthostatic hypotension may result from alpha$_1$ blockade. Tricyclic antidepressants also cause sedation, lower the seizure threshold, and can be fatal in overdose secondary to ventricular arrhythmias. For these reasons, most clinicians use serotonin-specific reuptake inhibitors instead of tricyclic antidepressants when possible.

664. The answer is C. (Psychiatry—General)

This woman is having a major depressive episode, which can be triggered by a stressful event or underlying illness (a classic atypical presentation of pancreatic cancer is depression). It is more common in women than men and is treated best by psychotherapy *and* medications. If you had to choose between the two treatments, medications alone are thought to be more effective than psychotherapy alone. Appetite classically is depressed but can be increased, just as insomnia is the classic sleep disturbance, but hypersomnia can occur (increased appetite and hypersomnolence are termed *atypical* depression symptoms). Severe depression can result in psychosis with mood-consistent hallucinations and delusions and may require antipsychotics in addition to antidepressants.

665. The answer is E. (Psychiatry—General)

Although there are no 100% predictors (i.e., bogus question), the most potent risk factors for suicide are age greater than 45, alcoholism, and past suicidal attempt (not gesture). Other strong risk factors are a history of violence, male sex, and a person unwilling to accept help. Depression is associated with suicide, as are single status, drug abuse, other psychiatric illnesses (especially schizophrenia), recent loss or separation, loss of physical health, debilitating chronic disease, and unemployment. Higher social status also is associated with an increased risk of suicide, as is a family history of suicide.

666. The answer is C. (Biostatistics)

The positive predictive value is calculated by dividing the number of true positives by the total number of people with a positive test result. In this case, there were 3000 true positives out of the 4000 people who tested positive for the disease: $3000/4000 = 0.75 = 75\%$.

667. The answer is C. (Medicine—Neurology)

This woman had the most common form of dementia: Alzheimer dementia. Neurofibrillary tangles and amyloid deposition are typical. With memory loss in dementia, recent memory is often the first to go, while distant memories are preserved. Affected patients can tell you about the "good old days," but can't remember yesterday. Most affected patients are over the age of 70 and minor histopathologic features of Alzheimer's are increasingly seen with age even in the absence of clinical dementia.

668. The answer is A. (Medicine—Geriatrics)

Lack of sexual desire and impotence are not normal and should be investigated. The other choices are recognized changes that occur in sexual functioning with age. Estrogen cream or lubricants may be used to improve the vaginal dryness that may occur in elderly women.

669. The answer is C. (Medicine—Neurology)

Despite the dramatic presentation of a tonic-clonic or grand mal seizure, most seizures stop on their own within a few minutes. Most treatment is supportive and includes putting the patient on his or her side to prevent aspiration, possibly inserting a soft (plastic) tongue blade to prevent tongue lacerations (be wary of putting your finger in a patient's mouth in this setting - you may lose the finger), giving oxygen, and starting an intravenous line to administer antiseizure medication. Although malingering is possible, the patient would have to be quite an actor to urinate on himself while having clonic muscular contractions. Death from seizure activity is rare and often due to complications of the seizure (aspiration, hypoxia) rather than primary brain damage, which is not thought to occur except in the rare case of prolonged, uninterrupted seizures (i.e., prolonged status epilepticus).

670. The answer is D. *(Medicine—Nutrition)*

Folate is not associated with peripheral neuropathy, an important differential diagnostic point when dealing with a megaloblastic anemia because vitamin B_{12} deficiency can cause neurologic symptoms. The peripheral neuropathy of thiamine (i.e., dry beri beri) and pyridoxine (patients taking long-term isoniazid) deficiency are classic nutrition questions and wrist or foot drop is a common presentation for lead toxicity in adults. Vitamin E and riboflavin deficiencies have also been listed as causes of peripheral neuropathy.

671. The answer is C. *(Medicine—Neurology)*

Benign causes of oculomotor nerve lesions, such as small vessel disease from hypertension, diabetes, or both, usually spare the pupil. More serious causes, such as tumor, aneurysm, or brain stem infarction, usually cause the pupil to be involved (dilated and nonreactive or *blown*). In hypoglossal nerve lesions, the tongue deviates toward the side of the lesion, and in spinal accessory nerve lesions, the person has trouble turning the head to the side opposite of the lesion. A vestibulocochlear lesion usually produces deafness, tinnitus, or both, not hyperacusis (i.e. an increased sensitivity to sound that causes everything to sound loud).

Proximal facial nerve lesions may cause hyperacusis as a result of stapedial muscle paralysis and lack of dampening as sound enters the middle ear. Upper versus lower motor facial nerve lesions are differentiated by the fact that upper motor neuron lesions spare the forehead on the affected side, whereas lower motor neuron lesions do not. Facial nerve lesions do not cause bilateral findings (unless both the left and right facial nerves are involved).

672. The answer is D. *(Dermatology)*

The patient has acne vulgaris or acne for short. Blockage of pilosebaceous glands and the bacteria *Propionibacterium acnes* are thought to be partially responsible for acne. Acne has not been proved to be associated with food, exercise, sex, or masturbation. The first treatment usually is topical benzoyl peroxide, then topical or oral antibiotics to help eliminate *P. acnes*. Topical vitamin A derivatives are used for more resistant cases. A last resort is oral isotretinoin, which is highly effective but can result in liver damage, muscle and joint pain, dry skin and mucosae, and teratogenesis.

673. The answer is C. *(Pediatrics—Infectious Disease)*

Thrush is a form of *Candida* infection that usually responds to topical therapy (such as a nystatin oral rinse) but is resistant to griseofulvin. Thrush is a normal occurrence in children, and *Candida* vulvovaginitis is extremely common in pregnant women and women who are given antibiotics. These conditions represent an alteration in normal flora, not a transmissible infection. If thrush or other *Candida* infection occurs in other populations (i.e., adult men), you should think of diabetes or a possible immune deficiency. Being able to scrape the white patches off makes you confident that you are dealing with *Candida* and not leukoplakia or another more worrisome condition.

674. The answer is C. *(Medicine—Infectious Disease)*

Pseudomonas aeruginosa colonies produce a bluish pigment and give off a fruity aroma. This organism is one of the most common causes of a burn wound infection, along with *Staphylococcus* and *Streptococcus* (which do not produce bluish pigments or a fruity aroma).

675. The answer is D. *(Medicine—Infectious Disease)*

This woman most likely has developed pseudomembranous colitis from overgrowth of toxin producing *Clostridium difficile*. Any broad-spectrum antibiotic can cause this phenomenon, not just the classically described clindamycin. The treatment of choice is metronidazole; the second-line agent is oral vancomycin. Pseudomembranes can be seen during sigmoidoscopy and are confirmatory if seen, though a positive stool test for *C. difficile* toxin provides enough evidence to begin treatment in the appropriate setting.

676. The answer is B. *(Medicine—Infectious Disease)*

Bacillus cereus classically is associated with reheated fried rice. The spores survive on the reheated rice and produce an enterotoxin that resembles staphylococcal food poisoning. Because a preformed toxin is involved, symptoms start within several hours of eating the contaminated food. *Salmonella* and hepatitis A involve a longer incubation period.

677. The answer is D. *(Preventive Medicine)*

Schistosoma is a genus of trematode referred to as a *blood fluke* that is common in the Middle East and Africa. *S. haematobium* resides in the veins draining the urinary bladder and lays its eggs into the wall of the bladder, resulting in chronic inflammation and scarring of the bladder. This condition may lead to squamous cell carcinoma of the bladder. Smoking is estimated to cause roughly 30-50% of all bladder cancer in the United States. Aniline dye commonly is used in the rubber and dye industries, and exposure has been linked to bladder cancer. Chronic cyclophosphamide and phenacetin (an analgesic, prodrug of acetaminophen not available in the United States) use have been linked to bladder cancer, but alcohol use has not.

678. The answer is C. *(Pediatrics—Infectious Disease)*

Viral causes, notably rotavirus and the Norwalk virus, are thought to be more common causes of gastroenteritis in children than bacterial causes.

679. The answer is D. *(Medicine—Oncology)*

Metastatic tumors account for about half of all intracranial tumors in adults. The most common offenders are lung, breast, and melanoma, accounting for about 75% of all cases. The most common primary brain tumors are gliomas, of which astrocytomas are by far the most common (oligodendrogliomas and ependymomas are the other two less common glial neoplasms). Astrocytomas range from low grade (well-differentiated) to highly aggressive (glioblastoma multiforme). The other choices—meningiomas (arise from dura), acoustic neuromas (8th cranial nerve), and choroid plexus papillomas (ventricles)—are not only less common but occur outside the brain parenchyma.

680. The answer is A. *(Preventive Medicine)*

Oral contraceptive pills have been shown to decrease the incidence of ovarian and endometrial cancer. Maternal folate reduces neural tube defects, but not Down syndrome, in offspring. A thin body habitus, smoking, and sedentary lifestyle increase the risk of osteoporosis, while obesity lowers the risk. Cryptorchidism increases the risk of testicular cancer regardless of whether or not surgical correction is performed, though some think a mild reduction in cancer risk exists. High parity increases the risk of cervical cancer, but decreases the risk of breast and endometrial cancer.

681. The answer is E. *(Gynecology)*

The role of human papillomavirus and possibly herpes simplex virus and others is thought to be the primary factor associated with cervical cancer. Epidemiologic studies have shown that multiple partners and sleeping with promiscuous persons are the most potent risk factors. The peak incidence of cervical cancer is in the 35 to 55 age group, declining after this peak. Alcohol abuse has not been associated with cervical cancer, but smoking, birth control pills, and low socioeconomic status have been. Nulliparity protects against cervical cancer, whereas it increases the risk of breast and endometrial cancer.

682. The answer is A. *(Ophthalmology)*

The appearance of the fundus is highly characteristic and classic for central retinal artery occlusion, which presents with sudden, painless, unilateral blindness. The cause often is an embolism or thrombosis. Treatment rarely is satisfactory. Make sure to watch for symptoms of cranial or temporal arteritis if a patient presents with this condition because steroids can prevent the condition from becoming progressing and/or becoming bilateral. Acute glaucoma (i.e., attack of closed-angle glaucoma) usually causes severe pain with nausea and headaches.

683. The answer is C. *(Ophthalmology)*

The time frame and highly purulent appearance make gonococcal conjunctivitis the most likely diagnosis. Chemical conjunctivitis usually occurs in the first 24 hours of life and almost always is gone by 48 hours. It is due to a reaction to prophylactic eye drops that may be instilled to prevent gonococcal conjunctivitis and does not generally cause purulence. Chlamydial (inclusion) conjunctivitis usually presents 5 to 14 days after birth. Gonococcal conjunctivitis usually presents 2 to 5 days after birth. Treatment includes systemic antigonococcal antibiotics (e.g., ceftriaxone) and adjuvant topical antibiotic ointment, such as erythromycin. Allergic and viral conjunctivitis are unlikely to produce significant purulence.

684. The answer is E. *(Surgery—General)*

A Nissen fundoplication and other procedures for reflux involve reinforcement of the lower esophageal sphincter to prevent reflux from occurring. Endoscopic treatments have shown promise and may be used more in the future. Vagotomy and antrectomy are used for peptic ulcer disease, myotomy is used for achalasia and esophageal spastic disorders, and esophagectomy is used for esophageal cancer or severe esophageal strictures.

685. The answer is C. *(Pediatrics—Neonates)*

Necrotizing enterocolitis almost always is seen in the first month of life, rarely in the second month, and almost never after that. Onset of symptoms after the second month of life should prompt a search for an alternative diagnosis. The more premature the child and the less he or she weighs, the higher the risk of necrotizing enterocolitis. The sickest infants in the neonatal ICU with cardiac defects, respiratory distress syndrome, sepsis, and other severe health problems are the classic victims of this life-threatening condition. Abdominal distention, vomiting, or blood in the stool usually are present. The bowel loops become distended on abdominal radiograph, and pneumatosis intestinalis, which is air within the walls of the bowel, is considered essentially pathognomonic in the appropriate patient population. Shock and death may occur, especially in severe forms of this condition. Surgical resection of bowel may be needed for bowel perforation or subsequent stricture development.

686. The answer is D. *(General Knowledge and Principles)*

This patient is "in good spirits" and able to speak at length, not characteristics of someone needing intubation. A trial of nasal cannula oxygen is appropriate. Antibiotics may be appropriate later in the work-up, but the shortness of breath may be due to lung cancer, in which case, antibiotics would not do any good. A chest radiograph should be obtained first given the absence of specific infectious symptoms. In *chronic lungers*, arterial blood gases may reveal dangerous-looking numbers, but these patients often are used to living at this level. In other words, treat the patient, not the laboratory value.

687. The answer is A. *(Medicine—Cardiology)*

Asymptomatic premature ventricular complexes should not be treated, even in the setting of a myocardial infarction. Should these become symptomatic or should ventricular tachycardia develop, amiodarone or lidocaine is the preferred treatment.

688. The answer is C. *(Medicine—Pulmonology)*

This patient most likely has sleep apnea and has developed cor pulmonale, or right-sided heart pathology secondary to lung disease. His cardiac findings indicate a hypertrophied, noncompliant right ventricle with probable pulmonary hypertension. These patients often have a respiratory acidosis at night (and sometimes during the day with significant obesity) secondary to apnea. Primary pulmonary hypertension is an idiopathic disorder that usually appears in women age 20 to 40 who have no discernible cause for pulmonary hypertension.

689. The answer is B. *(Medicine—Cardiology)*

Digoxin is not a first-line agent in the treatment of mild CHF because it has failed to show a survival benefit and has significant toxicities. All patients with CHF should be on an angiotensin-converting enzyme inhibitor if they can tolerate it because of the demonstrated reduction in mortality in controlled clinical trials. β-blockers also are first-line agents if they can be tolerated because they are thought to protect the heart from the toxicity of a chronic high catecholamine state that is thought to exist in CHF. Salt restriction, exercise, and smoking cessation are inexpensive adjuncts that improve outcomes. Diuretics may be needed if salt restriction fails to prevent fluid retention and edema. Digoxin usually is reserved for moderate-to-severe CHF and is thought to reduce hospitalizations without improving survival. Venous and arterial dilators are used in moderate-to-severe CHF to reduce preload and afterload.

690. The answer is C. *(Obstetrics)*

This woman is developing uterine hyperstimulation, probably from the oxytocin infusion. Additional uterine-stimulating measures should be avoided (e.g., increasing oxytocin, prostaglandin E_2 gel), and there is no indication for a cesarean section at this time. Oxytocin has an antidiuretic hormone-like effect; hypotonic solutions should be avoided in women receiving oxytocin to prevent dangerous levels of hyponatremia.

691. The answer is D. *(Gynecology)*

This is a classic description of endometriosis, an idiopathic condition that tends to affect reproductive-age women older than 30 and may cause infertility, dyspareunia (painful intercourse), dyschezia (painful defecation), dysmenorrhea, perimenstrual spotting, tender adnexa, retroversion of the uterus, and nodularities of the broad and uterosacral ligaments. The gold standard for diagnosis is laparoscopy, with visualization of the endometrial gland implants on the surface of pelvic organs or the peritoneal surface. Treatment involves oral contraceptive pills, danazol, or gonadotropin-releasing hormone agonists. Destruction of endometrial implants by surgery or cautery may restore fertility in women wishing to conceive. An ovarian teratoma (choice **B**), which is not consistent with this case description, commonly has hair or teeth within it.

692. The answer is B. *(Gynecology)*

Gardnerella generally is not considered a sexually transmitted disease; it is a disturbance in the normal vaginal flora. The other choices accurately describe *Gardnerella* vaginosis. Clue cells are seen on a normal saline preparation and represent epithelial cells with a granular appearance because of bacterial adherence to the cell surface. Choice **C** describes the *whiff* test and is a hallmark of *Gardnerella* vaginosis.

693. The answer is D. *(Medicine—Infectious Disease)*

Primary syphilis usually causes a genital chancre that is painless. The causative agent is *Treponema pallidum*, a thin-walled spiral rod that cannot be seen with Gram staining but can be seen using dark field microscopy. *Haemophilus ducreyi* is a gram-negative coccobacillus that causes the sexually-transmitted disease *chancroid*. A maculopapular rash involving the palms and soles is highly suggestive of secondary syphilis in the right setting. Screening for syphilis is done with non-specific, easy-to-perform nontreponemal antigen tests that look for an antibody reaction to cardiolipin. The most common examples of this test are the VDRL (Venereal Disease Research Laboratory) and RPR (rapid plasmin reagin). Specific serologic tests, such as FTA-ABS or MHA-TP (microhemagglutination test for antibodies to *Treponema pallidum*), are confirmatory tests done if the screen is positive. The VDRL and RPR often gradually become normal after treatment (agent of choice is still penicillin) of syphilis, whereas the FTA-ABS and MHA-TP typically remain positive for life, losing their diagnostic value after the first case of syphilis.

694. The answer is E. *(Biostatistics)*

The negative predictive value is defined as the number of true negatives divided by the total number of people who tested negative for the disease. In this case, 96,000 people tested negative for the disease, but only 94,000 of those were true negatives: $94,000/96,000 = 0.98 = > 95\%$.

695–699. *(General Knowledge and Principles)*

The answers are the following: 695. A   696. D   697. B   698. F   699. A.

This is an exercise in applying clinical likelihood or pretest probability to real situations. Diabetics are much more likely to have atypical chest pain (or none at all) with coronary disease, and the two examples given with choice **A** as an answer describe patients with numerous cardiac risk factors and relation to exertion and stress. Esophageal spasm or nutcracker esophagus can cause severe chest pain, and a history of precipitation by different temperatures is highly suggestive, especially in someone at low risk for heart disease. The 37-year-old man with pericarditis does not have a family history strong enough to consider it a cardiac risk factor, and the sudden onset with minimal exertion is not characteristic of angina. The history of a sore throat a week prior is important historically. The patient who gets chest pain when lying down at night has classic symptoms of reflux disease. The patient with peptic ulcer has a gnawing sensation, a classic description of peptic ulcer disease, accompanied by improvement with food (characteristic of duodenal ulcers). These questions may test one's patience with the phrase "best possible answer" because there is definite overlap and more than one possible right answer.

700. The answer is E. *(Medicine—Infectious Disease)*

The figure and clinical description are consistent with scabies, which is caused by the mite *Sarcoptes scabei*. It is contagious and can be acquired from persons that are household or sexual contacts. Treatment is typically with topical permethrin or lindane (less commonly used due to neurotoxicity concerns). Decontamination of bed sheets and linens and treatment of at-risk contacts are important measures to help prevent recurrence.

ANSWERS AND EXPLANATIONS

701. The answer is C. *(Psychiatry—General)*

This patient is acutely suicidal and needs inpatient psychiatric treatment, against her will if necessary. If patients are a danger to themselves or others, they can (and should) be admitted temporarily against their will for treatment. If you let this patient leave the emergency department, she may go out and commit suicide. Prescribing an antidepressant and scheduling an outpatient appointment is not enough in this setting.

702. The answer is E. *(Pediatrics—Infectious Disease)*

This child most likely has croup, also known as *acute laryngotracheitis*. Croup usually affects children age 1 to 2 in the fall or winter, and about 50% to 75% of cases are caused by the parainfluenza virus, with most of the other cases caused by the influenza virus. Treatment is largely supportive, with humidified oxygen and bronchodilators. The *steeple* sign (narrowing of the subglottic trachea) on frontal chest radiograph is classic but nonspecific. The diagnosis is typically clinical.

703. The answer is C. *(Pediatrics—Infectious Disease)*

This infant is quite sick and may have bacterial meningitis. The ABCs come first. Questions such as this can be frustrating because you want to choose two different answers. The infant should have a lumbar puncture, but initial therapy is more important than initial diagnosis in some situations. Lumbar puncture may give you a diagnosis but does not immediately help the infant survive the next 24 hours, whereas intravenous fluids and empirical antibiotics may.

704. The answer is C. *(Obstetrics)*

Fetal heart monitoring is done routinely, but is controversial in terms of the benefit gained. At term, the normal fetal heart rate is 120 to 160 beats/min. Outside this range is worrisome. Basic fetal heart strips with accompanying uterine contraction patterns have shown up on previous USMLE administrations. *Early decelerations*, when the peaks match up (fetal heart deceleration nadir and uterine contraction peak), usually signify head compression (probable vagal response) and are normal. *Variable decelerations*, meaning the decelerations are variable with relation to uterine contractions, are the most commonly encountered type and usually signify cord compression. *Late decelerations*, in which the fetal heart decelerations come after uterine contractions, usually signify uteroplacental insufficiency. This is the most worrisome pattern.

Short-term variability (beat-to-beat variability) reflects the interval between successive heart beats. Normal is 5 to 25 beats/min. When variability is consistently less than 5 beats/min, this is worrisome, especially when combined with decelerations. Increased variability is not usually a problem and is not particularly worrisome as an isolated occurrence. *Long-term variability* means that when looking over a 1-minute strip, there are normally changes in the baseline heart rate. Less than three cycles per minute is worrisome, especially when combined with decelerations. Long-term variability is decreased normally during fetal sleep.

705. The answer is A. *(Pediatrics—Neonates)*

A fairly common complication of maternal diabetes is fetal hypoglycemia in the postpartum period. This is due to fetal islet-cell hypertrophy caused by maternal and fetal hyperglycemia during the pregnancy. After birth, the infant is cut off from the mother's glucose supply, and the hyperglycemia goes away, but the hypertrophied islet cells still overproduce insulin and cause hypoglycemia. Although classically associated with fetal macrosomia, advanced diabetes with vascular complications can result in a microsomic (i.e., intrauterine growth retardation or small for gestational age) fetus. Polyhydramnios and preeclampsia are increased in mothers with diabetes. Other fetal complications of maternal diabetes include respiratory distress syndrome and an increased risk of congenital abnormalities (common are cardiac, colon, craniofacial, and neural tube defects; caudal regression rare but classic).

706. The answer is A. *(Obstetrics)*

Prostaglandin E_2 gel, also known as *dinoprostone*, commonly is used in conjunction with oxytocin to augment or hasten labor. Amniotomy also may be used, but carries a risk of infection if labor does not occur. Ritodrine, oxygen, and fluids often are used in an attempt to arrest labor or premature contractions. Indomethacin is generally avoided in late pregnancy because of concerns over premature ductus arteriosus closure.

707. The answer is B. *(Surgery—General)*

Adhesions are the most common cause of small bowel obstruction in adults overall in the United States. Adhesions are unlikely in the absence of previous surgery or trauma, however, and incarcerated hernia is the most likely cause in such a group (probably the second most common cause overall as well). Small bowel neoplasms are a less common cause of small bowel obstruction, whereas colonic neoplasm is a common cause of *large* bowel obstruction. Peritonitis can cause an ileus, but does not itself generally cause bowel obstruction. Malrotation with midgut volvulus, Meckel diverticuli and intussusception are more common causes of small bowel obstruction in the pediatric age group, though they can sometimes occur in adults.

708. The answer is D. *(Surgery—General)*

Endoscopic decompression can be used to treat sigmoid or gastric volvulus, but is not generally used to manage small bowel obstruction. The other choices describe standard small bowel obstruction management tools. If the obstruction is not relieved by medical or conservative management, surgical intervention generally is required to relieve the obstruction.

709–716. *(General Knowledge and Principles)*

The answers are the following: 709. A 710. B 711. A 712. C 713. A 714. B 715. A 716. C.

In many diseases, using epidemiology can help you concentrate your efforts toward specific diseases. For example, in 90% of cases, systemic lupus erythematosus affects women. Between the ages of 20 and 50, urinary tract infections are at least 20 times more common in women than men. Hirschsprung disease is 5 times more common in males. This type of striking difference in sex-related incidence can make certain differential diagnoses less likely. Hemophilia is X-linked, so it is much more likely in men. AIDS is still more common in men in the United States, although the rate of HIV seropositivity in women is increasing because of heterosexual spread. Alcoholism is about 2 times more likely in males compared with females and depression is twice as common in females. Phenylketonuria follows autosomal recessive inheritance patterns and so has no sex predilection. Schizophrenia does not have a gender predilection, but symptoms begin roughly 10 years earlier in men (commonly at 15–25) compared with women (classically at 25–35).

717. The answer is B. *(Medicine—Gastroenterology)*

This patient has celiac disease (or celiac sprue) and the related dermatitis herpetiformis. Both are related to a dietary intolerance to the gliadin portion of gluten (a wheat protein), not herpes. Antigliadin antibodies are often present in those affected and HLA studies have suggested a genetic predisposition (e.g., higher incidence of HLA-DR3 in those with celiac disease). The disease results in the histopathological appearance described in choice **A**, which leads to malabsorption and diarrhea with steatorrhea (abnornmally high fat content in the stool). Choice **C** is true.

718. The answer is C. *(Dermatology)*

This patient has findings consistent onychomycosis (i.e., tinea unguium), a fungal infection of the nails, as well as an infection between his toes (tinea pedis or "athlete's foot"), which are commonly seen together. Most cases are caused by *Trichophyton* species and treatment with oral antifungals (e.g., terbinafine, itraconazole, fluconazole) for at least 2 months is typically needed to clear the infection.

719. The answer is B. *(Biostatistics)*

Prevalence is defined as the ratio of the number of people with a given condition to the number of people in the population of interest. It can be expressed in different formats (e.g., 1/250, 4/1000). In this case, because 5000 out of 100,000 people have the disease, one way to express the prevalence would be 50/1000.

720. The answer is D. *(Biostatistics)*

The patient has a lesion that is most suggestive of squamous cell carcinoma (SCC), which does occasionally (≤ 5% of cases) metastasize. Like other skin cancers, SCC tends to affect sun-exposed, light-skinned persons. Actinic keratosis is a precursor to SCC and is classically described as reddish-brown papules and/or plaques with dry, rough, adherent scales. More severe cases often need biopsy to exclude SCC and destruction of the affected skin is part of the management to prevent malignant transformation. Once people have developed one skin cancer, they should be examined periodically for life to detect new lesions due to their significantly increased risk.

721. The answer is C. *(Medicine—Neurology)*

Kernig's and *Brudzinski's* signs are the hallmark physical findings in meningitis, although often absent in young children. The most common headaches are tension headaches, which most normal people experience at one point in their lives. These are thought to be related mainly to stress, are often bilateral, and generally respond to acetaminophen or aspirin and stress reduction. Cluster headaches are so called because they occur in temporal clusters, not in relation to the time of day, but related to the fact that they may not occur for months, then occur several times a day. They often are unilateral with symptoms of vasodilation on the affected side. Migraines often are associated with a family history, aura (e.g., seeing shimmering lights before the headache begins), and nausea and vomiting and may be unilateral (classic) or bilateral.

722. The answer is E. *(Medicine—Neurology)*

A normal arousal and attention level usually indicates dementia and should steer you away from a diagnosis of delirium. HIV can make things confusing because HIV-induced dementia is a well-recognized clinical entity, but severe illness can result in episodes of delirium. The other choices occur in both delirium and dementia and are not useful in differentiating the two. Acute onset and reversibility are much more common with delirium.

723. The answer is D. *(Medicine—Neurology)*

Transient ischemic attacks and strokes rarely cause syncope unless the vertebrobasilar system is involved, and in these cases, there are usually other symptoms that coexist and make the diagnosis more apparent. The exact cause of syncope is rarely found. The most common cause of syncope is labeled as vasovagal and classically occurs in the setting of fatigue and/or an unpleasant emotional experience (e.g., fear, stress). The other choices are uncommon causes for syncope, but history is often the best aid in determining the cause. For example, vasovagal syncope often has symptoms just before the loss of consciousness (e.g., nausea, weakness, dizziness), whereas some cardiac arrhythmias may cause more abrupt onset of syncope.

724. The answer is A. *(Gynecology)*

Although all of the choices are possibilities, *Candida* is the most likely, especially given the history of recent antibiotic use, diabetic status, and the whitish color of the discharge. Some physicians give reliable female patients an antifungal prescription to be used if needed when they prescribe antibiotics because the likelihood is fairly high that candidiasis will develop in this setting.

725. The answer is A. *(Gynecology)*

This patient meets the criteria for pelvic inflammatory disease (PID), including abdominal pain, adnexal tenderness, and cervical motion tenderness. She also has a low-grade temperature and leukocytosis, which are minor diagnostic criteria for PID. The most common cause is *Chlamydia*, but these infections frequently can be polymicrobial with coexisting gonorrhea, *E. coli*, or others. *Actinomyces* is associated with intrauterine device (IUD) use.

Although IUDs increase the risk of PID, most women with PID have never used an IUD. IUDs are generally avoided in younger women because of the increased PID risk. The bone marrow is normal in this condition. Methotrexate sometimes is used to induce abortion in the setting of ectopic pregnancy, but this patient has a negative pregnancy test, and methotrexate is not used to treat PID. Treatment usually involves the use of more than one antibiotic in an attempt to cover multiple organisms (e.g., levofloxacin plus metronidazole, cefotetan plus doxycycline), often on an inpatient basis in adolescents and more severe cases.

726. The answer is C. *(Dermatology)*

This patient has the classic lesions of psoriasis, which is much more common in whites. Lesions classically appear on the extensor surfaces of the elbows, knees, or both. Family history often is positive, and the condition generally begins between the ages of 10 and 40. Pitting of the nails and arthritis that clinically resembles rheumatoid arthritis may occur (although rheumatoid factor is negative). Biopsy can provide a diagnosis if needed, but appearance alone often is sufficient to make a diagnosis. Treatment involves UV light, keratolytics (e.g., coal tar, salicylic acid), lubricants, and steroids.

727. The answer is D. *(Dermatology)*

Chronic liver disease and cirrhosis often are associated with decreased body hair. The other choices have well-characterized associations with hirsutism.

728. The answer is D. *(Medicine—Oncology)*

Bowel obstruction is one of the major causes of death in ovarian cancer. Krukenberg's and Meigs' syndrome definitions were reversed in choices **A** and **B**, Ovarian Sertoli-Leydig cell tumors usually cause virilization (granulosa/theca cell tumors cause feminization and precocious puberty), and most ovarian malignancies arise from ovarian epithelium (not germ cells). The most common type is the serous cystadenocarcinoma, which often contains *psammoma bodies* histologically.

729. The answer is C. *(Medicine—General)*

This question tries to trick you by describing a dramatic health care worker, which should make you suspicious of factitious disorder. The numbers do not lie in this case, however—an elevated c-peptide level at the same time as an elevated insulin level means a likely insulinoma. Surreptitious insulin use would cause a decreased to normal c-peptide level, and chlorpropamide abuse would show up on the sulfonylurea screen. Glucagonomas and somatization disorder do not produce hypoglycemia.

730. The answer is C. *(Medicine—Hematology)*

Hereditary spherocytosis usually causes increased red blood cell fragility (or positive osmotic fragility test) and does not cause a positive Coombs' test. Antibody-mediated autoimmune hemolysis, in which cells often are destroyed in the spleen, may cause spherocytes to be seen on the peripheral smear as a result of incomplete phagocytosis of the red blood cells.

731. The answer is D. *(Medicine—Hematology)*

This patient has developed anemia secondary to severe renal insufficiency and will probably need to go on hemodialysis soon. Her creatinine clearance is in the range of 15, when renal failure is commonly diagnosed. Her kidneys are no longer able to manufacture the required erythropoietin. Although chronic disease is a possibility, you would expect the ferritin to be elevated and the iron-binding capacity to be decreased. There is little to support a diagnosis of iron or folate deficiency with a normocytic anemia and a normal peripheral smear. Corticosteroids may help with an autoimmune anemia, for which there is no evidence.

732. The answer is D. *(Medicine—Hematology)*

This woman is stable with fatigue as her only complaint and does not need a transfusion at this time. Do not transfuse based on a number—there is no such thing as a *trigger* value that mandates transfusion. Because the underlying cause has presumably been corrected, oral iron therapy is all that is required. Intravenous iron therapy can be dangerous and carries a risk of anaphylaxis; simple oral replacement is adequate. The duration of therapy usually is at least 3 months to replete the body's iron stores; a reticulocytosis will occur and hemoglobin will start to rise within a week or two.

733. The answer is D. *(Medicine—Hematology)*

This patient has most likely developed myelophthisic anemia, or anemia caused by invasion or infiltration of the bone marrow, in this case from breast cancer. The peripheral smear is classic for this condition, especially with a history of breast cancer that was treated partly with chemotherapy, usually implying tumor spread to at least one axillary lymph node. Although acute leukemia is possible and could present like this, it would be less likely given the history of breast cancer. Chemotherapy can increase the risk of future blood dyscrasias, but this would be uncommon with a single, short course of chemotherapy. A bone marrow biopsy should be performed next to confirm the diagnosis.

734. The answer is B. *(Medicine—General)*

This patient needs dialysis given his severe metabolic acidosis, hyperkalemia with dangerous electrocardiographic changes, and congestive heart failure evidenced by bilateral crackles in the lung fields. In the meantime, oral potassium binders are not the best measure in a severely hyperkalemic patient because they take too long to work—they would not be harmful, just not the best immediate treatment. The patient should have more immediate measures for hyperkalemia, including intravenous calcium gluconate (cardioprotective), intravenous insulin (with glucose to prevent hypoglycemia), or possibly nebulized beta agonists, both of which drive potassium intracellularly. The patient has only "mild" respiratory distress, thus a trial of oxygen via nasal cannula or face mask should be instituted before proceeding to intubation.

735. The answer is C. *(Medicine—General)*

Wegener's granulomatosis often results in nasal or sinus and kidney damage (as well as lung damage) and is characterized by the presence of positive cytoplasmic antineutrophil cytoplasmic antibody titers. Treatment involves immunosuppression with cyclophosphamide, corticosteroids, or other medications. The other choices (including Goodpasture syndrome) don't have sinonasal involvement or a positive cytoplasmic-type antineutrophil cytoplasmic antibody (i.e., C-ANCA) titer.

736. The answer is C. *(Radiology)*

Intravenous contrast material may precipitate acute renal failure, especially in patients with preexisting renal disease. Oral and intravenous hydration before and after administration of contrast material can help to prevent this dreaded complication. In the absence of a suggestive history of allergy to iodine or contrast material, pretreatment with antihistamines or corticosteroids or testing for an iodine allergy is not indicated.

737. The answer is A. *(Medicine—Nephrology)*

This patient most likely has primary hyperaldosteronism, also called *Conn's syndrome*, secondary to an adrenal adenoma. Renin is low in the presence of hypokalemia, hypernatremia, new-onset hypertension, and increased volume status (as evidenced by the ankle edema). Congestive heart failure, renal artery stenosis (which may cause an abdominal bruit), and dehydration should cause an elevated level of renin. Nephrotic syndrome should cause hypoalbuminemia.

738. The answer is A. *(Medicine—Endocrinology)*

This patient probably has Cushing syndrome. This diagnosis is best confirmed by a 24-hour urine cortisol test or a dexamethasone suppression test. Random cortisol is not as good a test because there is wide intraperson and interperson variability, making interpretation of results more difficult.

739. The answer is A. *(Pharmacology)*

Long-term steroids often are prescribed for severe idiopathic thrombocytopenia. Steroids do not generally affect platelet numbers negatively, may increase red blood cell counts, and can cause lymphopenia with increased neutrophil counts. The other choices are known side effects of steroids.

740. The answer is A. *(Obstetrics)*

Pituitary infarction classically occurs during childbirth complicated by postpartum hemorrhage and hypotension. Prolactin (women often note an inability to breast-feed) and/or other pituitary hormones (e.g., TSH in this case) are not produced, leading to presenting symptoms. Affected patients often require hormone supplementation for life. Turner syndrome patients are sterile; Noonan syndrome is best thought of as the male form of Turner syndrome. Trousseau syndrome is migratory thrombophlebitis seen with a visceral malignancy.

741. The answer is A. *(Medicine—Endocrinology)*

The thyroid gland usually takes up excessive amounts of iodine in a diffuse pattern, resulting in a *hot* scan. The other findings are common in Graves' disease.

742. The answer is B. *(Medicine—Gastroenterology)*

If the solutes that are not being absorbed are no longer ingested, the diarrhea generally should stop when the cause is malabsorption. Colon cancer can cause diarrhea. Giardiasis characteristically involves the small bowel, causing steatorrhea. White blood cells in the stool usually mean an invasive or inflammatory diarrhea, not secretory diarrhea. Diarrhea, especially in children, can be a nonspecific manifestation of any systemic disorder and when infectious, is often viral.

743. The answer is E. *(Medicine—Gastroenterology)*

Although external hemorrhoids may bleed in the absence of pain, there is commonly at least a history of pain from inflamed hemorrhoids and often pain during the acute episode. The other choices characteristically cause painless bleeding.

744. The answer is D. *(Medicine—Gastroenterology)*

Achlorhydria, or lack of hydrochloric acid in the stomach, is associated with pernicious anemia because the acid-secreting cells of the fundus are destroyed by antiparietal cell antibodies. The other conditions are generally associated with normal or increased gastric acid secretion.

745. The answer is C. *(Medicine—Gastroenterology)*

Duodenal ulcers are associated strongly with *H. pylori,* and eradication of this organism improves cure rates and decreases recurrences of this disorder. Duodenal ulcers have a peak incidence in middle age and are three times as common as gastric ulcers. The pain of duodenal ulcers classically improves with eating, then worsens again 2 to 3 hours later.

746. The answer is C. *(Surgery—General)*

Although not totally responsible, hiatal hernias are thought to increase the risk of gastroesophageal reflux. In this common condition, the esophageal junction and a portion of the stomach slide above the diaphragm, often intermittently. This is in contrast to less common paraesophageal hernias, in which the gastroesophageal junction remains below the diaphragm and a part of the stomach herniates into the thorax. Paraesophageal hernias are prone to strangulation and often are corrected surgically if discovered, whereas hiatal hernias usually are benign. Strangulation of sliding-type hernia can occur, but is rare.

747. The answer is A. *(Medicine—Cardiology)*

Though choice **A** is correct, on the USMLE exam, make sure to rule out the other choices as the cause of a congestive heart failure exacerbation before settling on diet or medication noncompliance as the cause.

748. The answer is A. *(Medicine—Cardiology)*

Left-sided heart failure causes orthopnea, paroxysmal nocturnal dyspnea, pulmonary rales, and other respiratory symptoms as fluid backs up into the lungs. Right-sided heart failure causes fluid to back up into the peripheral systemic circulation, causing jugular venous distention, peripheral edema, hepatomegaly, and abdominal fullness or ascites. Fatigue, weakness, and anorexia are nonspecific symptoms that occur in either left-sided or right-sided heart failure. Often, patients have a combination of left-sided and right-sided heart failure because the most common cause of right-sided heart failure is left-sided heart failure.

749. The answer is B. *(Medicine—Cardiology)*

The murmur of aortic stenosis is a harsh systolic ejection murmur that radiates into the carotid arteries, not the axilla, which is where the murmur of mitral regurgitation radiates. Angina, syncope, and congestive heart failure are ominous signs in the setting of aortic stenosis and generally mandate a valve replacement. First hypertrophy occurs as a result of left ventricular enlargement (often not detectable on chest x-ray), then failure and dilation/cardiomegaly occur as the disease progresses. A left-sided S_3 is common in left-sided heart failure.

750. The answer is A. *(Ophthalmology)*

This patient has background diabetic retinopathy, which is treated best with tight diabetic control to slow progression of the ocular disease. Panretinal photocoagulation is used for neovascularization, the most severe form of diabetic retinopathy. Retinal surgery, CT or MRI, and lumbar puncture are not indicated. Steroid drops are not effective in treating this condition. Diabetes is a leading cause of acquired blindness in the United States.

Master Answer Key

1. D	47. F	93. D	139. A	185. E	231. A	277. B	323. A
2. B	48. E	94. B	140. D	186. D	232. A	278. D	324. A
3. A	49. B	95. D	141. C	187. A	233. A	279. C	325. C
4. E	50. C	96. E	142. B	188. D	234. C	280. B	326. C
5. E	51. A	97. B	143. A	189. D	235. C	281. A	327. A
6. A	52. B	98. A	144. C	190. D	236. B	282. E	328. D
7. C	53. B	99. D	145. C	191. J	237. E	283. C	329. C
8. E	54. C	100. C	146. H	192. D	238. B	284. E	330. B
9. B	55. B	101. C	147. G	193. I	239. D	285. A	331. E
10. C	56. A	102. C	148. E	194. B	240. E	286. A	332. A
11. D	57. A	103. B	149. A	195. H	241. B	287. C	333. A
12. C	58. D	104. E	150. F	196. G	242. D	288. D	334. E
13. D	59. B	105. C	151. A	197. C	243. D	289. C	335. E
14. C	60. B	106. A	152. C	198. D	244. C	290. A	336. A
15. A	61. A	107. C	153. C	199. A	245. D	291. D	337. D
16. A	62. A	108. A	154. B	200. B	246. B	292. A	338. A
17. C	63. A	109. B	155. B	201. B	247. A	293. C	339. C
18. D	64. D	110. A	156. D	202. E	248. A	294. E	340. D
19. E	65. A	111. D	157. B	203. D	249. D	295. G	341. H
20. E	66. F	112. C	158. D	204. C	250. A	296. C	342. A
21. C	67. E	113. A	159. B	205. C	251. C	297. A	343. B
22. E	68. B	114. A	160. C	206. B	252. D	298. E	344. G
23. C	69. E	115. E	161. E	207. E	253. D	299. I	345. H
24. B	70. D	116. E	162. E	208. D	254. B	300. G	346. E
25. D	71. A	117. C	163. B	209. A	255. B	301. D	347. A
26. C	72. B	118. E	164. D	210. C	256. B	302. C	348. B
27. A	73. A	119. E	165. D	211. D	257. A	303. D	349. D
28. A	74. C	120. C	166. C	212. C	258. C	304. B	350. C
29. D	75. C	121. E	167. C	213. B	259. D	305. A	351. A
30. E	76. A	122. E	168. C	214. A	260. D	306. B	352. A
31. A	77. E	123. D	169. C	215. C	261. D	307. A	353. B
32. D	78. D	124. B	170. D	216. B	262. A	308. A	354. D
33. A	79. A	125. A	171. B	217. A	263. D	309. D	355. D
34. E	80. D	126. B	172. B	218. B	264. B	310. A	356. A
35. B	81. B	127. B	173. B	219. C	265. D	311. B	357. A
36. A	82. A	128. B	174. B	220. D	266. A	312. C	358. A
37. A	83. D	129. B	175. E	221. D	267. E	313. D	359. E
38. A	84. C	130. B	176. C	222. C	268. E	314. A	360. A
39. I	85. C	131. B	177. B	223. C	269. D	315. A	361. B
40. J	86. C	132. A	178. A	224. C	270. C	316. A	362. D
41. E	87. C	133. D	179. D	225. B	271. E	317. E	363. A
42. G	88. E	134. C	180. A	226. D	272. C	318. A	364. D
43. I	89. C	135. A	181. D	227. A	273. D	319. B	365. E
44. A	90. A	136. A	182. B	228. D	274. C	320. D	366. D
45. E	91. D	137. D	183. E	229. A	275. D	321. B	367. D
46. B	92. B	138. C	184. A	230. A	276. B	322. B	368. A

369. D	417. D	465. C	512. C	560. B	608. A	656. D	704. C
370. A	418. G	466. B	513. C	561. C	609. D	657. A	705. A
371. E	419. P	467. E	514. A	562. D	610. B	658. A	706. A
372. A	420. H	468. D	515. B	563. A	611. B	659. D	707. B
373. A	421. K	469. C	516. B	564. D	612. B	660. C	708. D
374. E	422. A	470. D	517. C	565. C	613. C	661. A	709. A
375. B	423. C	471. C	518. A	566. A	614. D	662. C	710. B
376. A	424. C	472. B	519. C	567. E	615. D	663. E	711. A
377. B	425. B	473. A	520. C	568. E	616. A	664. C	712. C
378. E	426. A	474. B	521. E	569. B	617. C	665. E	713. A
379. E	427. B	475. A	522. C	570. A	618. A	666. C	714. B
380. B	428. C	476. E	523. C	571. A	619. D	667. C	715. A
381. E	429. C	477. B	524. D	572. D	620. C	668. A	716. C
382. E	430. A	478. D	525. D	573. E	621. C	669. C	717. B
383. E	431. C	479. C	526. B	574. D	622. B	670. D	718. C
384. B	432. A	480. A	527. A	575. C	623. E	671. C	719. B
385. A	433. C	481. B	528. E	576. B	624. A	672. D	720. D
386. D	434. A	482. A	529. E	577. E	625. A	673. C	721. C
387. C	435. D	483. D	530. E	578. C	626. A	674. C	722. E
388. E	436. B	484. A	531. E	579. A	627. A	675. D	723. D
389. B	437. D	485. C	532. B	580. A	628. A	676. B	724. A
390. D	438. A	486. D	533. D	581. A	629. C	677. D	725. A
391. A	439. C	487. D	534. E	582. B	630. C	678. C	726. C
392. E	440. D	488. A	535. D	583. D	631. C	679. D	727. D
393. A	441. D	489. C	536. C	584. B	632. A	680. A	728. D
394. A	442. D	490. C	537. A	585. B	633. A	681. E	729. C
395. H	443. B	491. D	538. A	586. A	634. D	682. A	730. C
396. F	444. A	492. E	539. A	587. A	635. D	683. C	731. D
397. E	445. B	493. B	540. B	588. E	636. A	684. E	732. D
398. C	446. B	494. B	541. D	589. C	637. E	685. C	733. D
399. A	447. E	495. C	542. A	590. D	638. A	686. D	734. B
400. C	448. A	496. A, G,	543. A	591. D	639. C	687. A	735. C
401. E	449. B	H, I	544. A	592. C	640. D	688. C	736. C
402. D	450. C	497. G, K	545. C	593. A	641. C	689. B	737. A
403. E	451. D	498. M	546. A	594. A	642. C	690. C	738. A
404. A	452. E	499. D	547. O	595. A	643. A	691. D	739. A
405. C	453. D	500. B	548. J	596. A	644. E	692. B	740. A
406. B	454. A	501. C	549. A	597. C	645. B	693. D	741. A
407. B	455. C	502. B	550. L	598. D	646. C	694. E	742. B
408. D	456. C	503. A	551. C	599. A	647. A	695. A	743. E
409. E	457. B	504. D	552. A	600. B	648. I	696. D	744. D
410. A	458. C	505. B	553. D	601. D	649. B	697. B	745. C
411. D	459. B	506. D	554. D	602. A	650. E	698. F	746. C
412. A	460. E	507. D	555. D	603. C	651. C	699. A	747. A
413. A	461. A	508. A	556. A	604. A	652. A	700. E	748. A
414. O	462. D	509. B	557. C	605. E	653. C	701. C	749. B
415. E	463. A	510. D	558. C	606. B	654. D	702. E	750. A
416. S	464. B	511. E	559. B	607. A	655. D	703. C	

Subject Item Index

BIOSTATISTICS

167–169, 319, 436, 437, 463, 464, 528, 529, 565–567, 642–645, 666, 694, 719, 720

DERMATOLOGY

90, 91, 189, 190, 208, 240, 241, 400, 438, 444, 466, 479, 503, 527, 672, 726, 727

EAR, NOSE, AND THROAT SURGERY

76, 130, 207

EMERGENCY MEDICINE

88, 106, 107, 176, 185, 291, 401

ETHICS

74, 101, 413, 451, 551, 624, 625

GENERAL KNOWLEDGE AND PRINCIPLES

23, 81, 87, 138, 152, 158, 206, 223, 243–250, 261, 279, 282, 286, 317, 323, 328, 329, 356, 414–423, 485, 532, 574, 584, 686, 695–699, 709–716. *See also* Medicine, General

GYNECOLOGY

24, 44, 85, 143, 294, 327, 363, 372, 373, 391, 410, 411, 434, 435, 439, 470, 483, 518, 536, 537, 562, 590–593, 618, 619, 681, 691, 692, 724, 725

LABORATORY MEDICINE

75, 78, 79, 120, 225, 359

MEDICINE—CARDIOLOGY

8, 97, 112, 128, 129, 255, 260, 304, 305, 330, 442, 443, 478, 506, 507, 587, 620, 687, 689, 747–749

MEDICINE—ENDOCRINOLOGY

229, 230, 284, 473, 508, 581, 607, 738, 741

MEDICINE—GASTROENTEROLOGY

32, 182, 234–238, 285, 469, 474, 488, 509, 510, 523, 582, 583, 588, 601, 609, 610, 742–745

MEDICINE—GENERAL

12, 21, 27, 29, 31, 35, 53, 55, 59, 80, 89, 115, 136, 155, 181, 183, 218, 228, 267–269, 271, 272, 274, 276, 283, 292, 293, 302, 312, 350, 351, 358, 368, 369, 512, 580, 585, 586, 608, 611, 621, 622, 729, 734, 735. *See also* General knowledge and principles.

MEDICINE—GERIATRICS

172, 568, 668

MEDICINE—HEMATOLOGY

67, 72, 73, 94–96, 210, 212, 219, 303, 337, 371, 471, 511, 578, 579, 604, 730–733

MEDICINE—IMMUNOLOGY

14, 124, 175

MEDICINE—INFECTIOUS DISEASE

2, 10, 61–66, 117, 121, 133, 173, 174, 187, 188, 202–204, 215, 224, 251–253, 270, 288, 316, 370, 407, 460, 467, 468, 475, 487, 520, 571, 612, 674–676, 693, 700

MEDICINE—NEPHROLOGY

220, 226, 280, 281, 472, 513, 514, 606, 737

MEDICINE—NEUROLOGY

1, 9, 125, 131, 134, 144, 177–179, 197–200, 309, 465, 525, 526, 569, 570, 646–649, 667, 669, 671, 721–723

MEDICINE—NUTRITION

93, 353–355, 496–500, 546–550, 670

MEDICINE—ONCOLOGY

46–50, 92, 205, 209, 277, 278, 313, 318, 357, 360, 361, 366, 394–398, 449, 450, 489, 575, 577, 602, 603, 623, 679, 728

MEDICINE—PATHOLOGY

33, 287, 600

MEDICINE—PULMONOLOGY

265, 367, 476, 490, 505, 613, 614, 650, 688

USMLE Step 2 Mock Exam Answer Sheet

BLOCKS 1–3

Block 1

1	A B C D E
2	A B C D E
3	A B C D E
4	A B C D E
5	A B C D E
6	A B C D E
7	A B C D E
8	A B C D E
9	A B C D E
10	A B C D E
11	A B C D E
12	A B C D E
13	A B C D E
14	A B C D E
15	A B C D E
16	A B C D E
17	A B C D E
18	A B C D E
19	A B C D E
20	A B C D E
21	A B C D E
22	A B C D E
23	A B C D E
24	A B C D E
25	A B C D E
26	A B C D E
27	A B C D E
28	A B C D E
29	A B C D E
30	A B C D E
31	A B C D E
32	A B C D E
33	A B C D E
34	A B C D E
35	A B C D E
36	A B C D E
37	A B C D E
38	A B C D E
39	A B C D E F G H I J
40	A B C D E F G H I J
41	A B C D E F G H I J
42	A B C D E F G H I J
43	A B C D E F G H I J
44	A B C D E
45	A B C D E
46	A B C D E F G H
47	A B C D E F G H
48	A B C D E F G H
49	A B C D E F G H
50	A B C D E F G H

Block 2

51	A B C D E
52	A B C D E
53	A B C D E
54	A B C D E
55	A B C D E
56	A B C D E
57	A B C D E
58	A B C D E
59	A B C D E
60	A B C D E
61	A B C D E F
62	A B C D E F
63	A B C D E F
64	A B C D E F
65	A B C D E F
66	A B C D E F
67	A B C D E
68	A B C D E
69	A B C D E
70	A B C D E
71	A B C D E
72	A B C D E
73	A B C D E
74	A B C D E
75	A B C D E
76	A B C D E
77	A B C D E
78	A B C D E
79	A B C D E
80	A B C D E
81	A B C D E
82	A B C D E
83	A B C D E
84	A B C D E
85	A B C D E
86	A B C D E
87	A B C D E
88	A B C D E
89	A B C D E
90	A B C D E
91	A B C D E
92	A B C D E
93	A B C D E
94	A B C D E
95	A B C D E
96	A B C D E
97	A B C D E
98	A B C D E
99	A B C D E
100	A B C D E

Block 3

101	A B C D E
102	A B C D E
103	A B C D E
104	A B C D E
105	A B C D E
106	A B C D E
107	A B C D E
108	A B C D E
109	A B C D E
110	A B C D E
111	A B C D E
112	A B C D E
113	A B C D E
114	A B C D E
115	A B C D E
116	A B C D E
117	A B C D E
118	A B C D E
119	A B C D E
120	A B C D E
121	A B C D E
122	A B C D E
123	A B C D E
124	A B C D E
125	A B C D E
126	A B C D E
127	A B C D E
128	A B C D E
129	A B C D E
130	A B C D E
131	A B C D E
132	A B C D E
133	A B C D E
134	A B C D E
135	A B C D E
136	A B C D E
137	A B C D E
138	A B C D E
139	A B C D E
140	A B C D E
141	A B C D E
142	A B C D E
143	A B C D E
144	A B C D E
145	A B C D E F G H I J K
146	A B C D E F G H I J K
147	A B C D E F G H I J K
148	A B C D E F G H I J K
149	A B C D E F G H I J K
150	A B C D E F G H I J K

Block 4

151	A B C D E
152	A B C D E
153	A B C D E
154	A B C D E
155	A B C D E
156	A B C D E
157	A B C D E
158	A B C D E
159	A B C D E
160	A B C D E
161	A B C D E
162	A B C D E
163	A B C D E
164	A B C D E
165	A B C D E
166	A B C D E
167	A B C D E
168	A B C D E
169	A B C D E
170	A B C D E
171	A B C D E
172	A B C D E
173	A B C D E
174	A B C D E
175	A B C D E
176	A B C D E
177	A B C D E
178	A B C D E
179	A B C D E
180	A B C D E
181	A B C D E
182	A B C D E
183	A B C D E
184	A B C D E
185	A B C D E
186	A B C D E
187	A B C D E
188	A B C D E
189	A B C D E
190	A B C D E
191	A B C D E F G H I J
192	A B C D E F G H I J
193	A B C D E F G H I J
194	A B C D E F G H I J
195	A B C D E F G H I J
196	A B C D E F G H I J
197	A B C D E
198	A B C D E
199	A B C D E
200	A B C D E

Block 5

201	A B C D E
202	A B C D E
203	A B C D E
204	A B C D E
205	A B C D E
206	A B C D E
207	A B C D E
208	A B C D E
209	A B C D E
210	A B C D E
211	A B C D E
212	A B C D E
213	A B C D E
214	A B C D E
215	A B C D E
216	A B C D E
217	A B C D E
218	A B C D E
219	A B C D E
220	A B C D E
221	A B C D E
222	A B C D E
223	A B C D E
224	A B C D E
225	A B C D E
226	A B C D E
227	A B C D E
228	A B C D E
229	A B C D E
230	A B C D E
231	A B C D E
232	A B C D E
233	A B C D E
234	A B C D E
235	A B C D E
236	A B C D E
237	A B C D E
238	A B C D E
239	A. B C D E
240	A B C D E
241	A B C D E
242	A B C D E
243	A B C D
244	A B C D
245	A B C D
246	A B C D
247	A B C D
248	A B C D
249	A B C D
250	A B C D

Block 6

251	A B C D E
252	A B C D E
253	A B C D E
254	A B C D E
255	A B C D E
256	A B C D E
257	A B C D E
258	A B C D E
259	A B C D E
260	A B C D E
261	A B C D E
262	A B C D E
263	A B C D E
264	A B C D E
265	A B C D E
266	A B C D E
267	A B C D E
268	A B C D E
269	A B C D E
270	A B C D E
271	A B C D E
272	A B C D E
273	A B C D E
274	A B C D E
275	A B C D E
276	A B C D E
277	A B C D E
278	A B C D E
279	A B C D E
280	A B C D E
281	A B C D E
282	A B C D E
283	A B C D E
284	A B C D E
285	A B C D E
286	A B C D E
287	A B C D E
288	A B C D E
289	A B C D E
290	A B C D E
291	A B C D E
292	A B C D E
293	A B C D E
294	A B C D E
295	A B C D E F G H I J
296	A B C D E F G H I J
297	A B C D E F G H I J
298	A B C D E F G H I J
299	A B C D E F G H I J
300	A B C D E F G H I J

Block 7

301	A B C D E
302	A B C D E
303	A B C D E
304	A B C D E
305	A B C D E
306	A B C D E
307	A B C D E
308	A B C D E
309	A B C D E
310	A B C D E
311	A B C D E
312	A B C D E
313	A B C D E
314	A B C D E
315	A B C D E
316	A B C D E
317	A B C D E
318	A B C D E
319	A B C D E
320	A B C D E
321	A B C D E
322	A B C D E
323	A B C D E
324	A B C D E
325	A B C D E
326	A B C D E
327	A B C D E
328	A B C D E
329	A B C D E
330	A B C D E
331	A B C D E
332	A B C D E
333	A B C D E
334	A B C D E
335	A B C D E
336	A B C D E
337	A B C D E
338	A B C D E
339	A B C D E F G H
340	A B C D E F G H
341	A B C D E F G H
342	A B C D E F G H
343	A B C D E F G H
344	A B C D E F G H
345	A B C D E F G H I
346	A B C D E F G H I
347	A B C D E F G H I
348	A B C D E F G H I
349	A B C D E F G H I
350	A B C D E F G H I

Block 8

351	A B C D E
352	A B C D E
353	A B C D E
354	A B C D E
355	A B C D E
356	A B C D E
357	A B C D E
358	A B C D E
359	A B C D E
360	A B C D E
361	A B C D E
362	A B C D E
363	A B C D E
364	A B C D E
365	A B C D E
366	A B C D E
367	A B C D E
368	A B C D E
369	A B C D E
370	A B C D E
371	A B C D E
372	A B C D E
373	A B C D E
374	A B C D E
375	A B C D E
376	A B C D E
377	A B C D E
378	A B C D E
379	A B C D E
380	A B C D E
381	A B C D E
382	A B C D E
383	A B C D E
384	A B C D E
385	A B C D E
386	A B C D E
387	A B C D E
388	A B C D E
389	A B C D E
390	A B C D E
391	A B C D E
392	A B C D E
393	A B C D E
394	A B C D E F G H I J
395	A B C D E F G H I J
396	A B C D E F G H I J
397	A B C D E F G H I J
398	A B C D E F G H I J
399	A B C D E
400	A B C D E

Block 9

401	A B C D E F
402	A B C D E
403	A B C D E
404	A B C D E
405	A B C D E
406	A B C D E
407	A B C D E
408	A B C D E
409	A B C D E
410	A B C D E
411	A B C D E
412	A B C D E
413	A B C D E
414	A B C D E F G H I J K L M N O P Q R S
415	A B C D E F G H I J K L M N O P Q R S
416	A B C D E F G H I J K L M N O P Q R S
417	A B C D E F G H I J K L M N O P Q R S
418	A B C D E F G H I J K L M N O P Q R S
419	A B C D E F G H I J K L M N O P Q R S
420	A B C D E F G H I J K L M N O P Q R S
421	A B C D E F G H I J K L M N O P Q R S
422	A B C D E F G H I J K L M N O P Q R S
423	A B C D E F G H I J K L M N O P Q R S
424	A B C D E
425	A B C D E
426	A B C D E
427	A B C D E
428	A B C D E
429	A B C D E
430	A B C D E
431	A B C D E
432	A B C D E
433	A B C D E
434	A B C D E
435	A B C D E
436	A B C D E
437	A B C D E
438	A B C D E
439	A B C D E
440	A B C D E
441	A B C D E
442	A B C D E
443	A B C D E
444	A B C D E
445	A B C D E
446	A B C D E
447	A B C D E
448	A B C D E
449	A B C D E
450	A B C D E

USMLE Step 2 Mock Exam Answer Sheet

BLOCKS 10–12

Block 10	Block 11	Block 12
451 A B C D E	501 A B C D E	551 A B C D E
452 A B C D E	502 A B C D E	552 A B C D E
453 A B C D E	503 A B C D E	553 A B C D E
454 A B C D E	504 A B C D E	554 A B C D E
455 A B C D E	505 A B C D E	555 A B C D E
456 A B C D E	506 A B C D E	556 A B C D E
457 A B C D E	507 A B C D E	557 A B C D E
458 A B C D E	508 A B C D E	558 A B C D E
459 A B C D E	509 A B C D E	559 A B C D E
460 A B C D E	510 A B C D E	560 A B C D E
461 A B C D E	511 A B C D E	561 A B C D E
462 A B C D E	512 A B C D E	562 A B C D E
463 A B C D E	513 A B C D E	563 A B C D E
464 A B C D E	514 A B C D E	564 A B C D E
465 A B C D E	515 A B C D E	565 A B C D E
466 A B C D E	516 A B C D E	566 A B C D E
467 A B C D E	517 A B C D E	567 A B C D E
468 A B C D E	518 A B C D E	568 A B C D E
469 A B C D E	519 A B C D E	569 A B C D E
470 A B C D E	520 A B C D E	570 A B C D E
471 A B C D E	521 A B C D E	571 A B C D E
472 A B C D E	522 A B C D E	572 A B C D E
473 A B C D E	523 A B C D E	573 A B C D E
474 A B C D E	524 A B C D E	574 A B C D E
475 A B C D E	525 A B C D E	575 A B C D E
476 A B C D E	526 A B C D E	576 A B C D E
477 A B C D E	527 A B C D E	577 A B C D E
478 A B C D E	528 A B C D E	578 A B C D E
479 A B C D E	529 A B C D E	579 A B C D E
480 A B C D E	530 A B C D E	580 A B C D E
481 A B C D E	531 A B C D E	581 A B C D E
482 A B C D E	532 A B C D E	582 A B C D E
483 A B C D E	533 A B C D E	583 A B C D E
484 A B C D E	534 A B C D E	584 A B C D E
485 A B C D E	535 A B C D E	585 A B C D E
486 A B C D E	536 A B C D E	586 A B C D E
487 A B C D E	537 A B C D E	587 A B C D E
488 A B C D E	538 A B C D E	588 A B C D E
489 A B C D E	539 A B C D E	589 A B C D E
490 A B C D E	540 A B C D E	590 A B C D E
491 A B C D E	541 A B C D E	591 A B C D E
492 A B C D E	542 A B C D E	592 A B C D E
493 A B C D E	543 A B C D E	593 A B C D E
494 A B C D E	544 A B C D E	594 A B C D E F G H I
495 A B C D E	545 A B C D E	595 A B C D E F G H I
496 A B C D E F G H I J K L M N O	546 A B C D E F G H I J K L M N O	596 A B C D E F G H I
497 A B C D E F G H I J K L M N O	547 A B C D E F G H I J K L M N O	597 A B C D E F G H I
498 A B C D E F G H I J K L M N O	548 A B C D E F G H I J K L M N O	598 A B C D E F G H I
499 A B C D E F G H I J K L M N O	549 A B C D E F G H I J K L M N O	599 A B C D E F G H I
500 A B C D E F G H I J K L M N O	550 A B C D E F G H I J K L M N O	600 A B C D E

USMLE Step 2 Mock Exam Answer Sheet

BLOCKS 13–15

Block 13

601 A B C D E
602 A B C D E
603 A B C D E
604 A B C D E
605 A B C D E
606 A B C D E
607 A B C D E
608 A B C D E
609 A B C D E
610 A B C D E

611 A B C D E
612 A B C D E
613 A B C D E
614 A B C D E
615 A B C D E
616 A B C D E
617 A B C D E
618 A B C D E
619 A B C D E
620 A B C D E

621 A B C D E
622 A B C D E
623 A B C D E
624 A B C D E
625 A B C D E
626 A B C D E
627 A B C D E
628 A B C D E
629 A B C D E
630 A B C D E

631 A B C D E
632 A B C D E
633 A B C D E
634 A B C D E
635 A B C D E
636 A B C D E
637 A B C D E
638 A B C D E
639 A B C D E
640 A B C D E

641 A B C D E
642 A B C D E
643 A B C D E
644 A B C D E
645 A B C D E
646 A B C D E F G H I
647 A B C D E F G H I
648 A B C D E F G H I
649 A B C D E F G H I
650 A B C D E

Block 14

651 A B C D E
652 A B C D E
653 A B C D E
654 A B C D E
655 A B C D E
656 A B C D E
657 A B C D E
658 A B C D E
659 A B C D E
660 A B C D E

661 A B C D E
662 A B C D E
663 A B C D E
664 A B C D E
665 A B C D E
666 A B C D E
667 A B C D E
668 A B C D E
669 A B C D E
670 A B C D E

671 A B C D E
672 A B C D E
673 A B C D E
674 A B C D E
675 A B C D E
676 A B C D E
677 A B C D E
678 A B C D E
679 A B C D E
680 A B C D E

681 A B C D E
682 A B C D E
683 A B C D E
684 A B C D E
685 A B C D E
686 A B C D E
687 A B C D E
688 A B C D E
689 A B C D E
690 A B C D E

691 A B C D E
692 A B C D E
693 A B C D E
694 A B C D E
695 A B C D E F G H
696 A B C D E F G H
697 A B C D E F G H
698 A B C D E F G H
699 A B C D E F G H
700 A B C D E

Block 15

701 A B C D E
702 A B C D E
703 A B C D E
704 A B C D E
705 A B C D E
706 A B C D E
707 A B C D E
708 A B C D E
709 A B C
710 A B C

711 A B C
712 A B C
713 A B C
714 A B C
715 A B C
716 A B C
717 A B C D E
718 A B C D E
719 A B C D E
720 A B C D E

721 A B C D E
722 A B C D E
723 A B C D E
724 A B C D E
725 A B C D E
726 A B C D E
727 A B C D E
728 A B C D E
729 A B C D E
730 A B C D E

731 A B C D E
732 A B C D E
733 A B C D E
734 A B C D E
735 A B C D E
736 A B C D E
737 A B C D E
738 A B C D E
739 A B C D E
740 A B C D E

741 A B C D E
742 A B C D E
743 A B C D E
744 A B C D E
745 A B C D E
746 A B C D E
747 A B C D E
748 A B C D E
749 A B C D E
750 A B C D E